Neuropsychological Neurology

The Neurocognitive Impairments of
Neurological Disorders

Second Edition

Neuropsychological Neurology

The Neurocognitive Impairments of Neurological Disorders

Second Edition

A. J. Larner

Consultant Neurologist
Cognitive Function Clinic
Walton Centre for Neurology and Neurosurgery
Liverpool, UK

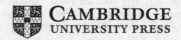

CAMBRIDGE
UNIVERSITY PRESS

University Printing House, Cambridge CB2 8BS, United Kingdom

Cambridge University Press is part of the University of Cambridge.

It furthers the University's mission by disseminating knowledge in the pursuit of education, learning and research at the highest international levels of excellence.

www.cambridge.org
Information on this title: www.cambridge.org/9781107607606

Second edition © A. J. Larner 2013
First edition © A. J. Larner 2008

Second edition first published 2013
First edition first published 2008

A catalogue record for this publication is available from the British Library

Library of Congress Cataloguing in Publication data
Larner, A. J.
Neuropsychological neurology : the neurocognitive impairments
of neurological disorders / A.J. Larner. – 2nd ed.
    p.   ;   cm.
Includes bibliographical references and index.
ISBN 978-1-107-60760-6 (pbk.)
I. Title.
[DNLM: 1. Nervous System Diseases – complications.   2. Cognition Disorders – physiopathology.   3. Neuropsychology – methods.   WL 140]
RC553.C64
616.8 – dc23   2013006091

ISBN 978-1-107-60760-6 Paperback

To Thomas and Elizabeth

Disorders of intellect . . . happen much more often than superficial observers will easily believe.

Samuel Johnson: *The History of Rasselas, Prince of Abyssinia* (1759)

Contents

Foreword

Timothy D. Griffiths

Professor of Cognitive Neurology,
Newcastle University, UK

This impressive single-author work sets out the psychological features of all of the common (and a number of not-so-common) neurological and medical disorders.

Neurologists often regard the psychological examination as a bit of a black art. However, the psychological examination can be regarded as a similar tool to the standard neurological examination as a means to establish "profiles" of deficits that implicate particular parts of the nervous system. I see the principal utility of this work as being the demystification of cognitive profiles to enable neurologists to have an idea of what to expect and what not to expect in a large number of disorders. The book includes both conventional cognitive disorders, such as acute and chronic memory disorders, and also neurological disorders in which cognitive deficits are not the most striking manifestations, in which it will serve as a useful reference. If you survey patients and their families that suffer from cognitive symptoms, what they appreciate most in the cognitive clinic is a clear explanation of the nature and effect of their disorder. This work provides a basis for such explanation.

Neuropsychological neurology is by definition a two-way street that requires a close collaboration between neurology and neuropsychology. A number of cognitive clinics in the UK, including my own, are run as joint clinics that cross between the two disciplines. Many neurologists, however, do not have the luxury of spending time with neuropsychology colleagues and this work will help them to know what to ask neuropsychology colleagues about in given disorders. This book will also be helpful to neuropsychologists who might need to demystify, for example, peculiar genetic conditions with ack-ack names and understand what cognitive deficits should be expected and sought. If the book helps neurologists and neuropsychologists to talk to each other more usefully that will be a valuable outcome in itself.

Preface to the second edition

The aim of the second edition of this book remains the same as in the first, namely to review what is known about the neuropsychological or neurocognitive impairments that occur in neurological disorders and in some general medical conditions that may be seen by neurologists. A phenomenological perspective is presented, using an etiological classification of neurological disorders (in the absence of a comprehensive pathogenic/molecular classification), an approach which at least has the advantage of being familiar to practising neurologists. The volume may be seen as the theoretical companion to a prior, practical volume that attempted to summarize the author's clinical experience of working in a cognitive disorders clinic over more than a decade [1].

There are two major changes from the first edition, one omission and one addition. The omission is the long section devoted to "Bedside neuropsychological test instruments" (first edition, Section 1.8, pp. 22–32), because these issues have since been covered in greater detail elsewhere [1,2]. The addition has been two further chapters, devoted to sleep-related disorders (Chapter 11) and psychiatric disorders (Chapter 12), respectively, both of which may be encountered in cognitive disorders clinics. All the pre-existing chapters have been thoroughly revised and updated, and there has been some reordering to make the text more logical.

As in the first edition, detailed discussions of the neurological features of the disorders covered and of neurological signs are not included, further concise information on which may be obtained elsewhere [3,4].

REFERENCES

[1] Larner AJ. *Dementia in Clinical Practice: A Neurological Perspective. Studies in the Dementia Clinic.* London: Springer, 2012.

[2] Larner AJ (ed.). *Cognitive Screening Instruments. A Practical Approach.* London: Springer, 2013.

[3] Larner AJ, Coles AJ, Scolding NJ, Barker RA. *A-Z of Neurological Practice. A Guide to Clinical Neurology* (2nd edn.). London: Springer, 2011.

[4] Larner AJ. *A Dictionary of Neurological Signs* (3rd edn). New York, NY: Springer, 2011.

Acknowledgments

Thanks are due to many colleagues with whom I have worked in Liverpool since the first edition of this book was published in 2008, including Mark Doran, Eric Ghadiali, Pavla Hancock, Atik Baborie, and Rhys Davies.

Positive feedback on the first edition from two clinical neuropsychologists, Ian Baker (Oxford) and Rupert Noad (Plymouth), both encountered at the Practical Cognition Course in Newcastle, was greatly appreciated. Thanks are due to Tim Griffiths, one of the organizers of this excellent annual course, who has kindly agreed to write the foreword.

I also thank colleagues and friends who have offered either advice on particular topics in the book or general encouragement, including Alasdair Coles, Crispin Fisher, Anu Jacob, Alex Leff, Michael and Sally Mansfield, Parashkev Nachev, and Sivaku-mar Sathasivam.

At Cambridge University Press, I thank Nicholas Dunton and Joanna Chamberlin for their continued faith in this project.

My principal debt of gratitude remains to Sue, my ever-supportive and endlessly forgiving partner.

All errors or misconceptions that remain are entirely my own work. I shall be pleased to hear from readers who detect errors or omissions.

Cognitive function, neuropsychological evaluation, and syndromes of cognitive impairment

1.1 Domains of cognitive function

Without necessarily subscribing to an explicitly modular concept of cerebral function, it is nonetheless convenient from the clinical standpoint to think in terms of cognitive domains or functional systems ("a congeries of mental faculties") in the brain, specifically attention, memory, language, perception, praxis, and executive function. These subdivisions, all working in concert not in isolation to produce in sum what we understand by consciousness, may direct a structured approach to the clinical assessment of cognitive function. Nowadays, a model of distributed neural networks with nodal points more specialized for certain functions has supplanted the idea of particular brain centers [1].

The neurocognitive domains may be described as either *localized*, implying lateralization to one hemisphere or part thereof, focal damage to which may impair that specific function; or *distributed*, implying a nonlocalized function often involving both hemispheres and/or subhemispheric structures (basal ganglia, brainstem), widespread damage being required to impair these functions [2]. Furthermore, particular domains may be subdivided, or fractionated, into subsystems or specific functions that may be selectively impaired, suggesting the existence of functionally distinct neuropsychological substrates.

1.1.1 Attention

It is surely redundant to point out that before any meaningful assessment of "higher cognitive function" can be made, it should be ascertained that "lower cognitive function" is intact, assuming that the workings of the nervous system are hierarchical (in the Jacksonian sense) in their operation. To indulge in *reductio ad absurdum*, it would not be reasonable to expect a comatose patient, or a sleeping subject, to perform well on tests of memory, although memory function may be intact or impaired on recovery from coma or awakening from sleep.

The nature of consciousness is an area of great interest to both neuroscientists and philosophers [3–7], but other than to assume that it is an emergent property of brain function, nothing further about its possible neuroanatomical and neurophysiological bases will be considered here, other than to note that dissociation between apparent preservation of consciousness and absence of cognitive function may occur, as in vegetative states [8], although this has been questioned on the basis of neuroimaging [9] and electroencephalography (EEG) studies [10].

Disturbance of consciousness may encompass both a quantitative and a qualitative dimension. Hence, one may speak of a "level" of consciousness, perhaps in terms of arousal, alertness, or vigilance, forming a continuum from coma to the awake state; and an "intensity" or quality of consciousness, in terms of clarity of awareness of the environment, and ability to focus, sustain, or shift attention. There are various clinical descriptors of states of impaired consciousness including coma [11], vegetative state [8], and minimally conscious state [12]. Coma implies a state of unresponsiveness from which a patient cannot be roused by verbal or mechanical stimuli. Lesser degrees of impaired consciousness, sometimes labeled clinically as stupor, torpor, or obtundation (although these terms lack precision, their meaning often varying between different observers), may also interfere with cognitive assessment. These states may be obvious clinically, such as drowsiness, or difficulty rousing the patient, but may also be occult, perhaps manifesting as increased distractibility. Impairments in level of consciousness are a *sine qua non* for the diagnosis of delirium, as enshrined in the diagnostic criteria of the *Diagnostic and Statistical Manual* (DSM-IV) and the *International Classification of Diseases* (ICD10), although these deficits may be subtle and not immediately obvious at the bedside but yet sufficient to impair attentional mechanisms. These attentional deficits may be responsible for the impaired cognitive function that is also a diagnostic feature of delirium (Section 12.1) [13,14].

Attention, or concentration, is a nonuniform, distributed cognitive function. It may be defined as that component of consciousness which distributes awareness to particular sensory stimuli. The nervous system is bombarded with stimuli in multiple sensory domains, only some of which reach awareness or salience while many percepts are not consciously noticed. Attentional resources, which are finite, are devoted to some channels but not to others. Attention is thus effortful, selective, and closely linked to intention. Distinction may be made between different types of attentional mechanism: sustained attention implies devotion of most attentional resources to one particular stimulus, whereas selective attention is the directing of attentional resources to one stimulus among many (the "cocktail party phenomenon"); divided attention implies a division of attentional resources between competing stimuli. Various neuroanatomical structures are thought to be important in mediating attention, including the ascending reticular activating system in the brainstem, the thalamus, and prefrontal cerebral cortex of multimodal association type, particularly in the right hemisphere, as damage to any of these areas may result in impairments of attention [15]. Dopaminergic and cholinergic tracts are thought to be the important neurotransmitter pathways mediating attention [16].

The term "working memory" is used by neuropsychologists to describe a limited capacity store for retaining and manipulating information over a short term, one to two minutes, and for "online" manipulation of that information. This system has a limited capacity wherein information rapidly degrades unless continuously rehearsed (hence "unstable," compared to longer-term memory). Working memory may be fractionated into a number of subsystems: verbal (phonological or articulatory loop) and visual (visuospatial sketch pad) components, governed by a supervisory central executive, as well as a postulated episodic buffer that acts as a multimodal temporary store to interface with perception and long-term memory [17]. Working memory function is dissociable from "long-term memory" function (Section 1.1.3); for example, in patients with amnesia as a consequence of Wernicke–Korsakoff syndrome, working memory is preserved (Section 8.3.1.1). Working memory is perhaps better envisaged as a component of the selective attention system (the "specious present" of William James), and is certainly not congruent with the usage of the term "short-term memory" by patients, which generally refers to recent long-term memory. Grammatical complexity, for example in sentence construction, is associated with working memory capacity, which mediates the need to keep many elements in play and not lose the train of thought before completing the sentence.

Another clinical phenomenon related to attentional processes is neglect. Sometimes also known as inattention, neglect is a failure to orient to, respond to, or report novel or meaningful stimuli in the absence of sensory or motor deficits (such as hemiparesis or hemianopia), which could explain such behavior. Extinction, the failure to respond to a novel or meaningful sensory stimulus on one side when a homologous stimulus is given simultaneously to the contralateral side (i.e., double simultaneous stimulation), sometimes called "suppression," may be a lesser degree of neglect. In the visual domain, neglect may be categorized as a disorder of spatial attention, which is more common after right-sided rather than left-sided brain damage, usually of vascular origin. This observation may be accounted for by the ability of the right hemisphere to attend to both sides of space whereas the left hemisphere attends to the right side of space only (i.e., there is some lateralization of function). The angular gyrus and parahippocampal gyrus may be the critical neuroanatomical substrates underpinning the development of visual neglect [18,19].

In terms of clinical assessment, the Glasgow Coma Scale (GCS) is the instrument most commonly used for monitoring the level of consciousness [20]. Introduced originally to assess the severity of traumatic head injuries, it has subsequently been applied in other clinical situations (e.g., delirium, stroke), although its validity in some of these circumstances remains to be confirmed. In the individual patient, use of the individual components of the GCS (best eye, verbal, and motor response or EVM) is more useful than the summed score (out of 15), although for the purposes of demographic research use of the summed score is preferable. It should be noted that a GCS score of 15/15 does not guarantee intact attention, as deficits may be subtle, and therefore it may be necessary to undertake other tests of attentional function before other neuropsychological instruments are administered.

Many tests of attention are available. Examples included the Trail Making Test, the Continuous Performance Test, the Paced Auditory Serial Addition Test (PASAT) and its visual equivalent (PVSAT), and the Symbol Digit Modalities Test. Simple bedside tests that tap attentional mechanisms include orientation in time and place, digit span forward and/or backward (also WAIS-R Digit Span subtest), reciting the months of the year or the days of the week backward, or counting back from 30 down to 1. Distractibility may be evident if the patient loses his or her way, or starts the more automatic forward recital. In the Mini-Mental State Examination (MMSE), the most commonly administered "bedside" or office test of cognitive function [21], subtracting 7 from 100 repeatedly (serial sevens:

93,86,79,72,65, etc.) or spelling the word "world" backward are labeled as tests of attention or concentration, but it should be realized that failure in these tests may be for reasons other than impaired attention (e.g., poor mental arithmetic abilities in serial sevens).

Neglect may be clinically obvious, for example if a patient fails to dress one side of the body, but it is sometimes more subtle, in which case its presence may be sought using cancelation tests (e.g., stars in an unstructured array, or letters in a structured array), figure copying (e.g., the Rey–Osterrieth complex figure), line bisection tasks, numbering a clock face, or drawing from memory.

1.1.2 General intelligence (IQ)

Formal neuropsychological assessment often involves testing of general intelligence (IQ) before any specific assessment of the individual domains of cognitive function. This is legitimate as a general intelligence factor "g" seems to account for a significant proportion of the individual differences among test scores for groups of people [22]. General intellectual function is most often measured by administration of one of the Wechsler Intelligence Scales, most often the Wechsler Adult Intelligence Scale-Revised (WAIS-R) [23] or the Wechsler Adult Intelligence Scale-III (WAIS-III) [24]. Updating of these tests is required periodically because of changes in the abilities of the normative group from which standardized scores are derived [22]. Studies over time and from around the world suggest that IQ is rising at the rate of three points every decade, the "Flynn effect" [25].

Administration of these tests may take up to two hours or more, sometimes necessitating more than one testing session to avoid patient fatigue. Subtests in these batteries fall into two categories, verbal and performance, the former including tests of general knowledge, vocabulary, comprehension, and verbal abstract thinking (e.g., digit span, arithmetic, similarities), and the latter including tests of perceptual organization, complex visuospatial function, and psychomotor speed (e.g., digit symbol, picture completion and arrangement, block design, object assembly). These subtests yield an index of verbal intelligence, verbal IQ (VIQ), and of performance intelligence, performance IQ (PIQ), as well as an overall full scale IQ (FSIQ). Based on extensive normative data from healthy North Americans and Europeans, these measures have a mean score of 100 with a standard deviation of 15 such that 95% of the population will fall within the range 70–130. Generally VIQ and PIQ are correlated, but occasional discrepancies may be seen in normal individuals. The belief that the VIQ–PIQ split can be reliably used to infer the lateralization of brain pathology (VIQ more impaired in left-sided lesions, PIQ with right-sided lesions) should be viewed with some caution [26].

When assessing individuals complaining of cognitive disorders, especially memory disorders, an IQ score per se may not be particularly helpful. However, change in IQ, possibly reflecting cognitive decline, is more useful, but it is seldom the case that an individual patient will have undergone previous testing with which a comparison may be made. Previous educational and occupational history may give clues to premorbid intelligence, as may performance on verbal subtests of the WAIS batteries. This difficulty may also be partially circumvented by administering a test specifically designed to estimate premorbid intellectual abilities, such as the National Adult Reading Test (NART) [27], because the overlearned ability to read a series of words with irregular spelling-to-sound correspondences is relatively preserved in a number of neurodegenerative disorders (there are exceptions such as frontotemporal lobar degenerations causing linguistic syndromes; Sections 2.2.2 and 2.2.3). The NART IQ may then be compared with the Wechsler FSIQ to give some indication of whether general intellectual function is stable or has declined. A difference of 20 points is probably significant, 40 points certainly so.

Nonverbal tests of general intelligence are also available, such as the Progressive Matrices described by Raven [28,29]. Other tests examining general cognitive functioning by means of neuro-psychological batteries and assessment of premorbid intelligence are available.

1.1.3 Memory

Memory is a nonuniform, distributed cognitive function or "subassembly" [30]. In other words, subdivisions in memory function may be differentiated, which involve various neuroanatomical substrates.

Current taxonomies of memory propose a distinction between declarative (also known as explicit or conscious memory) and nondeclarative memory (implicit, procedural, unconscious memory). Declarative or explicit memories are intentional or conscious recollections of previous experience. Declarative memory may be subdivided further into episodic memory and semantic memory. Episodic memories are specific personal events, sometimes known as autobiographical memories, which are time and place (context) specific, whereas semantic memories are facts, a database of culturally approved knowledge independent of any specific context. A distinction may also be drawn between anterograde memory, the laying down of new memories, and retrograde memory, the store of previously encoded material. An autobiographical–semantic dissociation of retrograde memory loss may be noted. In contrast with explicit memory, implicit memories refer to a heterogeneous collection of faculties, such as skill learning, priming, and conditioning, which are not available to conscious thought or report [31–33].

In clinical practice, lay observers and primary care physicians frequently distinguish between problems with "short-term memory" and "long-term memory," most usually referring to material learned recently or in the more distant past, respectively. Such a division persists in professional terminology, although the meanings are different. Professional "short-term memory" is analogous to "working memory," best conceptualized as an attentional function (Section 1.1.1). Patient "short-term memory" is in fact one component of

professional "long-term memory" (which encompasses all the subdivisions previously mentioned), specifically that for the learning of new information. Amnesia is the syndrome of impaired memory and new learning, which may be variously characterized as anterograde or retrograde and acute/transient or chronic/persistent. Anterograde amnesia may be clinically manifested as repeated questioning about day-to-day matters, inability to carry out simple chores, or repeating the same information. A better distinction may be between "recent" and "remote" memory.

The neuroanatomical substrates of explicit memory are partially understood, based on studies of experimental animals and of patients developing memory problems as a consequence of focal brain lesions that may be examined by means of neuro-psychological testing and, more recently, neuro-imaging. The literature makes reference to hippocampal, diencephalic, and frontal and basal forebrain amnesia, largely based on lesion and neuropathological studies. Structures in the medial temporal lobe, centered on the hippocampus, and in the diencephalon surrounding the third ventricle are thought to be crucial to episodic memory. Lesions anywhere along the circuit originally described by Papez (entorhinal area of the parahippocampal gyrus, perforant and alvear pathways, hippocampus, fimbria and fornix, mammillary bodies, mammillothalamic tract, anterior thalamic nuclei, internal capsule, cingulate gyrus, and cingulum) may lead to anterograde and retrograde amnesia. Furthermore, memory functions are lateralized in a material-specific manner, with verbal memory functions being associated with the dominant (usually left-sided) structures, and visual memory with the nondominant (usually right) side [34,35].

The experience of the patient known as HM was a key indicator of the importance of these structures for memory function (Section 4.1). Because of his medically refractory epilepsy, HM underwent bilateral medial temporal lobectomy, encompassing the amygdala, entorhinal cortex, anterior dentate gyrus, hippocampus, and subiculum. Surgery was followed by a dense anterograde amnesia, and retrograde amnesia covering about a decade prior to the surgery [36]. Similar outcomes have been reported, following unilateral surgery, presumably because of subclinical contralateral pathology [37]. Evocative terms used to describe the predicament of HM and other similarly affected patients include "marooned in the moment," "fossilized in the past," and living in a "world of isolated impressions." HM was followed up for many years with essentially no improvement in his neuropsychological deficits. His importance in the field of memory research continues to be emphasized [38].

There are many causes of memory disorder [32,39,40]. Impairment of episodic memory is the most common presenting feature of Alzheimer's disease (AD; Section 2.1), sometimes occurring in isolation although other cognitive deficits may be apparent on clinical or neuropsychological assessment. For this reason, and because AD is the most common cause of dementia, neuropsychological test batteries, particularly "bedside" tests, are often weighted toward memory testing, to the relative exclusion of other cognitive domains such as executive function, which has consequences when using such tests to try to identify other neurocognitive disorders in which memory is not the principal domain affected. Anterograde amnesia may also occur as a consequence of open or closed head injury (posttraumatic amnesia), Wernicke–Korsakoff syndrome (Section 8.3.1.1), herpes simplex encephalitis (Section 9.1.1), limbic encephalitis of paraneoplastic or nonparaneoplastic origin (Sections 6.12.1 and 6.12.2, respectively), strategic brain infarcts (Section 3.2), and surgery to remove temporal lobe or third ventricle lesions (Section 7.2.3). Transient amnesias may be of epileptic origin (transient epileptic amnesia; Section 4.3.1) or, in transient global amnesia, of probable vascular etiology (Section 3.6.2). Psychogenic amnesia may also enter the differential diagnosis of transient amnesia (Section 12.5.1). In addition, a temporal gradient of retrograde amnesia may be present in some of these conditions, but rare cases of focal retrograde amnesia with relative sparing of anterograde memory have been described,

sometimes following head injury or an encephalitic illness [41].

Many tests are available to neuropsychologists to probe the specific areas of episodic and semantic long-term memory. The Wechsler Memory Scale, now in its third edition (WMS-III), is a battery testing auditory and visual declarative (and working) memory. Other specific tests of episodic memory sometimes deployed include the Buschke Selective Reminding Test [42], the California Verbal Learning Test [43], the Hopkins Verbal Learning Test [44], the Camden Recognition Memory Test and the Topographical Recognition Memory Test [45,46], and the Rey Auditory Verbal Learning Test. Recall of the Rey–Osterrieth Complex Figure may be used as a test of visual memory. Retrograde memory may be investigated using the Autobiographical Memory Interview [47], which covers both personal semantic information and autobiographical incidents, although this may underestimate the true extent of retrograde amnesia, missing "islands" of memory loss unique to the individual. The Famous Faces Test may be used to study remote memory [48]. Integrity of the semantic network, including semantic memory, may be tested using category (or semantic) fluency tests (Section 1.1.7). Reading words with irregular sound-to-spelling correspondence may produce surface dyslexia (regularization errors) in patients with impaired access to or breakdown of semantic networks. Other tests accessing associative semantic networks include the Pyramids and Palm Trees Test [49].

Of the frequently used "bedside" neuropsychological test instruments, some are specific cognitive tests for memory, such as the Memory Impairment Screen (MIS) [50] and the Free and Cued Selective Reminding (or Five Words) Test [51]. General, multidomain, cognitive screening instruments (e.g., MMSE [21], Addenbrooke's Cognitive Examination [52,53], and Montreal Cognitive Assessment [54]) test memory to a greater or lesser extent; for example, the MMSE has only perfunctory examination of memory function (registration of the names of three objects, e.g., ball, flag, tree, and recall after distractor items). Longer (supraspan) word lists are used in the

DemTect [55] and the Hopkins Verbal Learning Test [44], and the latter includes both recall and recognition paradigms to try to ascertain whether failures result from encoding or retrieval defects. Generally, examination of implicit memory functions is not undertaken in clinical practice.

Rather less has been written about forgetting, as opposed to remembering, but this is presumably also a physiological memory function [56]. It was Nietzsche's belief that "For healthy and effective action, it is as important to forget as to remember, and forgetting, even more than memory, must be an effect of time rather than will" (*On the Uses and Disadvantages of History for Life*). The phenomenon of accelerated long-term forgetting has attracted increasing attention in recent times, whereby memory tests applied at extended intervals (usually greater than 24 hours) may disclose anterograde memory impairments not seen in standard test paradigms. This may be of particular relevance to some of the memory disorders seen in the context of epilepsy (Chapter 4).

1.1.4 Language

Language, "the wind-swift motion of the brain" (Sophocles *Antigone*, line 355), historically provided the first unequivocal evidence that loss of a higher brain function could be ascribed to damage to a specific brain region, based on the work of Paul Broca and, possibly, Marc Dax in the mid-nineteenth century [57]. The work of Carl Wernicke was also seminal in establishing the neural substrates of language function, indicating that language is a localized function. Every medical student now knows that most individuals, whether left- or right handed, have language in the dominant hemisphere, although around 30% of left handers and less than 1% of right handers have language in the nondominant hemisphere.

Aphasia, a primary disorder of language, is often mirrored by similar defects in reading (alexia) and writing (agraphia), all of which are amenable to clinical localization, within certain limitations [58], often on the basis of simple bedside examination.

In addition to the Broca (nonfluent, anterior, motor, "expressive") and Wernicke (fluent, posterior, sensory, "receptive") types of aphasia, clinical distinctions may be drawn between conduction aphasia (impaired repetition) and transcortical aphasias (preserved repetition). A classification of aphasias as perisylvian (Broca, Wernicke, conduction), and extrasylvian has also been proposed [59].

It may be necessary to test auditory comprehension before undertaking any other neuropsychological testing of language; for example, using the Token Test [60] in which commands of increasing length and complexity are given for manipulating a deck of colored tokens of differing size and shape (some have objected to the word "token," preferring "item" [61]). Sentence comprehension skills may be ascertained by performance of the Test for the Reception of Grammar [62]. Wernicke-type aphasia typically has marked comprehension impairments, with fluent speech output but often with poverty of content, sometimes reduced to a meaningless jumble of words (jargon aphasia). Although Broca-type aphasia is often characterized as having preserved comprehension, this in fact may be impaired for more complex syntax.

There are many tests of language available to neuropsychologists. Comprehensive batteries include the Boston Diagnostic Aphasia Examination (BDAE) [63], the Western Aphasia Battery (WAB) [64], the Psycholinguistic Assessment of Language Processing in Aphasia (PALPA) [65], and the Comprehensive Aphasia Test [66]. Specific tests of naming often deployed include the Graded Naming Test [67] and the Boston Naming Test [68].

At the bedside, listening to speech output will generally permit a simple classification of aphasia as fluent or nonfluent, and also detect paraphasias (phonemic or semantic) and neologisms. From questioning or instructing the patient during history taking and clinical examination, comprehension difficulties may be evident. Testing of repetition may differentiate aphasias in which this ability is relatively preserved (transcortical aphasias) or impaired (conduction aphasia). Naming skills have less localizing value, although marked anomia should raise the suspicion of semantic problems, either degradation of or access to semantic stores. Reading and writing function should also be examined, even if spoken language function seems intact, as various syndromes of alexia and agraphia are described. Idea density in written material reflects language processing ability.

Of the frequently used "bedside" neuropsychological test instruments, most are heavily weighted for language function, such that patients with primarily linguistic disorders (e.g., semantic dementia, aphasic presentations of AD) may find it difficult or impossible to complete them.

1.1.5 Perception

That perceptions are not a faithful brain response to external stimuli but are to some extent constructed by the brain, based on the expectations of time and culture, has been known by philosophers since Kant, and perception as illusion has been implicitly understood by artists such as Magritte ("the treachery of images") and manifested by artists such as Escher in certain of his graphical works (e.g., *Ascending and Descending, Belvedere*).

Higher-order deficits of sensory processing, not explicable in terms of failure of primary sensory function, or a disorder of attention, intellectual decline, or a failure to name the stimulus (anomia), are known as agnosias, a term coined by Sigmund Freud in 1891 and literally meaning "not knowing" or "without knowledge" [69]. Before this, Lissauer in 1890 [70] (abridged translation by Shallice and Jackson [71]), speaking of *Seelenblindheit*, literally "soul-blindness" or technically "psychic blindness," drew a distinction between apperceptive deficits and associative deficits. In the former, a defect of higher-order complex perceptual processing was deemed to be present, whereas in the latter, perception was held to be intact but a defect in giving meaning to the percept was present. The debate continues as to whether all agnosias, although clinically distinguishable as apperceptive or associative, are in fact attributable to faulty perception [72].

Although auditory and tactile agnosias are described, they seem to be relatively rare in comparison with visual agnosia, which has certainly been more extensively studied. The visual agnosias may be relatively selective; for example, an inability to recognize previously known human faces or equivalent stimuli, known as prosopagnosia. This may be developmental or acquired in origin, the latter usually a consequence of cerebrovascular disease causing bilateral occipitotemporal lesions, but occasionally it occurs as a feature of neurodegenerative disease, sometimes in relative isolation, associated with focal right temporal lobe atrophy (progressive prosopagnosia [73]). Pure alexia or pure word blindness is an agnosia for words that results in a laborious letter-by-letter reading strategy to arrive at a word's identity. Pure alexia may be conceptualized as a consequence of damage to a brain region mediating whole word recognition that may be located in the medial left occipital lobe and posterior fusiform gyrus [74]. The rare syndrome of pure word deafness (Section 1.3.4) may be a form of auditory agnosia. Finger agnosia, the inability to identify which finger has been touched despite knowing that a finger has been touched, is a form of tactile agnosia, which may be seen as one feature of Gerstmann syndrome although it may occur in isolation [75]. Likewise, Braille alexia may, in some instances, be a form of tactile agnosia [76].

The existence of two visual processing pathways within the brain was first proposed by Ungerlieder and Mishkin [77]: an occipitoparietal dorsolateral ("where") visual processing stream and an occipitotemporal ventromedial ("what") stream. In rare cases, these pathways may be affected selectively; for instance, the ventral stream, specifically the lateral occipital area, in a famous patient with "visual-form agnosia" following carbon monoxide poisoning. Her perceptual identification of shape and form was lost, although she could still perceive color and the fine detail of surfaces (visual texture), and her visuomotor ("vision for action") skills were strikingly preserved [78]. Optic ataxia, impaired voluntary reaching for a visually presented target with misdirection and dysmetria, is the sign typically evident in dorsal stream lesions. The workings of the visuomotor control system are not available to consciousness ("unconscious vision"), unlike the visual identification of objects.

A specific inability to see objects in motion, akinetopsia or cerebral visual motion blindness, despite preserved perception of other visual attributes such as color, form, and depth, has been described in association with selective lesions to area V5 of the visual cortex [79]. Although exceptionally rare, such cases suggest a distinct neuroanatomical substrate for movement vision, as do cases in which motion vision is selectively spared in a scotomatous area (Riddoch's syndrome [80]). Perception within a "blind" visual field without conscious awareness has been termed blindsight [81].

Cases of isolated progressive visual agnosia were presented by De Renzi [82], and Benson *et al.* [83] drew attention to a disorder comprising alexia, agraphia, visual agnosia, with or without components of Balint and Gerstmann syndromes, and transcortical sensory aphasia, but with relative preservation of memory until late in the course, a disorder they named posterior cortical atrophy (PCA) in the absence of neuropathological data. It is now believed that most PCA cases have AD pathology, although other pathologies have been described including dementia with Lewy bodies (DLB), corticobasal degeneration (CBD), and prion disease [84].

Various means may be used by neuropsychologists specifically to test visual perceptual and visuo-constructive functions. These may be individual tests such as Judgment of Line Orientation (thought to tap right occipital lobe function); copy of the Rey–Osterrieth Complex Figure ([85,86]; translation by Corwin and Bylsma [87]) or the Taylor Figure [88]; decoding embedded (Poppelreuter) figures [89]; or parts of test batteries, such as the WAIS-R Block Design (visuospatial construction); or dedicated batteries such as the Visual Object and Space Perception Battery (VOSP) [90].

Of the frequently used "bedside" neuropsychological test instruments, the MMSE has only perfunctory examination of visuospatial function, requiring copying a drawing of intersecting pentagons [21]. Clock Drawing is, at least in part, a visuospatial test, but requires other skills. The Addenbrooke's Cognitive Examination (ACE) adds copying a wire (Necker) cube and clock drawing [52], and ACE-R adds counting dots and identifying fragmented letters [53].

1.1.6 Praxis

The term apraxia was coined by Steinthal in 1871 but the phenomena of higher-level motor control disorders were first systematically studied by Liepmann [91], who defined apraxia as an inability to perform purposeful skilled movements as a result of neurological dysfunction, usually associated with left-sided lesions. Part of the definition of apraxia is one of exclusion, as the observed motor difficulties should not be caused by sensory loss, weakness, tremors, dystonia, optic ataxia, chorea, ballismus, athetosis, myoclonus, ataxia, or epileptic seizures. For example, deficits previously labeled as "constructional apraxia" or "dressing apraxia" are better explained as visuoperceptual and/or visuospatial deficits, as is the misdirected reaching for visual targets typical of optic ataxia. Traditionally, a distinction has been drawn between ideational and ideomotor apraxias, although both are often present in left hemisphere damage [92–95]. Ideomotor apraxia in Broca's aphasia may be conceptualized as a disconnection syndrome (Section 1.3.4).

Cases of isolated progressive apraxia were presented by De Renzi [82]. Apraxia may be a feature of neurodegenerative disease, classically CBD (Section 2.4.4), although AD can present with a similar phenotype (biparietal atrophy; Section 2.1), even with alien limb behavior.

Praxic difficulties may be tested for in various ways, including gesture naming, decision and recognition; gesture to verbal command, to visual or tactile tools; imitation of real or nonsense gestures; and tool selection. There are also test batteries for apraxia assessment [95].

1.1.7 Executive function

The term executive function is used to encompass various cognitive abilities, including the formulation of goals; organization, planning, execution, and monitoring of a sequence of actions; problem solving; and abstract thinking. It also overlaps with sustained attention. The term "dysexecutive syndrome" may be used to describe dysfunction in any or all of these areas, which is most often associated with pathological processes in the frontal lobes [96,97]. Because of the heterogeneity of these functions, some authors dislike the umbrella term of "executive function," and prefer to describe the specific function impaired. Moreover, frontal lobe damage may result in various clinical phenotypes, in which behavioral change is often the most salient feature. Orbitofrontal injury may result in disinhibition, as described in Phineas Gage, one of the most famous patients in the annals of clinical neuropsychology, who sustained marked behavioral change following traumatic frontal lobe injury [98], although other patterns of clinical and cognitive change may be observed with frontal lobe injury; for example, apathetic (frontal convexity) and akinetic (medial frontal) syndromes are also described. Because most tests of executive function probe planning and strategy, mediated by dorsolateral prefrontal cortex, some patients with exclusive orbitofrontal damage, for example with behavioral (frontal) variant frontotemporal dementia (Section 2.2.1), may complete these tests without conspicuous errors.

Because of the overarching nature of the construct of "executive function," no single test is adequate to assess its integrity [99]. Many tests known to be sensitive to aspects of executive dysfunction are available. Perhaps the most frequently used are the Stroop Test and the Modified Wisconsin Card Sorting Test (MWCST). In the Stroop Test, patients are required to read a list of color names, printed in colors that differ from the name, followed by reading the colors in which each name is printed, thus having to inhibit the reading of each color name (i.e., inhibition of inappropriate responses)

[100]. MWCST uses a set of cards marked with symbols of different shape, color, and number, which may be sorted in various ways. Sorting rules are changed by the examiner without informing the subject, requiring problem solving skills. Difficulty switching category is typical of frontal lobe damage, leading to perseveration with previous categories [101]. Clearly MWCST, unlike the Stroop Test, calls for novel responses. MWCST may not be specific to frontal lobe dysfunction, as patients with hippocampal lesions may commit perseverative errors [102].

Oral tests of verbal fluency, or controlled oral word association tests (COWAT), may be divided into those testing phonological, letter, or lexical fluency (naming to letter), such as the FAS test (name as many words beginning with the letters *F, A,* or *S* as possible in one minute each), and those testing semantic or category fluency (naming to set; in one minute name as many animals, fruits, or musical instruments as possible). Letter fluency has been characterized as a test of mental flexibility (as well as of expressive language) probing executive function, which is particularly impaired ("defective exemplification" [103]) with left frontal lesions (without aphasia), whereas category fluency examines the integrity of the semantic network. Design fluency, a visual analog of verbal fluency, may be more impaired with right frontal lesions [104]. Verbal fluency tasks are attractive because they are brief (one minute each) and require no special equipment, but account may need to be taken of patient age and education when considering test norms [105].

There are many other tests available to neuropsychologists to probe executive functions, sometimes along with other domains. These include Raven's Progressive Matrices, the Porteus Mazes, Tower tests (London, Hanoi), Trail-Making Test (especially Part B), the Halstead–Reitan Category Test, the Weigl Color Form Sorting Test [106], the Cognitive Estimates Test [107], and the Verbal Switching Test [108]. The Hayling and Brixton Tests for sentence completion and spatial anticipation are tests of rule following and verbal suppression of a familiar response [109]. Certain WAIS-R subtests are sensitive to aspects of executive/frontal lobe function, such as the Similarities test of verbal abstraction and the Digit Symbol test of psychomotor speed. Tests of decision making and risk taking, faculties which may also be encompassed under the rubric of executive function [110] and mediated by prefrontal cortex and the amygdala, include the Iowa Gambling Test [111] and the Cambridge Gamble Task [112].

There are also batteries of tests such as the Behavioral Assessment of the Dysexecutive Syndrome (BADS) [113] and the Delis–Kaplan Executive Function System (D-KEFS) [114], but because these take some time to administer, they are best reserved for specific investigation of known frontal problems. The Frontal Lobe Personality Change Questionnaire (FLOPS) may be used to assess behavioral change and includes a carer version, useful for gaining collateral information; likewise the Iowa Rating Scale of Personality Change [115]. Verbal fluency tests are incorporated into test batteries such as the Dementia Rating Scale [116] and the CERAD Battery [117].

At the bedside or in the clinic, "Go–No Go" tests may be applied to assess failure of inhibitory responses, or stimulus–boundedness; for example, asking the patient to tap twice in response to a single tap given by the examiner, and once in response to two taps. Repeating alternating sequences, for example of hand gestures (fist–palm) or of writing (*m n m n m n*) may be used to similar purpose. The Trails A and B Test also requires a sequence of letters or numbers to be followed (one of these is incorporated in the Montreal Cognitive Assessment [54]). Interpretation of proverbs is a popular bedside test, "concrete" interpretation suggesting frontal lobe problems. Of the "bedside" neuropsychological test instruments, the MMSE has been criticized for its lack of assessment of executive function [21], one shortcoming which the Addenbrooke's Cognitive Examination seeks to address by using letter and category verbal fluency tests [52,53]. Other batteries that tap executive function include the Frontal Assessment Battery [118], the

Frontal Behavioral Inventory [119], and the Middelheim Frontality Score [120].

1.2 Neuropsychological assessment

1.2.1 Formal neuropsychological assessment

There are many tests available to the neuropsychologist for the evaluation of cognitive function, either global function or individual domains [121–123]. Of course, it must be remembered that any neuropsychological test may have multiple sensory, motor, perceptual and cognitive demands, and hence "pure" tests of any single cognitive domain are the exception rather than the rule. The variety of tests available may bewilder the nonspecialist. Moreover, the choice of different test instruments in different studies may make direct comparisons difficult: variable test sensitivity to a particular cognitive domain may explain discrepancies between studies.

Neuropsychologists insist, rightly, that specialist training is required for the correct administration and interpretation of neuropsychological tests. Clinical neurologists, therefore, will rely on their neuropsychologist colleagues for the performance and interpretation of these "formal" tests, as they fall outside neurologists' expertise and may take substantial time to administer, being incompatible with clinical schedules. Nonetheless, some form of neuropsychological testing, often labeled as "bedside" to distinguish it from "formal" testing, is within the scope of neurologists and may be of diagnostic use.

1.2.2 "Bedside" neuropsychological assessment

Numerous tests and test batteries that may be applied within one to 30 minutes are available, encompassing not only cognitive function but also functional, behavioral, and global assessment [21,52–55,124–126]. Because of the brevity that makes them clinically applicable, these instruments often have certain shortcomings, which neurologists need to bear in mind: a raw score derived from a series of tests is not necessarily "diagnostic," although it may increase the likelihood of a particular diagnosis. The potential for incongruous or anomalous performance of tests in a medicolegal setting has been noted [127]. Many other situational influences may also impact on testing of cognitive skills, such as fatigue, emotional status, medication use, pain, and stress [128]. These also need to be taken into account when considering the results of cognitive testing, as do factors such as educational and background experience. Many norms are also culturally weighted.

It is outside the scope of this volume to discuss frequently used "bedside" or office cognitive screening instruments, for which information the reader is referred elsewhere [124–126]. When evaluating possible cognitive disorders, particularly those involving memory impairment, in addition to history taking and examination, it is also important to obtain some collateral history from a relative, friend, or carer familiar with the subject as part of the evaluation [129,130]. Simple clinical observations may also assist with diagnosis. A patient who attends the clinic alone despite having been instructed to bring a relative or friend is very unlikely to have a cognitive disorder [131]. Looking to a relative, friend, or carer for assistance when asked to volunteer information or answer questions, the "head-turning sign," is suggestive of the presence of a cognitive disorder [132,133].

1.3 Syndromes of cognitive impairment

1.3.1 Normal aging

Various motor, sensory, and cognitive changes in neurological function occur with increasing age [134]. To what extent these changes reflect "normal aging," however that may be defined, or to what extent they reflect an increasing burden of age-related neurological disease, remains uncertain. In consequence, the inevitable physiological changes that occur in cognition with increasing age may be difficult to distinguish from the earliest stages of pathological brain disorders causing cognitive impairments.

A distinction may be drawn between "crystallized intelligence," characterized by practical problem solving skills, knowledge gained from experience, and vocabulary, and "fluid intelligence," characterized by the ability to acquire and use new information, as measured by the solution of abstract problems and speeded performance [135]. Crystallized intelligence is assumed to be cumulative; longitudinal studies of vocabulary, for example, show no decline through old age. By contrast, fluid intelligence does change with age; performance on tests such as Raven's Progressive Matrices and Digit Symbol Substitution decline marginally up to the age of 40 years and then more rapidly. Such physiological cognitive decline may be evident in early middle age (45–49 years) [136]. There is general consensus that typical cognitive aging involves losses in processing speed, cognitive flexibility, and the efficiency of working memory (sustained attention). In other words, it may take more time and/or more trials to learn new information. Cognitive domains such as access to remotely learned information, including semantic networks, and retention of well-encoded new information are spared with typical aging; this may permit testing of these domains to be used as sensitive indicators of disease processes. It may be that memory decline in healthy aging is secondary to decline in processing speed and efficiency, as controlling for processing speed may attenuate or eliminate age-related differences in memory performance, unlike the situation with memory impairment in dementia.

Longitudinal studies of neuropsychological function indicate that there is considerable variability in normal older adults across different skills, and consistency across different domains may not necessarily be observed. Clearly this needs to be taken into account when assessing whether perceived cognitive decline is pathological or normal, that is in defining neuropsychological norms for aging.

Furthermore, norms for IQ are increasing over time [22,25]. Likewise, norms may need to be age-weighted rather than age-corrected to detect cognitive impairment related to AD, the prevalence of which increases exponentially with increasing age.

Notwithstanding these difficulties, the definition of a syndrome (or syndromes) of cognitive impairment greater than expected for age, often termed mild cognitive impairment, which is (are) the harbinger of progressive cognitive decline, the prodromal phases of neurodegenerative disorder may now be identifiable, with consequent implications for potential therapeutic intervention.

1.3.2 Mild cognitive impairment (MCI)

Age-related cognitive decline insufficient to fulfil validated criteria for the diagnosis of AD has attracted a variety of labels over the past 50 years, including benign senescent forgetfulness, age-associated memory impairment (AAMI), age-associated cognitive decline (AACD), cognitive decline no dementia (CIND), and mild cognitive impairment (MCI). A degree of consensus has developed around the concept of MCI [137–141], although there is not unanimity [142,143]. MCI may be defined by the presence of a subjective memory complaint, preferably corroborated by an informant; evidence of objective memory impairment for age and level of education; largely normal general cognitive function; essentially intact activities of daily living (ADL); and failure to fulfil criteria for dementia [137]. Global rating scales have been used to define MCI, such as a Clinical Dementia Rating (CDR) [144] score of 0.5 or a Global Deterioration Scale (GDS) [145] score of 3, but MCI remains a clinical diagnosis. Complex ADL may be impaired in MCI [146].

MCI may be clinically and etiologically heterogeneous. At presentation, memory complaint is the most common feature, so-called amnestic MCI. Other variants have been described, specifically single nonmemory domain MCI and multiple domain MCI. Multiple domain MCI might reflect single or multiple etiologies [138]. The possibility that MCI may reflect conditions such as dysphoria, vascular disease, and miscellaneous disorders that may cause cognitive impairment such as obstructive sleep apnea, alcohol misuse, head injury, and metabolic or nutritional deficiencies, some of them treatable, has been emphasized by several authors [143]. A category of MCI in Parkinson's disease, PD-MCI, has been described [147], and vascular cognitive impairment (VCI) may be differentiated from vascular dementia (Section 3.1). The neuropsychological profile of AD-related MCI is discussed in Section 2.1.2.

1.3.3 Dementia

The diagnosis of dementia is currently based on fulfilment of clinical diagnostic criteria, for example those in the generic DSM, the ICD, or the dedicated criteria for specific dementia subtypes. DSM-IV-TR [148], for example, requires for a dementia diagnosis the development of multiple cognitive deficits that include memory impairment, of gradual onset and progressive course, sufficiently severe to cause impairment in occupational or social functioning, not better accounted for by another diagnosis. Application of such diagnostic criteria to large cohorts of patients may classify different numbers of patients as having dementia, with differences up to a factor of 10 found in one study [149]. One reason for this variability is that many diagnostic criteria are heavily weighted toward memory impairment. Because memory impairment is the most salient feature in AD, the most common cause of dementia, many diagnostic criteria, for example those for vascular dementia, have been inadvertently "Alzheimerized," with undue emphasis placed on memory loss at the expense of other cognitive features [150]. A "type 2 dementia" which, unlike "type 1 dementia," is lacking cortical features such as amnesia, has been proposed, and in which demonstrable executive control function impairments are sufficient to cause disability [151].

Another potentially confusing outcome of the emphasis of diagnostic criteria on memory is tautology: syndromes with a diagnostic label of dementia, such as frontotemporal dementia and DLB, which may not necessarily fulfil diagnostic criteria for dementia in their early stages, for example in the case of frontotemporal dementia, because the initial features are executive (frontal) dysfunction and noncognitive behavioral change [152]. Unequivocal cognitive deficits may not be sufficient to meet criteria for dementia, requiring a lexicon of other terms [153].

Other diagnoses entering the differential diagnosis of dementia include delirium (Section 12.1) and depression (Section 12.3.1).

1.3.3.1 Cortical versus subcortical dementia

Albert *et al.* [154] first used the term "subcortical dementia" to describe the cognitive impairments seen in progressive supranuclear palsy (PSP; Section 2.4.3): forgetfulness, slowness of thought processes (bradyphrenia), alteration of personality with marked apathy and depression, and an impaired ability to manipulate acquired knowledge. These deficits were felt to be qualitatively distinct from those seen in cortical dementias, typically AD, which included impairments in memory (amnesia), language (aphasia), perception (agnosia), and skilled learned movements (apraxia). The term "limbic dementia" has sometimes been used for syndromes with marked amnesia and evidence for limbic system pathology such as AD. Whereas in subcortical dementias cueing or recognition paradigms may improve performance in delayed recall memory tests, suggesting ineffective retrieval but with relatively preserved encoding of material, in cortical dementias such strategies may be ineffective, suggesting impaired encoding as well as retrieval. The term "subcortical" was selected because of the resemblance of the deficits to those seen with bifrontal lobe disease, also reflected in the concurrent emotional and movement deficits in the two types: subcortical dementias tended to be associated with apathy and depression and prominent disorders of muscle tone, posture, and gait, whereas cortical dementias were attended with cognitive

anosognosia and disinhibition and an absence of movement disorder [155].

Objections to the concept of subcortical dementia have been raised [156]. Cortical and subcortical areas are not functionally independent, but overlapping. Because white matter has an essentially integrative function, reciprocally linking cortical and subcortical structures, white matter pathology might be expected to result in functional disconnection of brain areas, and disordered brain function at a site distant from a lesion (diaschisis) is a well recognized phenomenon (Section 1.3.4). This may be seen, for example, with frontal lobe dysfunction in multiple sclerosis (MS) (Section 6.1) [157], and has also been suggested in X-linked adrenoleukodystrophy (Section 5.5.2.2) [158]. Identical or similar clinical phenotypes may result from pathologies affecting either gray matter or subjacent white matter (e.g., subcortical aphasias [59]). Against this argument, however, false localization of neurological signs usually deemed indicative of higher, cortical cognitive function (e.g., agnosia, neglect) is rarely reported [159].

Cognitive impairment and/or dementia in a variety of disorders has been labeled as subcortical, including Huntington's disease (HD; Section 5.1.1) [160], Parkinson's disease (PD; Section 2.4.1) [161], multiple sclerosis (Section 6.1) and other white matter disorders [162,163], and certain forms of vascular cognitive impairment (subcortical ischemic vascular dementia; Section 3.1.2) [164]. In the case of the movement disorders PSP, HD, and PD, it has been hypothesized that the basal ganglia, in addition to their role in control of movement, support a basic attentional mechanism, facilitating the synchronization of cortical activity underlying the selection and promulgation of an appropriate sequence of thoughts; this "focused attention" differs from arousal, vigilance, or alertness. Basal ganglia damage thus results in a failure of synchronization, manifested as abulia and bradyphrenia [165].

Whatever the precise physiological relationship of cortex and subcortex in supporting cognitive function, the cortical/subcortical terminology may still have some clinical utility in the differential diagnosis of dementia syndromes [166,167].

1.3.3.2 Thalamic dementia; brainstem and cerebellar cognitive impairment

An entity called thalamic dementia is also mentioned in the literature, which refers to cognitive impairments in conditions with relatively selective thalamic damage [168]. Most commonly this is a result of vascular lesions, focal infarction (Section 3.2.3), hypoperfusion related to a dural arteriovenous fistula (Section 3.4.2) [169], or neoplasia. In addition, relatively selective degeneration of the thalamus may occur. This may be due to a prion disease (Section 2.5) [170] such as fatal familial insomnia (Section 2.5.3) [171], although cases of selective thalamic degeneration with the pathology of multiple system atrophy [170] or motor neuron disease [172], or without evidence of prion disease [173], have been reported. The neuropsychological features may include forgetfulness, apathy, and hypersomnia.

Cognitive impairment may also occur in patients with isolated brainstem lesions of vascular, inflammatory, neoplastic, infective, or metabolic origin (for examples: Sections 3.2.8, 8.2.3.2, and 9.4.3) [174–178].

Although traditionally viewed as a component of the motor system, a cognitive role for the cerebellum has been recognized increasingly, with a specific "cerebellar cognitive affective syndrome" being delineated by some authors [179], and characterized by executive dysfunction (in set-shifting, planning, verbal fluency, abstract reasoning, working memory) and difficulties with spatial cognition, memory, and language, as well as personality change, associated with posterior lobe and vermis lesions. Cognitive impairment may occur in patients with isolated cerebellar lesions of vascular or neurodegenerative origin (Sections 3.2.8, 3.3.3, and 5.2). Studies of relative pure cerebellar degenerations such as spinocerebellar ataxia (SCA) type 6 (Section 5.2.1.4) have allowed the delineation of cerebellar

subregions that may play a role in verbal working memory [180].

1.3.4 Disconnection syndromes; callosal dementia

Disconnection syndromes may be defined as conditions in which there is an interruption of inter- and/or intrahemispheral fiber tracts. The concept was originally advanced in the 1890s, but has subsequently been revived and developed, perhaps most notably by Norman Geschwind in the 1960s [181–183].

Disconnection syndromes result essentially either from interruption of fibers within the corpus callosum or commissures (interhemispheric disconnection syndromes), or of fibers within a hemisphere (intrahemispheric disconnection syndromes). Interhemispheric disconnection is most graphically seen in patients who have undergone surgical commissurotomy for intractable seizure disorders, so-called "split-brain" patients [184,185]. Intrahemispheric disconnection syndromes are best described in the domain of language. Although mass lesions and iatrogenesis (surgery) are obvious causes of disconnection, functional disconnection may also result from inflammatory disorders of white matter. A "callosal dementia" has been postulated, characterized by callosal disconnection, Balint's syndrome, gaze apraxia, and neurobehavioral features such as alternating apathy and agitation [186].

With complete interhemispheric disconnection, for example with a tumor or following surgical section of the corpus callosum, a blindfolded patient can correctly name objects placed in the right hand, but not those in the left, and objects in the left visual hemifield cannot be named or matched to a similar object in the right hemifield. With posterior callosal section at the splenium, a partial interhemispheric disconnection, for example following left posterior cerebral artery occlusion, patients cannot read or name colors, as information cannot pass to the left hemispheric language areas. Copying of words and writing, both spontaneously and to dictation, is intact as information may pass to the left hemisphere anterior to the site of damage: the syndrome of aphasia without agraphia first described by Dejerine in 1892.

Various intrahemispheric disconnection syndromes have been described. In conduction aphasia, patients have fluent but paraphasic speech and writing, with greatly impaired repetition despite relatively normal comprehension of the spoken and written word. This has been explained traditionally as being due to a lesion in the arcuate fasciculus/supramarginal gyrus disconnecting the sensory (Wernicke) and motor (Broca) language areas. Ideomotor apraxia in Broca's aphasia, an apraxia of left hand movements to command, is ascribed to lesions disconnecting the cortical motor areas anterior to the primary motor cortex. In pure word deafness, a form of auditory agnosia (Section 1.1.5), patients are able to hear and identify nonverbal sounds but unable to understand spoken language, due to lesions in the white matter of the left temporal lobe that isolate Wernicke's area from the auditory cortex.

AD has sometimes been conceptualized as a disconnection syndrome [187,188]. AD pathology effectively isolates the hippocampus from association cortices, basal forebrain, thalamus, and hypothalamus [189]. A multiple disconnection model is currently favored to explain the cognitive dysfunction seen in MS, in which lesions of subcortical periventricular white matter fiber pathways effectively disconnect cortical and subcortical regions (Section 6.1) [190]. Cognitive impairment associated with carotid artery occlusive disease (Section 3.1.1.1) may be a consequence of disconnection of cortical regions caused by white matter lesions and cerebral atrophy [191].

REFERENCES

[1] Mesulam MM. Large-scale neurocognitive networks and distributed processing for attention, language, and memory. *Ann Neurol* 1990; 28: 597–613.

[2] Hodges JR. *Cognitive Assessment for Clinicians* (2nd edn.). Oxford: Oxford University Press, 2007.

[3] Dennett DC. *Consciousness Explained*. London: Penguin, 1993.

[4] Penrose R. *Shadows of the Mind*. London: Vintage, 1995.

[5] Searle JR. Consciousness. *Annu Rev Neurosci* 2000; 23: 557–78.

[6] Zeman A. *Consciousness: A User's Guide*. New Haven, CT: Yale University Press, 2002.

[7] Libet B. *Mind Time. The Temporal Factor in Consciousness*. Cambridge, MA: Harvard University Press, 2004.

[8] Jennett B. *The Vegetative State. Medical Facts, Ethical and Legal Dilemmas*. Cambridge: Cambridge University Press, 2002.

[9] Monti MM, Coleman MR, Owen AM. Neuroimaging and the vegetative state: resolving the behavioural assessment dilemma? *Ann NY Acad Sci* 2009; 1157: 81–9.

[10] Cruse D, Chennu S, Chatelle C, *et al.* Bedside detection of awareness in the vegetative state: a cohort study. *Lancet* 2011; 378: 2088–94.

[11] Posner JB, Saper CB, Schiff ND, Plum F. *Plum and Posner's Diagnosis of Stupor and Coma* (4th edn.). Oxford: Oxford University Press, 2007.

[12] Giacino JT, Ashwal S, Childs N, *et al.* The minimally conscious state: definition and diagnostic criteria. *Neurology* 2002; 58: 349–53.

[13] Fong TG, Tulebaev SR, Inouye SK. Delirium in elderly adults: diagnosis, prevention and treatment. *Nat Rev Neurol* 2009; 5: 210–20.

[14] Gofton TE. Delirium: a review. *Can J Neurol Sci* 2011; 38: 673–80.

[15] Posner MI, Petersen SE. The attention system of the human brain. *Annu Rev Neurosci* 1990; 13: 25–42.

[16] Perry E, Ashton H, Young A (eds.). *Neurochemistry of Consciousness. Neurotransmitters in Mind*. Amsterdam: John Benjamins, 2002.

[17] Baddeley A. Working memory: theories, models, and controversies. *Annu Rev Psychol* 2012; 63: 1–29.

[18] Chatterjee A. Neglect: a disorder of spatial attention. In: D'Esposito M (ed.). *Neurological Foundations of Cognitive Neuroscience*. Cambridge, MA: MIT Press, 2003; 1–26.

[19] Husain M. Hemispatial neglect. *Handb Clin Neurol* 2008; 88: 359–72.

[20] Teasdale G, Jennett B. Assessment of coma and impaired consciousness: a practical scale. *Lancet* 1974; 2: 81–4.

[21] Folstein MF, Folstein SE, McHugh PR. "Mini-Mental State." A practical method for grading the cognitive state of patients for the clinician. *J Psychiatr Res* 1975; 12: 189–98.

[22] Deary IJ. *Intelligence. A very short introduction.* Oxford: Oxford University Press, 2001.

[23] Wechsler D. *Weschler Adult Intelligence Scale-Revised (WAIS-R).* San Antonio, TX: Psychological Corporation, 1981.

[24] Wechsler D. *Weschler Adult Intelligence Scale, Third Edition (WAIS-III).* San Antonio, TX: Psychological Corporation, 1997.

[25] Flynn JR. *Are We Getting Smarter? Rising IQ in the Twenty-first Century.* Cambridge: Cambridge University Press, 2012.

[26] Iverson GL, Mendrek A, Adams RL. The persistent belief that VIQ-PIQ splits suggest lateralized brain damage. *Appl Neuropsychol* 2004; 11: 85–90.

[27] Nelson HE, Willison J. *National Adult Reading Test (NART)* (2nd edn.). Windsor: NFER-Nelson, 1991.

[28] Raven JC. *Progressive Matrices: A Perceptual Test of Intelligence.* London: HK Lewis & Co. Ltd, 1938.

[29] Raven JC. *Advanced Progressive Matrices, Set 1.* London: HK Lewis & Co. Ltd, 1958.

[30] Von Neumann J. *The Computer and the Brain* (2nd edn.). New Haven, CT: Yale University Press [1958] 2000; 60, 68.

[31] Schacter DL, Tulving E. *Memory Systems.* Cambridge, MA: MIT Press, 1994.

[32] Kapur N. *Memory Disorders in Clinical Practice.* Hove: Lawrence Erlbaum, 1994.

[33] Baddeley A, Eysenck M, Anderson M. *Memory.* Hove: Psychology Press, 2009.

[34] Cohen NJ, Eichenbaum H. *Memory, Amnesia, and the Hippocampal System.* Cambridge, MA: MIT Press, 1993.

[35] Zola-Morgan S, Squire LR. Neuroanatomy of memory. *Annu Rev Neurosci* 1993; 16: 547–63.

[36] Scoville W, Milner B. Loss of recent memory after bilateral hippocampal lesions. *J Neurol Neurosurg Psychiatry* 1957; 20: 11–21.

[37] Kapur N, Prevett M. Unexpected amnesia: are there lessons to be learned from cases of amnesia following unilateral temporal lobe surgery? *Brain* 2003; 126: 2573–85.

[38] Moscovitch M. Memory before and after H.M.: an impressionistic historical perspective. In: Zeman A, Kapur N, Jones-Gotman M (eds.). *Epilepsy and Memory.* Oxford: Oxford University Press, 2012; 19–50.

[39] Kopelman MD. Disorders of memory. *Brain* 2002; 125: 2152–90.

[40] Papanicolaou AC. *The Amnesias: A Clinical Textbook of Memory Disorders.* Oxford: Oxford University Press, 2006.

[41] Kapur N. Focal retrograde amnesia in neurological disease. A critical review. *Cortex* 1993; 29: 219–34.

[42] Buschke H, Fuld PA. Evaluating storage, retention, and retrieval in disordered memory and learning. *Neurology* 1974; 24: 1019–25.

[43] Delis DC, Kramer JH, Kaplan E, Ober BA. *California Verbal Learning Test – Second Edition, Adult Version.* San Antonio, TX: Psychological Corporation, 2000.

[44] Brandt J. The Hopkins Verbal Learning Test: development of a new memory test with six equivalent forms. *Clin Neuropsychol* 1991; 5: 125–42.

[45] Warrington EK. *Recognition Memory Test.* Windsor: NFER-Nelson Publishing Co Ltd, 1984.

[46] Warrington EK. *The Camden Memory Tests Manual.* Hove: Psychology Press, 1996.

[47] Kopelman MD, Wilson BA, Baddeley AD. The Autobiographical Memory Interview: a new assessment of autobiographical and personal semantic memory in amnesic patients. *J Clin Exp Neuropsychol* 1989; 11: 724–44.

[48] Hodges JR, Salmon DP, Butters NA. Recognition and naming of famous faces in Alzheimer's disease: a cognitive analysis. *Neuropsychologia* 1993; 31: 775–88.

[49] Howard D, Patterson K. *Pyramids and Palm Trees: A Test of Semantic Access from Pictures and Words.* Bury St Edmunds: Thames Valley Test Company, 1992.

[50] Buschke H, Kuslansky G, Katz M, *et al.* Screening for dementia with the Memory Impairment Screen. *Neurology* 1999; 52: 231–8.

[51] Dubois B, Touchon J, Portet F, *et al.* "The 5 words": a simple and sensitive test for the diagnosis of Alzheimer's disease [in French]. *Presse Med* 2002; 31: 1696–9.

[52] Mathuranath PS, Nestor PJ, Berrios GE, Rakowicz W, Hodges JR. A brief cognitive test battery to differentiate Alzheimer's disease and frontotemporal dementia. *Neurology* 2000; 55: 1613–20.

[53] Mioshi E, Dawson K, Mitchell J, Arnold R, Hodges JR. The Addenbrooke's Cognitive Examination Revised

(ACE-R): a brief cognitive test battery for dementia screening. *Int J Geriatr Psychiatry* 2006; 21: 1078–85.

[54] Nasreddine ZS, Phillips NA, Bédirian V, *et al.* The Montreal Cognitive Assessment, MoCA: a brief screening tool for mild cognitive impairment. *J Am Geriatr Soc* 2005; 53: 695–9.

[55] Kalbe E, Kessler J, Calabrese P, *et al.* DemTect: a new, sensitive cognitive screening test to support the diagnosis of mild cognitive impairment and early dementia. *Int J Geriatr Psychiatry* 2004; 19: 136–43.

[56] Della Sala S (ed.). *Forgetting.* Hove: Psychology Press, 2010.

[57] Schiller F. *Paul Broca. Founder of French Anthropology, Explorer of the Brain.* Oxford: Oxford University Press, 1993.

[58] Willmes K, Poeck K. To what extent can aphasic syndromes be localized? *Brain* 1993; 116: 1527–40.

[59] Benson DF, Ardila A. *Aphasia: A Clinical Perspective.* New York, NY: Oxford University Press, 1996.

[60] De Renzi E, Faglioni P. Normative data and screening power of a shortened version of the Token Test. *Cortex* 1978; 14: 41–9.

[61] Critchley M. *The Divine Banquet of the Brain and Other Essays.* New York, NY: Raven Press, 1979; 68.

[62] Bishop DVM. *Test for the Reception of Grammar.* Great Britain: Chapel Press, 1983.

[63] Goodglass H, Kaplan E. *Boston Diagnostic Aphasia Examination (BDAE).* Philadelphia, PA: Lea & Fibiger, 1983.

[64] Shewan CM, Kertesz A. Reliability and validity characteristics of the Western Aphasia Battery (WAB). *J Speech Hear Disord* 1980; 45: 308–24.

[65] Kay J, Lesser R, Coltheart M. *Psycholinguistic Assessment of Language Processing in Aphasia.* Hove: Psychology Press, 1992.

[66] Swinburn K, Porter G, Howard D. *Comprehensive Aphasia Test.* Hove: Psychology Press, 2004.

[67] McKenna P, Warrington EK. *The Graded Naming Test.* Windsor: NFER-Nelson Publishing, 1983.

[68] Kaplan EF, Goodglass H, Weintraub S. *The Boston Naming Test* (2nd edn.). Philadelphia, PA: Lippincott Williams & Wilkins, 2001.

[69] Freud S. *Zur Auffassung der Aphasien, eine Kritische Studie.* Leipzig: Deuticke, 1891.

[70] Lissauer H. Ein Fall von Seelenblindheit nebst Einem Beitrag zure Theorie derselben. *Arch Psychiatr Nervenkr* 1890; 21: 222–70.

[71] Shallice T, Jackson M. Lissauer on agnosia. *Cogn Neuropsychol* 1988; 5: 153–92.

[72] Farah MJ. *Visual Agnosia: Disorders of Object Recognition and What They Tell us about Normal Vision.* Cambridge, MA: MIT Press, 1995.

[73] Evans JJ, Heggs AJ, Antoun N, Hodges JR. Progressive prosopagnosia associated with selective right temporal lobe atrophy. A new syndrome? *Brain* 1995; 118: 1–13.

[74] Leff AP, Spitsyna G, Plant GT, Wise RJS. Structural anatomy of pure and hemianopic alexia. *J Neurol Neurosurg Psychiatry* 2006; 77: 1004–7.

[75] Della Sala S, Spinnler H. Finger agnosia: fiction or reality? *Arch Neurol* 1994; 51: 448–50.

[76] Larner AJ. Braille alexia: an apperceptive tactile agnosia? *J Neurol Neurosurg Psychiatry* 2007; 78: 907–8.

[77] Ungerlieder LG, Mishkin M. Two cortical visual systems. In: Ingle DJ, Goodale MA, Mansfield RJW (eds.). *Analysis of Visual Behavior.* Cambridge, MA: MIT Press, 1982: 549–86.

[78] Goodale MA, Milner AD. *Sight Unseen: An Exploration of Conscious and Unconscious Vision.* Oxford: Oxford University Press, 2004.

[79] Zeki S. Cerebral akinetopsia (cerebral visual motion blindness). *Brain* 1991; 114: 811–24.

[80] Zeki S, Ffytche DH. The Riddoch syndrome: insights into the neurobiology of conscious vision. *Brain* 1998; 121: 25–45.

[81] Weiskrantz L. *Blindsight. A Case Study and Implications.* Oxford: Clarendon Press, 1986.

[82] De Renzi E. Slowly progressive visual agnosia or apraxia without dementia. *Cortex* 1986; 22: 171–80.

[83] Benson DF, Davis RJ, Snyder BD. Posterior cortical atrophy. *Arch Neurol* 1988; 45: 789–93.

[84] Crutch SJ, Lehmann M, Schott JM, *et al.* Posterior cortical atrophy. *Lancet Neurol* 2012; 11: 170–8.

[85] Rey A. L'examen psychologique dans les cas d'encephalopathie traumatique. *Archiv Psychol* 1941; 28: 286–340.

[86] Osterrieth PA. Le test de copie d'une figure complexe: contribution a l'étude de la perception et de la mémoire. *Archiv Psychol* 1944; 30: 286–356.

[87] Corwin J, Bylsma FW. "Psychological examination of traumatic encephalopathy" by A. Rey and "The complex figure copy test" by P.A. Osterrieth. *Clin Neuropsychol* 1993; 7: 3–21.

[88] Taylor LB. Localization of cerebral lesions by psychological testing. *Clin Neurosurg* 1969; 16: 269–87.

[89] Poppelreuter W. *Die psychischen Schädigungen durch Kopfschuss im Kriege 1914/17: mit besonderer Berücksichtigung der pathopsychologischen, pädagogischen, gewerblichen und sozialen Beziehungen* (Two volumes: Band 1: Die Störungen der niederen und höheren Sehleistungen durch Verletzungen des Okzipitalhirns; Band 2: Die Herabsetzung der körperlichen Leistungsfähigkeit und des Arbeitswillens durch Hirnverletzung im Vergleich zu Normalen und Psychogenen). Leipzig: Voss, 1917–1918.

[90] Warrington EK, James M. *The Visual Object and Space Perception Battery.* Bury St Edmunds: Thames Valley Test Company, 1991.

[91] Liepmann H. *Das Krankheitsbild der Apraxie ("motorischen Asymbolie").* Berlin: Karger, 1900.

[92] Jeannerod M. *The Cognitive Neuroscience of Action.* Oxford: Blackwell, 1997.

[93] Gonzalez Rothi LJ, Heilman KM (eds.). *Apraxia: The Neuropsychology of Action.* Hove: Psychology Press, 1997.

[94] Freund H-J, Jeannerod M, Hallett M, Leiguarda R (eds.). *Higher-Order Motor Disorders. From Neuroanatomy and Neurobiology to Clinical Neurology.* Oxford: Oxford University Press, 2005.

[95] Dovern A, Fink GR, Weiss PH. Diagnosis and treatment of upper limb apraxia. *J Neurol* 2012; 259: 1269–83.

[96] Filley CM. Clinical neurology and executive function. *Semin Speech Lang* 2000; 21: 95–108.

[97] Miller BL, Cummings JL (eds.). *The Human Frontal Lobes. Functions and Disorders* (2nd edn.). London: Guilford Press, 2007.

[98] Macmillan M. *An Odd Kind of Fame. Stories of Phineas Gage.* Cambridge, MA: MIT Press, 2000.

[99] Goldberg E, Bougakov D. Neuropsychologic assessment of frontal lobe dysfunction. *Psychiatr Clin N Am* 2005; 28: 567–80.

[100] Stroop J. Studies of interference in serial verbal reaction. *J Exp Psychol* 1935; 18: 643–62.

[101] Nelson HE. A modified card sorting test sensitive to frontal lobe defects. *Cortex* 1976; 12: 313–24.

[102] Corcoran R, Upton D. A role for the hippocampus in card sorting? *Cortex* 1993; 29: 293–304.

[103] Critchley M. *The Divine Banquet of the Brain and Other Essays.* New York, NY: Raven Press, 1979; 54.

[104] Jones-Gotman M, Milner B. Design fluency: the invention of nonsense drawings after focal cortical lesions. *Neuropsychologia* 1977; 15: 653–74.

[105] Mathuranath P, George A, Cherian P, *et al.* Effects of age, education and gender on verbal fluency. *J Clin Exp Neuropsychol* 2003; 25: 1057–64.

[106] Weigl E. On the psychology of so-called processes of abstraction. *J Norm Soc Psychol* 1941; 36: 3–33.

[107] Shallice T, Evans ME. The involvement of the frontal lobes in cognitive estimation. *Cortex* 1978; 14: 294–303.

[108] Warrington EK. Homophone meaning generation: a new test of verbal switching for the detection of frontal lobe dysfunction. *J Int Neuropsychol Soc* 2000; 6: 643–8.

[109] Burgess PW, Shallice T. *The Hayling and Brixton Tests.* Thurston, Suffolk: Thames Valley Test Company, 1997.

[110] Lehto JE, Elorinne E. Gambling as an executive function task. *Appl Neuropsychol* 2003; 10: 234–8.

[111] Bechara A, Damasio AR, Damasio H, Anderson SW. Insensitivity to future consequences following damage to human prefrontal cortex. *Cognition* 1994; 50: 7–15.

[112] Rogers RD, Everitt BD, Baldacchino A, *et al.* Dissociable deficits in the decision-making cognition of chronic amphetamine abusers, opiate abusers, patients with focal damage to prefrontal cortex, and tryptophan-depleted normal volunteers: evidence for monoaminergic mechanisms. *Neuropsychopharmacol* 1999; 20: 322–39.

[113] Wilson BA, Alderman N, Burgess PW, Emslie H, Evans JJ. *Behavioural Assessment of the Dysexecutive Syndrome.* Bury St Edmunds: Thames Valley Test Company, 1996.

[114] Delis D, Kaplan E, Kramer J. *Delis-Kaplan Executive Function System.* New York, NY: Psychological Corporation, 2001.

[115] Barrash J, Anderson SW. *The Iowa Rating Scales of Personality Change.* Iowa City, IA: University of Iowa, 1993.

[116] Mattis S. *Dementia Rating Scale.* Windsor: NFER-Nelson, 1992.

[117] Morris J, Heyman A, Mohs R, *et al.* The Consortium to Establish a Registry for Alzheimer's Disease (CERAD). Part I. Clinical and neuropsychological assessment of Alzheimer's disease. *Neurology* 1989; 39: 1159–65.

[118] Dubois B, Slachevsky A, Litvan I, Pillon B. The FAB: a Frontal Assessment Battery at bedside. *Neurology* 2000; 55: 1621–6.

[119] Kertesz A, Nadkarni N, Davidson W, Thomas AW. The Frontal Behavioural Inventory in the differential diagnosis of frontotemporal dementia. *J Int Neuropsychol Soc* 2000; 6: 460–8.

[120] De Deyn PP, Engelborghs S, Saerens J, *et al.* The Middelheim Frontality Score: a behavioural assessment scale that discriminates frontotemporal dementia from Alzheimer's disease. *Int J Geriatr Psychiatry* 2005; 20: 70–9.

[121] Mitrushina M, Boone KB, Razani J, D'Elia LF. *Handbook of Normative Data for Neuropsychological Assessment* (2nd edn.). Oxford: Oxford University Press, 2005.

[122] Strauss E, Sherman EMS, Spreen O. *A Compendium of Neuropsychological Tests: Administration, Norms, and Commentary* (3rd edn.). New York, NY: Oxford University Press, 2006.

[123] Lezak MD, Howieson DB, Bigler ED, Tranel D. *Neuropsychological Assessment* (5th edn.). New York, NY: Oxford University Press, 2012.

[124] Burns A, Lawlor B, Craig S. *Assessment Scales in Old Age Psychiatry* (2nd edn.). London: Dunitz, 2004.

[125] Tate RL. *A Compendium of Tests, Scales, and Questionnaires. The Practitioner's Guide to Measuring Outcomes After Acquired Brain Impairment.* Hove: Psychology Press, 2010.

[126] Larner AJ (ed.). *Cognitive Screening Instruments. A Practical Approach.* London: Springer, 2013.

[127] Trimble M. *Somatoform Disorders. A Medicolegal Guide.* Cambridge: Cambridge University Press, 2004; 109–39.

[128] Nicholson K, Martelli MF, Zasler ND. Does pain confound interpretation of neuropsychological test results? *NeuroRehabilitation* 2001; 16: 225–30.

[129] Knopman DS, DeKosky ST, Cummings JL, *et al.* Practice parameter: diagnosis of dementia (an evidence-based review). Report of the Quality Standards Subcommittee of the American Academy of Neurology. *Neurology* 2001; 56: 1143–53.

[130] Waldemar G, Dubois B, Emre M, *et al.* Recommendations for the diagnosis and management of Alzheimer's disease and other disorders associated with dementia. *Eur J Neurol* 2007; 14: e1–26.

[131] Larner AJ. Screening utility of the "attended alone" sign for subjective memory impairment. *Alzheimer Dis Assoc Disord* 2012 [Epub ahead of print]

[132] Fukui T, Yamazaki R, Kinno R. Can the "Head-Turning Sign" be a clinical marker of Alzheimer's disease? *Dement Geriatr Cogn Disord Extra* 2011; 1: 310–17.

[133] Larner AJ. Head turning sign: pragmatic utility in clinical diagnosis of cognitive impairment. *J Neurol Neurosurg Psychiatry* 2012; 83: 852–3.

[134] Larner AJ. Neurological signs of ageing. In: Sinclair A, Morley JE, Vellas B (eds.). *Pathy's Principles and Practice of Geriatric Medicine* (5th edn.). Chichester: Wiley, 2012; 609–16.

[135] Horn JL, Cattell RB. Age difference in fluid and crystallized intelligence. *Acta Psychol* 1967; 26: 107–29.

[136] Singh-Manoux A, Kivimaki M, Glymour MM, *et al.* Timing of onset of cognitive decline: results from Whitehall II prospective cohort study. *BMJ* 2012; 344: d7622.

[137] Petersen RC, Smith GE, Waring SC, *et al.* Mild cognitive impairment: clinical characterization and outcome. *Arch Neurol* 1999; 56: 303–8.

[138] Petersen RC (ed.). *Mild Cognitive Impairment. Aging to Alzheimer's Disease.* Oxford: Oxford University Press, 2003.

[139] Winblad B, Palmer K, Kivipelto M, *et al.* Mild cognitive impairment – beyond controversies, towards a consensus: report of the International Working Group on Mild Cognitive Impairment. *J Int Med* 2004; 256: 240–6.

[140] Gauthier S, Reisberg B, Zaudig M, *et al.* Mild cognitive impairment. *Lancet* 2006; 367: 1262–70.

[141] Mariani E, Monastero R, Mecocci P. Mild cognitive impairment: a systematic review. *J Alzheimers Dis* 2007; 12: 23–35.

[142] Ritchie K, Touchon J. Mild cognitive impairment: conceptual basis and current nosological status. *Lancet* 2000; 355: 225–8.

[143] Gauthier S, Touchon J. Mild cognitive impairment is not a clinical entity and should not be treated. *Arch Neurol* 2005; 62: 1164–6.

[144] Hughes CP, Berg L, Danziger WL, Coben LA, Martin RL. A new clinical scale for the staging of dementia. *Br J Psychiatry* 1982; 140: 566–72.

[145] Reisberg B, Ferris SH, de Leon MJ, Crook T. The Global Deterioration Scale (GDS) for assessment of primary degenerative dementia. *Am J Psych* 1982; 139: 1136–9.

[146] Perneczky R, Pohl C, Sorg C, *et al.* Impairment of activities of daily living requiring memory of complex reasoning as part of the MCI syndrome. *Int J Geriatr Psychiatry* 2006; 21: 158–62.

[147] Litvan I, Aarsland D, Adler CH, *et al.* MDS Task Force on mild cognitive impairment in Parkinson's disease: critical review of PD-MCI. *Mov Disord* 2011; 26: 1814–24.

[148] American Psychiatric Association. *Diagnostic and Statistical Manual of Mental Disorders, Fourth Edition, Text Revison (DSM-IV-TR)*. Washington, DC: American Psychiatric Association, 2000.

[149] Erkinjuntti T, Ostbye T, Steenhuis R, Hachinski V. The effect of different diagnostic criteria on the prevalence of dementia. *N Engl J Med* 1997; 337: 1667–74.

[150] Bowler JV, Hachinski V. Current criteria for vascular dementia – a critical appraisal. In: Bowler JV, Hachinski V (eds.). *Vascular Cognitive Impairment: Reversible Dementia.* Oxford: Oxford University Press, 2003; 1–11.

[151] Royall DR. Executive control function in "mild" cognitive impairment and Alzheimer's disease. In: Gauthier S, Scheltens P, Cummings JL (eds.). *Alzheimer's Disease and Related Disorders Annual 5.* London: Taylor & Francis, 2006: 35–62.

[152] Mendez MF, McMurtray A, Licht EA, Saul RE, Miller BL. Is early frontotemporal dementia a dementia? *Alzheimers Dement* 2006; 2: S548 (abstract P4-112).

[153] Dubois B, Feldman HH, Jacova C, *et al.* Revising the definition of Alzheimer's disease: a new lexicon. *Lancet Neurol* 2010; 9: 1118–27.

[154] Albert ML, Feldman RG, Willis AL. The "subcortical dementia" of progressive supranuclear palsy. *J Neurol Neurosurg Psychiatry* 1974; 37: 121–30.

[155] Cummings JL. *Subcortical Dementias.* London: Oxford University Press, 1990.

[156] Brown RG, Marsden CD. "Subcortical dementia": the neuropsychological evidence. *Neuroscience* 1988; 25: 363–87.

[157] Foong J, Rozewicz L, Quaghebeur G, *et al.* Executive function in multiple sclerosis. The role of frontal lobe pathology. *Brain* 1997; 120: 15–26.

[158] Larner AJ. Adult-onset dementia with prominent frontal lobe dysfunction in X-linked adrenoleukodystrophy with R152C mutation in ABCD1 gene. *J Neurol* 2003; 250: 1253–4.

[159] Larner AJ. A topographical anatomy of false-localising signs. *Adv Clin Neurosci Rehabil* 2005; 5(1): 20–1.

[160] McHugh PR, Folstein MF. Psychiatric symptoms of Huntington's chorea: a clinical and phenomenological study. In: Benson DF, Blumer D (eds.). *Psychiatric Aspects of Neurological Disease.* New York, NY: Raven Press, 1975: 267–85.

[161] Starkstein SE, Merello M. *Psychiatric and Cognitive Disorders in Parkinson's Disease.* Cambridge: Cambridge University Press, 2002: 59–66.

[162] Rao SM. White matter disease and dementia. *Brain Cogn* 1996; 31: 250–68.

[163] Filley CM. *The Behavioral Neurology of White Matter.* New York, NY: Oxford University Press, 2001.

[164] Menon U, Kelley RE. Subcortical ischemic cerebrovascular dementia. *Int Rev Neurobiol* 2009; 84: 21–33.

[165] Brown P, Marsden CD. What do the basal ganglia do? *Lancet* 1998; 351: 1801–4.

[166] Neary D, Snowden JS. Sorting out the dementias. *Pract Neurol* 2002; 2: 328–39.

[167] Bak TH, Crawford LM, Hearn VC, Mathuranath PS, Hodges JR. Subcortical dementia revisited: similarities and differences in cognitive function between progressive supranuclear palsy (PSP), corticobasal degeneration (CBD) and multiple system atrophy (MSA). *Neurocase* 2005; 11: 268–73.

[168] Stern K. Severe dementia associated with bilateral symmetrical degeneration of the thalamus. *Brain* 1939; 62: 157–71.

[169] Gonçalves MB, Maia Jr O, Correa JL, *et al.* Dural arteriovenous fistula presenting as thalamic dementia. *Arq Neuropsiquiatr* 2008; 66: 264–7.

[170] Petersen RB, Tabaton M, Berg L, *et al.* Analysis of the prion protein gene in thalamic dementia. *Neurology* 1992; 42: 1859–63.

[171] Gallassi R, Morreale A, Montagna P, *et al.* Fatal familial insomnia: behavioral and cognitive features. *Neurology* 1996; 46: 935–9.

[172] Deymeer F, Smith TW, De Girolami U, Drachman DA. Thalamic dementia and motor neuron disease. *Neurology* 1989; 39: 58–61.

[173] Janssen JC, Lantos PL, Al Sarraj S, Rossor MN. Thalamic degeneration with negative prion protein immunostaining. *J Neurol* 2000; 247: 48–51.

[174] Meador KJ, Loring DW, Sethi KD, *et al.* Dementia associated with dorsal midbrain lesion. *J Int Neuropsychol Soc* 1996; 2: 359–67.

[175] Garrard P, Bradshaw D, Jäger HR, *et al*. Cognitive dysfunction after isolated brainstem insult. An underdiagnosed cause of long tem morbidity. *J Neurol Neurosurg Psychiatry* 2002; 73: 191–4.

[176] Lee TM, Cheung CC, Lau EY, Mak A, Li LS. Cognitive and emotional dysfunction after central pontine myelinolysis. *Behav Neurol* 2003; 14: 103–7.

[177] van Zandvoort M, de Haan E, van Gijn J, Kappelle LJ. Cognitive functioning in patients with a small infarct in the brainstem. *J Int Neuropsychol Soc* 2003; 9: 490–4.

[178] Salgado JV, Costa-Silva M, Malloy-Diniz LF, Siqueira JM, Teixeira AL. Prefrontal cognitive dysfunction following brainstem lesion. *Clin Neurol Neurosurg* 2007; 109: 379–82.

[179] Schmahmann JD, Sherman JC. The cerebellar cognitive affective syndrome. *Brain* 1998; 121: 561–79.

[180] Cooper FE, Grube M, Von Kriegstein K, *et al*. Distinct critical cerebellar subregions for components of verbal working memory. *Neuropsychologia* 2012; 50: 189–97.

[181] Geschwind N. Disconnexion syndromes in animals and man. *Brain* 1965; 88: 237–94; 585–644.

[182] Absher JR, Benson DF. Disconnection syndromes: an overview of Geschwind's contributions. *Neurology* 1993; 43: 862–7.

[183] Catani M, Ffytche DH. The rises and falls of disconnection syndromes. *Brain* 2005; 128: 2224–39.

[184] Sperry RW. Some effects of disconnecting the cerebral hemispheres. *Science* 1982; 217: 1223–6.

[185] Zaidel E, Iacoboni M, Zaidel DW, Bogen JE. The callosal syndromes. In: Heilman KM, Valenstein E (eds.). *Clinical Neuropsychology* (4th edn.). Oxford: Oxford University Press, 2003; 347–403.

[186] Ghika Schmid F, Ghika J, Assal G, Bogousslavsky J. Callosal dementia: behavioral disorders related to central and extrapontine myelinolysis [in French]. *Rev Neurol Paris* 1999; 155: 367–73.

[187] Lakmache Y, Lassonde M, Gauthier S, Frigon JY, Lepore F. Interhemispheric disconnection syndrome in Alzheimer's disease. *Proc Natl Acad Sci USA* 1998; 95: 9042–6.

[188] Delbeuck X, van der Linden M, Collette F. Alzheimer's disease as a disconnection syndrome? *Neuropsychol Rev* 2003; 13: 79–92.

[189] Hyman BT, van Hoesen GW, Damasio AR, Barnes CL. Alzheimer's disease: cell-specific pathology isolates the hippocampal formation. *Science* 1984; 225: 1168–70.

[190] Dineen RA, Vilisaar J, Hlinka L, *et al*. Disconnection as a mechanism for cognitive dysfunction in multiple sclerosis. *Brain* 2009; 132: 239–49.

[191] Yamauchi H, Fukuyama H, Nagahama Y, *et al*. Atrophy of the corpus callosum associated with cognitive impairment and widespread cortical hypometabolism in carotid artery occlusive disease. *Arch Neurol* 1996; 53: 1103–9.

Neurodegenerative disorders

The term "neurodegenerative disease" has been criticized by some authors as virtually meaningless, because degenerative changes are seen as a consequence of diseases of differing etiology, such as vascular and inflammatory processes. "Proteinopathy" is an alternative, possibly better term, suggesting that abnormal protein metabolism and folding may be a common pathogenic event in the disorders listed here.

2.1 Alzheimer's disease (AD)

Alzheimer's disease (AD) is the archetypal neurodegenerative cognitive disorder [1]. The critical contribution made by Alois Alzheimer (1864–1915), which later prompted Emil Kraepelin to bestow the eponym upon the condition, was to link the clinical phenotype of cognitive decline with specific neuropathological findings, namely neurofibrillary tangles (NFTs) [2,3]. Initially thought to be a rare disease of the presenium, neuropsychological [4] and neuropathological [5,6] studies in the 1960s showed that most cases hitherto known as "senile dementia" were, in fact, identical to AD.

Epidemiological studies have shown that the prevalence of AD increases steeply with increasing age, with more than 50% of over 85-year-olds being affected. Early onset AD, that is, presenting at or before 65 years of age, may be differentiated from late-onset disease [7], although this distinction is probably arbitrary as the underlying pathobiology is identical. More useful, in terms of elucidating etiology, has been the distinction of sporadic AD where there is no family history of the condition from familial AD where at least one first-degree family relative is affected and autosomal dominant AD where at least three family members are affected in at least two generations [8]. Autosomal dominant AD is most usually of early onset type, sometimes manifesting as early as the third or fourth decade of life (Section 2.1.1).

Cognitive decline, usually memory dysfunction, is the dominant phenotypic manifestation of AD, but occasionally other cognitive, neurological, and behavioral or psychiatric features may be prominent, in some cases representing other variants of AD [9] (not subtypes [10]). From the cognitive perspective, slowly progressive aphasia has been reported to be the presenting feature of AD, rather than one of the focal frontotemporal lobar degeneration syndromes (Section 2.2), often with nonfluent aphasia but sometimes with fluent aphasia with the characteristics approximating a transcortical sensory aphasia [11–13]. Presentation with primarily visuoperceptual dysfunction is well recognized, described as posterior cortical atrophy (PCA) [14] or the visual variant of AD [15], although other pathologies can be the substrate of PCA [16]. Slowly progressive apraxia has been described as a presentation of AD, either bilateral with biparietal [13,17] or, rarely, unilateral [18] atrophy. AD cases that overlap clinically with corticobasal degeneration (CBD) are described [19], even occasionally with the alien limb phenomenon [20]. A frontal variant of AD (fvAD) has also been postulated, based on the retrospective finding of early and disproportionately severe impairments on tests of frontal lobe functioning in a subset of definite AD cases with higher NFT load in the frontal cortex [21]. Patients with the clinical phenotype of behavioral variant frontotemporal dementia (Section 2.2.1) but with pathologically proven AD are uncommonly reported [13,22]; this phenotype is probably more common in familial AD associated with presenilin-1 mutations (Section 2.1.1). The frequency of these AD clinical variants is uncertain, but may constitute up to 10% of AD presentations in a specialist cognitive disorders clinic with a particular interest in early onset cases, the agnosic (PCA) and aphasic presentations being the most common [23].

Other neurological features that may occur in AD include epileptic seizures [24,25] and movement disorders, particularly myoclonus [26], most often in the later stages of the disease. Extrapyramidal signs are reported [27], although concurrent Lewy body pathology (Sections 2.4.1 and 2.4.2) or use of neuroleptic medications may also be a cause of parkinsonism. Neurological signs may

Table 2.1. Typical neuropsychological deficits in Alzheimer's disease

Attention	↓ Selective, divided > sustained
General intelligence	↓ FSIQ vs. premorbid IQ; PIQ typically more impaired than VIQ
Memory	↓ Episodic memory (encoding, storage) with temporal gradient; +/− semantic memory impairment (category verbal fluency)
Language	Semantic naming errors, circumlocutions; phonology, syntax relatively spared. Aphasic presentations rare. (Logopenic progressive aphasia usually has AD pathology.)
Perception	Agnosic presentations may occur (PCA): Balint syndrome, topographical agnosia, dressing apraxia; object agnosia, pure alexia, prosopagnosia
Praxis	Ideomotor, ideational apraxia: modest. Apraxic presentations rare
Executive function	May be early impairments of judgment, abstract reasoning, and problem solving

particularly be a feature of familial AD associated with presenilin-1 mutations (Section 2.1.1). Sleep-related disorders may likewise become more common with disease progression [28]. Behavioral and psychiatric symptoms are very common as AD progresses [29,30].

AD is usually a slowly progressive disorder, with periods of relative stability and decline [31,32]. Occasionally, it may be rapidly progressive, mimicking sporadic prion disease [33] (Section 2.5.1), and acute postoperative presentation resembling a cerebrovascular event but with subsequent evolution to a typical AD picture may occur [34].

Diagnosis of AD rests on appropriate clinical features aided by ancillary investigations [35–37]. Clinical diagnostic criteria for AD developed by the National Institute of Neurologic and Communicative Disorders and Stroke and the Alzheimer's Disease and Related Disorders Association (NINCDS–ADRDA) workgroup in the 1980s required a binary approach to diagnosis, necessitating the presence of dementia before AD could be diagnosed, with definite, probable, and possible categories [7]. These clinical criteria were supported by neuropathological criteria based on quantitation and distribution of the hallmark pathological features: senile plaques and NFTs [38–40]. Neurofibrillary tangle dementia (NTD) may be a variant of AD (Section 2.2.4.3). More recent diagnostic criteria have abandoned the binary approach for a biological definition of AD, by incorporating into the criteria disease biomarkers including structural and functional imaging changes, cerebrospinal fluid (CSF) analysis, and neurogenetic testing in order to identify AD, even before dementia is apparent [41–44].

Neuropsychological profile (Table 2.1)

The neuropsychological features of AD have been studied extensively [45]. Disturbance of memory, particularly recent memory, is the most common presenting symptom, often manifested as repeating the same information or questions within a short space of time, accompanied by difficulty learning new information, for example use of new household appliances. Although this may be an isolated amnesic syndrome, usually with a temporal gradient with more recent information more significantly affected, other cognitive domains are often found to be affected when formally tested, particularly language and visuospatial function.

Attention

Both selective and divided attention are impaired in AD [46–48]. Tests of selective attention such as the Stroop Test show impairment early in the disease course, possibly reflecting pathological involvement of the cingulate gyrus and/or the basal forebrain cholinergic system [49]. Tests of divided attention such as dual-task performance tests also show impairment [50]. A review of studies of working memory function in early AD found relative preservation of the phonological loop but impairment of the visuospatial sketchpad and central executive system in mild AD, and possibly also in the preclinical stages [51]. There may be a reduced working memory capacity, as evidenced by the influence of information load on the performance of AD patients [52]. The relative preservation of attentional functions may be one feature assisting in the differential diagnosis of AD from dementia with Lewy bodies (DLB) (Section 2.4.2).

General intelligence (IQ)

Typically patients with AD show disparity between their current fullscale IQ (FSIQ) scores and estimates of premorbid IQ based on the National Adult Reading Test (NART) or educational/occupational achievement, especially for performance IQ (PIQ), indicating a decline in intellectual functioning. Estimates of premorbid IQ using the NART may be difficult or impossible if there is marked aphasia.

Memory

Memory decline is the most common complaint of patients and, more often, of their caregivers in AD. This is most commonly seen in the domain of anterograde episodic memory, that is the encoding, storage, retention, and recall of new information about day-to-day personal experiences, in other words memories with an autobiographical referent [53]. Tests requiring the learning and recall of supraspan word lists are very sensitive to the episodic memory impairment in early AD; examples include the Buschke Selective Reminding Test, the Rey Auditory Verbal Learning Test, the California Verbal Learning Test, and the Hopkins Verbal Learning Test (Section 1.1.3). With a word list containing only three items, the Mini-Mental State Examination (MMSE) represents a less stringent test of episodic memory, a deficiency that has been addressed in other bedside cognitive screening instruments such as the Addenbrooke's Cognitive Examination, DemTect, and Montreal

Cognitive Assessment. The learning curve is virtually flat (i.e., many trials are required to learn the new information), intrusion errors are common (i.e., reporting words that were not on the list to be remembered, although these may be semantically related), and recognition paradigms are little better than recall. There may be an accelerated rate of forgetting [54]. In other words, the findings are typical of a cortical as opposed to subcortical disorder: encoding and storage deficits are paramount rather than a primary deficit of memory retrieval (Section 1.3.3.1). The hippocampal origin of the AD memory deficit may be examined by controlling for the encoding phase using the "five-words" test [55]. Although it is a common clinical observation that AD patients' distant, long-term, (remote) memory is spared, evaluation shows retrograde memory is not entirely normal, with a temporal gradient such that more distant memories are most intact [56]. The deficits in episodic memory reflect pathological change in the mesial temporal regions, particularly the hippocampal formation, which is also evident on volumetric brain imaging. These are typically the earliest changes in the AD brain seen in presymptomatic individuals carrying deterministic genetic mutations for AD [57]. This is also the area earliest affected by neurofibrillary pathological change [39,58].

Semantic memory impairments may also be detected in AD [59]. On tests of verbal fluency, category fluency is more impaired than letter fluency indicating difficulty accessing the semantic lexicon of word meanings [60]. Naming difficulties may also be semantic in their origin [61].

The pattern of implicit memory impairments in AD differs from that in Huntington's disease, with verbal priming severely impaired but motor (pursuit rotor) skill normally acquired [62].

Language

Language deficits in AD have been studied extensively [61,63]. The language disorder of AD varies with the stage of the disease, initially remaining fluent with lexicosemantic deficits predominating, but ultimately evolving to global aphasia. Naming and fluency deficits are particularly evident.

Word-finding difficulties are common in the early stages of AD; circumlocution (the tip-of-the-tongue phenomenon) may be evident; for example, on picture naming the first letter or phoneme may be generated but not the rest of the word (anomia). Naming errors are largely semantic, rarely phonological or visual.

Progressive loss of the richness of language may be evident to the point that speech production may be described as "empty," lacking in specific content and impoverished in both conveying and obtaining information. Some semantic information about items that cannot be named may be generated; for example, "a beautiful thing that jumps" for kangaroo [64]. As previously mentioned (see earlier Memory section), verbal fluency is typically more impaired in the category (semantic) as compared to the letter (phonological) paradigm [60]. In comparison with the semantic aspects of language, phonological and syntactic abilities are relatively preserved early in AD, although they may breakdown as the disease progresses. Repetition and motor speech may be relatively intact while increasingly impaired comprehension of the spoken or written word is evident. Attempts have been made to fit the language disturbance of AD into established aphasia categories (e.g., anomic aphasia in the early stages, extrasylvian or transcortical sensory aphasia in the later stages), but the implication that AD-related language dysfunction is congruent with one of these "typical" aphasia syndromes may not be justified.

Slowly progressive aphasia has been reported occasionally as the presenting symptom of AD [11–13], which may be confused with the linguistic variants of frontotemporal lobar degeneration (Sections 2.2.2 and 2.2.3). Presence or absence of deficits in other cognitive domains may give clues to the correct diagnosis, as may structural and functional brain imaging. Sometimes, however, only with the passage of time and the evolution of symptoms, or even only at post-mortem, does diagnostic clarity emerge.

Within the rubric of primary progressive aphasia (PPA), Gorno-Tempini and colleagues have delineated a syndrome of logopenic progressive aphasia (LPA) or logopenic variant PPA [65,66]. This is characterized by deficits in word retrieval and sentence repetition but with spared semantic, syntactic, and motor speech abilities: there is no frank agrammatism, dysprosody, or motor speech errors as seen in progressive nonfluent aphasia (Section 2.2.2). Single word comprehension is spared and any confrontation naming impairment is less severe than in semantic dementia (Section 2.2.3). The most common pathological substrate in LPA is AD [65,66].

Perception

Various visual processing disorders may occur in AD [67], their exact nature depending upon the relative involvement of right or left hemisphere, and the two streams of visual processing (Section 1.1.5), namely dorsal (occipitoparietal, "where") or ventral (occipitotemporal, "what") [17]. Visuoperceptual and visuospatial deficits are seldom clinically evident in the early stages of AD, with the exception of those patients who present with visual agnosia, known as PCA or the visual variant of AD [14–16], with relative preservation of memory and language function. Dorsal stream involvement, the most commonly observed pattern in one series of PCA patients [68], results in Balint's syndrome and dressing apraxia, whereas ventral stream involvement may produce object agnosia, pure alexia, and prosopagnosia. Predominant right hemisphere involvement may produce left visual hemineglect, whereas predominant left hemisphere involvement is associated with Gerstmann syndrome, pure alexia, and right hemiachromatopsia. Cortical blindness and Anton's syndrome (visual anosognosia) have also been recorded.

Impaired naming is not thought to result from perceptual deficits. Tests that tap aspects of visual cognition, such as drawing the Rey–Osterrieth Complex Figure, overlapping pentagons (from the MMSE), the Necker cube, and clock drawing may be impaired early in AD, although performance may also be degraded by concurrent apraxia and/or planning difficulties.

Praxis

Both ideomotor and ideational apraxia may occur in AD, the prevalence increasing with disease severity [69]. However, this is usually inapparent or of modest severity, rarely producing symptoms in comparison with the cognitive impairments in other domains. Limb transitive actions (e.g., asking the patient to show how he/she would use a comb/toothbrush/pair of scissors) are most likely to show impairment; imitation of meaningless gestures may be a sensitive early measure of apraxia. Apraxia as the earliest symptom of AD is rare [13,17,70]. Apraxia sufficient to cause diagnostic confusion with CBD does occur rarely, AD being one cause of the "corticobasal syndrome" [19].

Conceptual apraxia, defined by Ochipa *et al.* [71] as impaired knowledge of what tools and objects are needed to perform a skilled movement, was reported to be common in AD.

Executive function

Executive abilities may be impaired in AD, producing impairments of judgment, abstract reasoning, and problem solving, as evidenced by difficulties with verbal fluency, Wisconsin Card Sorting Test (WCST), and trail-making tests. These changes may occur early in the disease course in some patients and are commonly observed when specifically sought [72,73].

Working memory deficits may be ascribed to central executive impairment (see earlier Attention section) [46,52]. Impairments in verbal fluency tests, which tap executive function, may in fact reflect semantic deficits in AD (category more affected than phonemic), and performance in tests of perceptual function may be reduced because of planning difficulties. Executive dysfunction may impact on activities of daily living in AD [74].

Treatment of neuropsychological deficits

Cholinesterase inhibitors (ChEIs) are licensed for the symptomatic treatment of mild to moderate AD in many jurisdictions, the rationale being that they help to restore the cholinergic deficits that are a neurochemical feature of the AD brain due to loss of the ascending cholinergic projection from the nucleus basalis of Meynert. The evidence base for their modest efficacy is relatively strong, as evidenced by meta-analyses [75–77]. These show stability or even improvement in cognitive scales such as the MMSE and ADAS-Cog as compared with placebo-treated patients over six- to twelve-month periods. Whether this reflects genuine mnemonic improvement or simply better attentional function is debatable. Behavioral improvements are also noted with ChEI, but cognitive domains other than attention and memory are little affected. Whether ChEIs have disease-modifying effects or alter the natural history of AD, for example by reducing the rate of nursing home placement [78–80], remain debatable subjects.

Memantine, an antagonist at the NMDA type of glutamate receptors, has also been shown to benefit cognitive domains [81] and is licensed for use in moderate to severe AD in some jurisdictions. Combined ChEI and memantine treatment may possibly have synergistic effects [82–84].

2.1.1 Familial AD

To date, mutations deterministic for familial AD have been discovered in three genes, encoding:
- amyloid precursor protein (APP) on chromosome 21q21.3 (OMIM#104300);
- presenilin-1 (PS1) on chromosome 14q24.2 (OMIM#607822);
- presenilin-2 (PS2) on chromosome 1q42.13 (OMIM#606889).

Multiple mutations have been identified in each gene [85], with around 200 in PS1, which is the most common site for genetic mutations causing AD [8]. Virtually all of these mutations appear to alter the metabolism of APP such that production of the amyloid β-peptide, the major protein component of amyloid plaques, is increased. These findings have raised hopes for the development of disease-modifying therapy for AD, particularly if cases can be identified early in the disease course. Studies of autosomal dominant AD have suggested that the disease cascade may commence 20 years before symptom onset [86]. Experimental therapies targeting the amyloid pathway have been developed [87], sometimes with impressive effects in animal models, but to date only symptomatic treatments for AD are available, namely cholinesterase inhibitors and memantine.

The clinical phenotype in PS1 mutations may include features not often seen in sporadic AD, including epileptic seizures, myoclonus, extrapyramidal features, spastic paraparesis, and cerebellar ataxia [88–90]. The cognitive profile is often typical of that in sporadic AD, but cases have been reported that present with aphasia [91], although naming may be relatively preserved in some instances [92,93]. Presentation with prominent behavioral features indicative of executive dysfunction, with a phenotype suggestive of the behavioral variant of frontotemporal dementia (Section 2.2.1), has been reported with a number of PS1 mutations [88,89,94].

2.1.2 Mild cognitive impairment (MCI)/prodromal AD

Mild cognitive impairment (MCI) may be clinically and etiologically heterogeneous (Section 1.3.2), but in some instances it is the forerunner of AD, and hence may be better called prodromal AD [95] (newer diagnostic criteria for AD eschew the MCI category altogether, preferring to identify AD at an early stage based on disease biomarkers [41]). The rate of conversion of MCI to AD varies in different studies but a meta-analysis of reports suggested it is probably around 5%–10% per year [96].

Criteria for MCI have been developed [43,97,98]. Various forms have been described depending on the most prominent clinical feature; hence, amnestic MCI is characterized by memory complaint.

Other variants include single nonmemory domain MCI and multiple domain MCI.

Studies of ChEI in MCI have failed to show evidence of prevention of conversion to AD [99–101]. Presumably the pathogenic cascade is too far advanced, even at the MCI stage, for neurotransmitter repletion to prevent progression.

2.1.3 Presymptomatic AD

AD may be conceptualized as having a presymptomatic or preclinical phase [44,95], predating MCI or prodromal AD. Reliable identification of such individuals would raise the prospect of preventive therapy for AD.

Community-based longitudinal follow-up studies have suggested that tests of both memory and executive function, and possibly perceptual speed, show the greatest declines over time in individuals destined to manifest AD, and these may be apparent several years prior to diagnosis [102–104]. Because these domains are similar to those that decline in "normal" cognitive aging (Section 1.3.1), use of other biomarkers to identify presymptomatic AD may be necessary.

Of these biomarkers, deterministic genetic mutations (Section 2.1.1) are the best since these are highly penetrant ("asymptomatic-at-risk AD" [95]). Longitudinal studies of presymptomatic individuals with AD mutations have shown episodic memory deficit to be the earliest change detected, along with decline in IQ, while perceptual, naming, and spelling skills were relatively preserved [57,86,105,106].

2.2 Frontotemporal lobar degenerations (FTLD)

Arnold Pick, in the 1890s, was the first clinician to describe syndromes related to focal lobar degeneration of the brain, both frontal degeneration associated with behavioral change and temporal degeneration associated with linguistic decline [107]. The term "Pick's disease" came later, based on the neuropathological finding (by Alzheimer) of ballooned achromatic neurons (Pick cells) and neuronal inclusions (Pick bodies) in some but not all cases of lobar degeneration.

Reported prevalence rates of FTLD are around 15/100 000, similar to AD in the early onset dementia age group [108,109].

FTLDs are characterized by heterogeneity at the clinical, pathological, and genetic levels [110,111]. Broadly, the clinical phenotype may be divided into behavioral or linguistic presentations, the former described as behavioral variant frontotemporal dementia (bvFTD) or frontal variant FTD (fvFTD) (Section 2.2.1). The linguistic or temporal variants of FTLD may be categorized as forms of "primary progressive aphasia" (PPA), of which two types were originally characterized, either fluent, semantic dementia (Section 2.2.3), or nonfluent, progressive nonfluent aphasia (Section 2.2.2). A more recent classification rebrands these disorders as semantic variant PPA and nonfluent/agrammatic variant PPA, respectively, as well as recognizing a third variant, logopenic variant PPA, which is most usually characterized as a form of AD (Section 2.1, Aphasia) [66]. Neuropsychiatric symptoms may also be prominent in FTLDs, but although psychosis is described, it is rare [112–114]. Perceptual functions are largely preserved in FTLDs, and indeed, enhancement of artistic abilities has been noted in temporal variant FTLD [115,116].

The cognitive deficits in FTLDs may occur in conjunction with other neurological features, such as motor neuron disease or amyotrophic lateral sclerosis (FTD/MND or FTD/ALS). Certain parkinsonian syndromes (Section 2.4), particularly CBD (Section 2.4.4) and progressive supranuclear palsy (PSP) (Section 2.4.3), may also have similar cognitive impairments and be subsumed under the rubric of FTLDs in some classifications ("Pick complex" [117]). Attempts have been made to develop diagnostic criteria for the clinical variants of FTLDs [66,118–120]. The neuropathological substrates of these clinical syndromes are variable, with an evolving classification based on abnormal proteins detected in FTLD brains, most commonly tau, transactive response DNA-binding protein (TDP), and fused in sarcoma protein (FUS) (Section 2.2.4) [121]. Likewise, the number of genetic mutations that may be deterministic for FTLDs continues to expand (Section 2.2.5) [85].

2.2.1 Behavioral variant frontotemporal dementia (bvFTD)

This syndrome is defined on the basis of a behavioral disorder, with decline in social interpersonal conduct and the regulation of personal conduct, emotional blunting, and loss of insight. Characteristics may include neglect of personal hygiene, transgression of social mores, mental rigidity and inflexibility (increased adherence to routines, rituals, clockwatching), changes in dietary habits with a predilection for sweet foods, motor and verbal perseverations, disinhibition, or inertia. The syndrome is not homogeneous and clinical subtypes may be defined on the basis of the most prominent behavioral and motor features: disinhibited type with predominant orbitofrontal lobe involvement; apathetic type with predominant dorsolateral convexity involvement, and stereotypic type with predominant striatal involvement [110,111].

Delayed diagnosis is common [122] because neuropsychological tests and structural and functional neuroimaging may not be sensitive to the very earliest changes in bvFTD. As a result of the behavioral phenotype, many patients present to psychiatrists rather than neurologists, who may be less familiar with this condition than with AD [123]. Use of highly sensitive diagnostic criteria developed by the International Behavioural Variant FTD Criteria Consortium (FTDC) [120] may facilitate case identification, as may use of an integrated care pathway [124]. bvFTD is the most frequent FTLD clinical phenotype, with a variable pathological correlate (tau, TDP, FUS).

Table 2.2. Typical neuropsychological deficits in behavioral variant frontotemporal dementia

Attention	↓ Sustained attention; distractibility, apathy, economy of effort, poor self-monitoring, impulsivity
General intelligence	FSIQ may be normal or ↓ due to lack of mental effort
Memory	Absence of amnesia may be a requirement for diagnosis; amnesia generally not prominent but reported in some cases; better performance with cueing, and specific as opposed to open-ended questions
Language	↓ Verbal fluency (letter and category)
Perception	Typically normal
Praxis	Generally preserved; imitation and utilization behavior may be seen
Executive function	Lack of insight, impaired planning, judgment, abstraction, organization, and problem solving; perseveration, failure to inhibit inappropriate responses

Neuropsychological profile (Table 2.2)

Attention

Poor sustained attention, manifested as distractibility or motor restlessness, may be an evident behavioral feature in bvFTD (cf. AD). "Don't know" responses may be frequent, especially for effortful tasks, one feature of the lack of mental application, or economy of effort, evident on clinical testing. Responses may be rapid and impulsive, with lack of attention to accuracy, or slowed in apathetic patients.

General intelligence (IQ)

Performance may be normal on test batteries such as the WAIS-R or MMSE, despite the change in behavior. More usually, however, performance is impaired. This sometimes may affect all areas, reflecting lack of mental application to tests, or may favor Performance over Verbal subtests.

Memory

Unlike the situation in AD, amnesia generally is not a prominent feature in FTLD cases, albeit the presenting complaint (often of relatives) may be "poor memory." Severe rapidly progressive anterograde amnesia has been recorded in pathologically confirmed FTD with prominent involvement of the hippocampi, and marked amnesia at presentation has been noted in other pathologically confirmed cases

[125–127]. Memory problems may be more evident in older persons with FTLD, perhaps related to the neuropathological finding of hippocampal sclerosis [128].

Performance on memory tests is often impaired for both recall and recognition, despite patients' ability to provide some autobiographical information and orientation in time (i.e., not evidently amnesic clinically). Autobiographical memory is impaired in bvFTD, with a reduced capacity to recall specific and contextually rich autobiographical memories across all life epochs [129]. Semantic memory is relatively preserved in bvFTD in comparison to semantic dementia (Section 2.2.3), although scores may be abnormal compared to those of controls [130].

Memory performance may benefit from cues and from use of specific as opposed to open-ended questions. Poor performance may be related to the generalized economy of effort in performing tests and poor sustained attention.

Language

In conversation, spontaneous speech output may be reduced, brief, and concrete in character in bvFTD. Stereotyped words or phrases ("catchphrases") and verbal perseverations may be evident; repetition is relatively preserved. Output is fluent although prosody may be lost. Comprehension is preserved at the individual word level but may be impaired on tests of more complex items, perhaps related to lack of mental effort or self-monitoring, and impulsive responding. Object naming is generally preserved, in contrast to difficulties with verbal fluency, both letter and category. Progression to mutism may eventually occur. Preservation of calculation skills despite dissolution of language has been reported [131]. Acute aphasic presentation of clinically diagnosed frontal variant FTD, following cardiac surgery, has been reported [34].

Perception

Perceptual skills are relatively preserved in bvFTD. Visual agnosia is not apparent, and spatial skills are intact. Patients may take long walks without becoming lost. Impaired performance on tests such as drawing the Rey–Osterrieth Complex Figure may reflect cursory performance with lack of attention to detail. Dot counting and line orientation, undemanding tasks of visuospatial function, are typically normal.

Praxis

Manual skills are generally well preserved. Tests of praxis may reveal perseveration of gestures, writing, and alternating hand movements or motor sequences, although copying of hand postures is generally performed better. Use of body part as object is typical when pantomiming actions. Contextually inappropriate use of objects, utilization behavior, may occur. Dependent upon the topographical distribution of pathology, a phenotype resembling CBD may occur occasionally [19].

Executive function

A dysexecutive syndrome is typical of bvFTD, manifested as lack of insight, impaired planning, judgment, abstraction, organization, and problem solving. Tests deemed sensitive to frontal lobe function are performed poorly. For example, in the WAIS-R, the Similarities subtest may be impaired due to difficulties in abstracting similarities between objects,

and Picture Arrangement to tell a story may not be completed although individual elements can be identified and described. Proverb interpretation is concrete and cognitive estimates may be wildly inaccurate. As previously mentioned, verbal fluency is impaired for both letter and category; design fluency, the visual analog of verbal fluency, is also impaired, with multiple rule violations. Sorting rules are not identified and perseverative errors are common in both the Weigl Color Form Sorting Test and the Wisconsin Card Sorting Test. Failure to inhibit inappropriate responses may be encountered on the Stroop Color Word Test. In mild bvFTD, however, risk-taking behavior with increased deliberation time may be the only finding, with other tests sensitive to frontal lobe function remaining normal [132]. bvFTD presenting with pathological gambling has been reported [133]. Tests of decision making and risk taking that involve gambling (Section 1.1.7) may be used to identify these patients.

Treatment of neuropsychological deficits

Currently, there are no licensed treatments for the neuropsychological deficits of bvFTD. Small studies looking at the use of cholinesterase inhibitors have been negative [134]. Empirical treatments for behavioral features (e.g., mood stabilizers for disinhibition) might temporarily improve some aspects of cognitive function. A trial of the serotonin reuptake inhibitor paroxetine showed impaired cognition in bvFTD [135].

2.2.2 Progressive nonfluent aphasia (PNFA); nonfluent/agrammatic variant PPA

Of the temporal variants of FTLD, progressive nonfluent aphasia (PNFA) is the more commonly encountered. The syndrome, first described in 1982 by Mesulam [136], who used the rubric of PPA [137], is characterized by progressive nonfluent aphasia with relative preservation of other cognitive functions and activities of daily living until late in the illness. As the PPA terminology may also encompass semantic dementia (Section 2.2.3) and the

Table 2.3. Typical neuropsychological deficits in progressive nonfluent aphasia or nonfluent/agrammatic variant of primary progressive aphasia

Attention	Essentially intact
General intelligence	↓ FSIQ; VIQ typically more impaired than PIQ due to linguistic impairment
Memory	Essentially intact; impaired scores may reflect linguistic impairment
Language	Agrammatic language production; effortful halting speech with inconsistent speech sound errors and distortions (apraxia of speech). Spared single word comprehension but impaired comprehension of syntactically complex sentences; spared object knowledge
Perception	Essentially intact
Praxis	Essentially intact
Executive function	↓ Verbal fluency (letter > category), otherwise intact

logopenic progressive aphasic variant of AD (Section 2.1), PNFA is preferred for this syndrome. Consensus criteria are available [66].

Most PNFA cases are sporadic. Although some familial cases have been reported [138], discordance in monozygotic twins has also been found [139], suggesting genetic heterogeneity. A PNFA phenotype may be seen in familial FTLD with progranulin mutations (Section 2.2.5.1) and with the C9ORF72 hexanucleotide repeat (Section 2.2.5.4). PNFA cases that evolve over time to the phenotype of CBD (Section 2.4.4) [140–142] or PSP (Section 2.4.3) [143,144] have been reported. Clinical diagnosis of PNFA is associated with tau-positive pathology (as is the case in CBD and PSP) [126,145]. PNFA has the best prognosis of any of the FTLD syndromes [146].

The neuroradiological signature of PNFA is predominant left posterior frontoinsular atrophy on structural neuroimaging and hypoperfusion/hypometabolism of this area on functional neuroimaging [66].

Neuropsychological profile (Table 2.3)

The description is for a "pure" case, without features of any other underlying neuropathological entity such as AD, CBD or PSP.

Attention

Attentional functions are preserved in PNFA.

General intelligence (IQ)

A verbal–performance discrepancy on the WAIS-R in favor of nonverbal tasks is found.

Memory

Functional memory skills appear intact although scores on memory tests may be impaired because of the language disorder, especially for verbal tests. Recognition memory for faces is typically well preserved. Likewise, impaired category verbal fluency is due to language deficits rather than impaired semantic memory.

Language

The proposed diagnostic criteria for PNFA [66] require at least one of two core features to be present; namely, agrammatism in language production and effortful halting speech with inconsistent speech sound errors and distortions (i.e., apraxia of speech; insula involvement had previously been implicated in this condition [147]). In addition, two of three other features must be present, specifically impaired comprehension of syntactically complex sentences, spared single word comprehension, and spared object knowledge.

There is progressive breakdown of phonological and syntactic processes in PNFA. Speech output is hesitant and effortful, with phonemic paraphasias and transpositional errors ("spoonerisms"). Comprehension is largely intact, at least initially; for example, in word–picture matching tasks, although complex syntax may prove difficult. Increasing comprehension problems develop with disease progression. Repetition is severely impaired, as is naming to confrontation or description, although semantic information about the item that cannot be named may be provided and the correct word can be selected from alternatives; hence, this is a problem of lexical access or phonological selection. Verbal fluency is typically better for category rather than for letter. Reading and writing deficits mirror those in spoken language. Loss of prosody, a telegraphic quality to speech output (agrammatism), and diminution of output to the point of mutism occurs over time.

Perception

Visuoperceptual and visuospatial function is essentially preserved in PNFA, any errors resulting from linguistic rather than perceptual dysfunction.

Praxis

Apraxia of speech is a core feature of PNFA [66]. Orofacial apraxia and limb apraxia have been recorded, in descending order of frequency, in PNFA [148].

Executive function

Any deficits on tests of executive function may be explicable in terms of language deficits.

2.2.3 Semantic dementia (SD); semantic variant PPA

Warrington, in 1975, was the first to report patients with selective impairment of semantic memory causing a progressive anomia [149]. The linguistic variant of FTD, which has come to be known as semantic dementia (SD) (also known as progressive fluent aphasia and semantic variant PPA), is characterized by a loss of the knowledge about, or the meaning of items, which affects naming, word comprehension, and object recognition but with

relatively stable attention and preserved executive function [150]. Activities of daily living are relatively well preserved, at least in the initial stages.

The neuroradiological signature of SD is asymmetric focal atrophy of all anterior temporal lobe structures, especially entorhinal cortex, amygdala, anterior medial and inferior temporal gyri, and anterior fusiform gyrus, with an anteroposterior gradient of atrophy (cf. AD: symmetrical atrophy, especially medial temporal lobe structures including hippocampus, with no anteroposterior gradient) [151]. Left-sided cases of semantic dementia are apparently more common than right-sided [152] but this may be artifactual, the profound anomia drawing attention to the former cases whereas progressive prosopagnosia associated with right-sided cases may not come to clinical attention. The most common neuropathological substrate is MND-type, ubiquitin-positive, tau-negative inclusions, although true Pick's disease and AD may also be seen [13,153,154].

Neuropsychological profile (Table 2.4)

Attention

In contrast to bvFTD, sustained attention to tasks is good in SD. Working memory is intact as assessed by digit span and by Corsi span, at least until the very late stages of the disease.

General intelligence (IQ)

Performance on the WAIS-R is typically impaired. For patients with a disorder of word meaning, a verbal–performance discrepancy favoring performance is evident with subtests scores reflecting the semantic component of each task, the most impaired being Vocabulary, Comprehension, Information, Similarities, Picture Completion, and Picture Arrangement, while Block Design remains intact.

Memory

Episodic memory is relatively preserved. Patients are not amnesic as they can relate details about

Table 2.4. Typical neuropsychological deficits in semantic dementia or semantic variant of primary progressive aphasia

Attention	Essentially intact
General intelligence	↓ FSIQ; VIQ typically more impaired than PIQ due to semantic deficit
Memory	Absence of amnesia for recent events; remote autobiographical memory may be impaired. Semantic memory severely impaired
Language	Impaired confrontation naming (anomia); impaired single word comprehension. Impaired object knowledge; surface dyslexia (regularization errors) or dysgraphia; spared repetition; spared grammar and motor speech production
Perception	Essentially intact
Praxis	Essentially intact
Executive function	↓ Verbal fluency; frontal features may gradually emerge

recent activities. However, autobiographical memory for remote epochs is more impaired, a reversal of the temporal gradient effect seen in AD, deficits that are related to compromised emotions/thoughts and spatiotemporal details [129].

Semantic memory is severely impaired, moreso than in AD or other FTLDs [130]; there is a breakdown in factual knowledge. Depending on the lateralization of brain atrophy, this may be more evident for verbal or visual material. Cued recall shows no advantage over free recall, indicating breakdown or impaired access to semantic knowledge.

Language

The proposed diagnostic criteria for semantic variant PPA [66] require both of two core features to be present; namely, impaired confrontation naming (anomia) and impaired single word comprehension. In addition, three of four other features must be present; specifically, impaired object knowledge, particularly for low frequency or low familiarity items; surface dyslexia or dysgraphia; spared repetition; and spared grammar and motor speech production.

There is a selective breakdown in the lexico-semantic aspects of language. "Loss of memory for words" is often the main presenting complaint, with relatives and carers providing examples of

the patient's loss of word meaning ("What's Coca-Cola?," "What's a hobby?"). Marked anomia is evident on testing; moreover, unlike the situation in AD, patients are often unable to provide any contextual information about objects they cannot name: a patient with AD unable to name a picture of a kangaroo may nonetheless be able to say that it jumps and is found in Australia, but such details are not available to the patient with SD with degradation of, or loss of access to semantic memory. Providing semantically related multiple choice alternatives is not helpful. Repetition is common; for example, of overlearned words and phrases or of the examiner's questions, although there may be inability to understand what is being repeated. Verbal fluency tasks are severely impaired, letter fluency generally being superior to category fluency as the latter is reliant upon access to semantic knowledge. There may also be difficulty recognizing familiar faces, the syndrome of progressive prosopagnosia [155].

Conversational speech is fluent, syntactically and grammatically correct, but may demonstrate anomia, and use of superordinate categories (e.g., all animals are called dogs). Reading often demonstrates regularization errors when reading words with irregular sound–spelling correspondence; for example, "pint" is read to rhyme with "mint," the phenomenon of surface dyslexia. As the disease progresses, utterances may become increasingly brief and stereotyped.

Perception

Visuoperceptual and visuospatial function is preserved. Tests such as Raven's Progressive Matrices,
Judgment of Line Orientation, copy of the Rey–
Osterrieth Complex Figure, and object matching are
intact. Impaired object recognition on visual and
tactile presentation, sometimes labeled associative
agnosia, reflects the breakdown in semantics.

Praxis

Praxis is generally intact in SD, although there may
be impaired recognition and production of motor
acts.

Executive function

As previously mentioned, tests of sustained attention are intact but tests thought sensitive in part
to frontal lobe function such as verbal fluency are
impaired. The Weigl Color Form Sorting Test may
be completed but patients may fail to understand
the instructions for the Wisconsin Card Sorting Test.
Behavioral features reminiscent of bvFTD may be
present in SD occasionally, such as apathy, irritability, and disinhibition. However, in contrast to the
impulsiveness that compromises bvFTD patients'
performance on gambling tasks, a patient with SD
who was still able to bet regularly on horse rac-
ing with moderate, better than breakeven success
despite being essentially mute, has been reported
[156].

2.2.4 Other FTLDs

A number of other FTLD syndromes have been
described, most usually based on neuropathological appearances. More recent classification of these
disorders has attempted to organize them according
to the abnormal proteins detected in neuropathological inclusions, the most common of which are
tau, TDP, and FUS [121]. Some of these entities
are tauopathies (e.g., argyrophilic grain disease,
neurofibrillary tangle dementia) while others are
FUS proteinopathy or FUSopathies (e.g., basophilic
inclusion body disease, neuronal intermediate filament inclusion disease).

The FTLD phenotype or a syndrome resembling
it has also been described in association with a
wide variety of other conditions, including AD associated with certain presenilin-1 gene mutations
(Section 2.1.1), familial Creutzfeldt–Jakob disease
(Section 2.5.3), neurodegeneration with brain iron
accumulation (NBIA; Section 5.4.3), metachromatic
leukodystrophy (MLD; Section 5.5.2.1), adult-onset
Alexander's disease (Section 5.5.2.3), hereditary diffuse leukoencephalopathy with spheroids (HDLS;
Section 5.5.2.8), cerebrotendinous xanthomatosis (CTX; Section 5.5.4), hemochromatosis (possibly chance concurrence; Section 5.5.5), Sjögren's
syndrome (Section 6.6), spontaneous intracranial
hypotension (SIH; Section 7.3.3), Whipple's disease
(Section 9.4.5), and a non-DM1 non-DM2 multisystem myotonic disorder (Section 10.1). Phenocopies
of bvFTD in which clinical and neuroradiological
progression does not occur have been described by
Davies *et al.* [157]; the exact nature of these cases is
uncertain, but some may have primary psychiatric
rather than a neurodegenerative disease.

2.2.4.1 Argyrophilic grain disease (AGD)

Argyrophilic grain disease (AGD) is defined neuropathologically by the presence of spindle-shaped
argyrophilic grains in neuronal processes and
coiled bodies in oligodendrocytes composed of tau
protein, mainly in limbic regions (hippocampus,
entorhinal and transentorhinal cortices, amygdala).
This is a tauopathy, shown by immunohistochemical and biochemical studies to be of four-repeat
(4R) type, as in PSP and CBD but unlike AD. AGD is
said to affect 5% of all patients with dementia, particularly the elderly [158,159].

Macroscopically there is atrophy of frontal
and temporal lobes with little or no atrophy
of the hippocampus and amygdala. Because of
the tau inclusions and frontotemporal atrophy,
AGD may be classified with the FTLDs with tau
inclusions.

A case with an MAPT mutation (Section 2.2.5.1) has been reported [160].

The clinical phenotype of AGD has been difficult to define because it is commonly associated with other tauopathies such as AD, PSP, and CBD and with synucleinopathies. AGD may be similar to the limbic dementias such as AD. One study comparing AGD with AD suggested that the impairments in memory, language, attention, and executive function were less severe in AGD [161]; another suggested that concurrence of AD and AGD lowered the threshold for AD-related cognitive deficits [162].

2.2.4.2 Basophilic inclusion body disease (BIBD)

Basophilic inclusion body disease (BIBD) was defined on the basis of tau-negative and inconsistently ubiquitin-immunoreactive neuronal cytoplasmic inclusions. The clinical presentation is with a cognitive phenotype of bvFTD with subsequent development of MND, or with a motor phenotype that may be MND-like or PSP-like. Neuropathological inclusions have now been shown to stain intensely for the fused in sarcoma (FUS) protein [163], so this disorder may be classified as a FUS proteinopathy or FTLD-FUS, as is the case for neuronal intermediate filament inclusion disease (NIFID) (Section 2.2.4.4) [121].

2.2.4.3 Neurofibrillary tangle dementia (NTD); diffuse neurofibrillary tangles with calcification (DNTC; Kosaka–Shibayama disease)

Neurofibrillary tangle dementia (NTD), also known as senile dementia with tangles or neurofibrillary tangle-predominant dementia (NFTPD), is a form of late-life dementia characterized by medial temporal lobe neurofibrillary tangles and neuropil threads but no or few isocortical tau lesions, absence of neuritic plaques, and scarcity of amyloid deposits. Tau is of 3R and 4R type, as in classical AD. The clinical phenotype is said to differ from AD in being of shorter duration and with less severe

cognitive impairment [164,165], although it has also been classified with the FTLDs [119].

Diffuse neurofibrillary tangles with calcification (DNTC), also known as Kosaka–Shibayama disease, is a condition that pathologically resembles NTD, mostly reported from Japan. It is characterized radiologically by temporal or temporofrontal atrophy, with pallidal and cerebellar calcification typical of that seen in Fahr's disease (bilateral striatopallidodentate calcinosis; Section 5.4.8), and pathologically by neuronal loss, astrocytosis, with massive neurofibrillary tangles and neuropil threads but without senile plaques. There is a high frequency of neuronal cytoplasmic accumulation of α-synuclein (80%) and TDP-43 (90%) [166,167]. The clinical phenotype is broad, including both presenile and senile dementia.

Neuropsychological assessment has shown decline in memory retention and intelligence, and anomic aphasia, with or without parkinsonian features [168,169]. Cases without dementia have also been reported [170]. Reduced blood flow and metabolism in the temporal lobes has been observed on functional imaging, without change in the basal ganglia or cerebellum, prompting the suggestion that the calcification and neurodegeneration occurred independently [168]. However, Fahr's disease presenting with a pure and progressive dementia has been reported [171], suggesting that brain calcification per se may not be innocuous for cognitive function.

2.2.4.4 Neuronal intermediate filament inclusion disease (NIFID)

Neuronal intermediate filament inclusion disease (NIFID) was initially characterized neuropathologically on the basis of intraneuronal cytoplasmic inclusions of variable morphology that immunostained for all class IV intermediate filament (IF) proteins, namely NF-H, NF-M, NF-L, and α-internexin [172–175], for which reason the term FTLD-IF was proposed [176]. NIFID has a heterogeneous phenotype including features resembling bvFTD, such as personality change, apathy, disinhibition, and blunted affect, as well as memory and language impairments. Cases without dementia are reported. Neurological features may also be present, including extrapyramidal signs, hyperreflexia, orofacial apraxia, supranuclear ophthalmoplegia, with or without clinical or subclinical signs of motor neuron disease. The phenotype may sometimes resemble CBD [177].

More recently it has been shown that a much larger proportion of the inclusions in NIFID are immunoreactive with the fused in sarcoma (FUS) protein than with IF [178], leading to a change in the suggested nomenclature to FTLD-FUS [121], as is the case for basophilic inclusion body disease (BIBD) (Section 2.2.4.2).

2.2.4.5 Progressive subcortical gliosis (of Neumann)

The term progressive subcortical gliosis (PSG) was first suggested by Neumann and Cohn in 1967 [179] to describe a rare dementing disorder with typical histopathological findings, namely frontotemporal atrophy with a distinctive distribution of fibrillary astrogliosis in the superficial and deep cerebral cortical layers, as well as in the subcortical white matter, the latter sometimes extending to the basal ganglia, thalamus, brainstem, and even to the ventral horns of the spinal cord. Amyloid plaques, neurofibrillary tangles, Pick cells, and Pick bodies were not seen. The clinical correlate of these neuropathological findings is variable. Some reported cases have the clinical features of prototypical FTD [179–181], including one family with an underlying tau gene mutation [182], which would be classified now as FTDP-17 (Section 2.2.5.1). Cases with the phenotype of AD [179,183], Creutzfeldt–Jakob disease [184], and PSP [185] have also been reported. The profile of neuropsychological deficits might be anticipated to vary accordingly.

2.2.4.6 Pure hippocampal sclerosis; hippocampal sclerosis dementia

Pure hippocampal sclerosis was initially defined on neuropathological grounds, specifically by neuronal loss in the CA1 region of the hippocampus, in association with the neuroradiological signature of hippocampal atrophy and the clinical correlate of dementia [186–188]. Clinical overlap with AD was emphasized initially, but many cases were reclassified subsequently as a subtype of FTLD based on the overlap of clinical and neuropsychological features with FTLD [189] and neuropathological findings of tau-negative, ubiquitin-positive inclusions typical of "MND-inclusion dementia" [190]. Specifically, decreased grooming, inappropriate behavior, decreased interest, and hyperorality were observed, with most patients meeting FTLD diagnostic criteria [119]. However, other authors did not see the core neuropathological features of FTD (prefrontal neuronal loss, microvacuolation, gliosis) in hippocampal sclerosis brains [191].

The potential heterogeneity of this condition has been demonstrated by a report of cases of hippocampal sclerosis dementia with pathological changes immunostaining for both tau and TDP-43 [192]. Hippocampal sclerosis may be seen as a feature in brains of older individuals with FTLD [128].

2.2.5 Familial FTLDs

To date, mutations deterministic for familial FTLD have been discovered in several genes [85], encoding:

- microtubule-associated protein tau (MAPT) on chromosome 17q21.31 (OMIM#600274);
- progranulin (GRN) on chromosome 17q21.31 (OMIM#607485);
- valosin-containing protein (VCP) on chromosome 9p13.3 (OMIM#167320);
- charged multivesicular body protein 2B (CHMP2B) on chromosome 3p11.2 (OMIM#600795), also known as chromosome 3-linked FTD or FTD3;
- TAR-DNA binding protein 43 (TDP-43) on chromosome 1p36.22 (OMIM#612069), also known as ALS10;

- fused in sarcoma protein (FUS) on chromosome 16p11.2 (OMIM#608030), also known as ALS6;
- ubiquilin 2 (UBQLN2) gene on chromosome Xp11.21 (OMIM#300857), also known as ALS15;
- C9ORF72 noncoding region hexanucleotide repeat on chromosome 9p21.2 (OMIM#105550), also known as FTDALS.

Of these, the most commonly encountered are mutations in MAPT and progranulin and the C9ORF72 hexanucleotide repeat (GGGGCC). The overlap with genetic mutations deterministic for familial ALS (Section 2.3.5) is evident.

2.2.5.1 FTDP-17: MAPT and progranulin mutations

Frontotemporal dementia with parkinsonism linked to chromosome 17 (FTDP-17) was the umbrella term coined by Foster *et al.* [193] to describe autosomal dominant kindreds linked to chromosome 17q21–22 with a highly penetrant clinical phenotype of frontotemporal dementia and parkinsonism. Prior to this, various clinical and clinicopathological labels had been used to describe such kindreds, including disinhibition–dementia–parkinsonism–amyotrophy complex (DDPAC), hereditary dysphasic disinhibition dementia (HDDD), pallido–ponto–nigral degeneration (PPND), progressive subcortical gliosis, and multiple system tauopathy with presenile dementia (MSTD).

Pathogenic mutations in the gene encoding the microtubule-associated protein tau deterministic for FTDP-17 were first described in 1998 [194–196], since when around 70 different sequence variants have been described, although many are not pathogenic or are of uncertain pathogenic significance [85].

Not all FTDP-17 families were found to have MAPT mutations, and in 2006 another mutation linked to chromosome 17q21 in the gene encoding progranulin (GRN) was defined in FTDP families [197,198]. Around 150 sequence variants

are now described, many not pathogenic or of uncertain pathogenic significance [85].

FTDP-17 associated with MAPT mutations (OMIM#600274) may have a variable clinical phenotype, including bvFTD, CBD syndrome, PSP, and an amnestic syndrome more suggestive of AD [199]. Intrafamilial clinical heterogeneity has also been observed with certain *MAPT* mutations [200]. Identification of tau mutation carriers has permitted presymptomatic testing of neuropsychological function, many years before expected disease onset. Asymptomatic members of a large French–Canadian kindred known to carry the P301L tau mutation were impaired in tasks testing frontal executive and attentional functions, such as verbal fluency, Wisconsin Card Sorting Test categories completed, Stroop interference test, WAIS-R similarities and digit span subtests, and Trails B, compared to those without tau mutations. However, verbal and spatial memory, language, and visuomotor constructive abilities were preserved in the mutation carriers. Hence, the deficits in the mutation carriers mirrored those seen at the onset of clinical disease, but many years before the expected age at onset. This observation raised the possibility that certain brain areas are more vulnerable due to reduced reserve, thus explaining the focal clinical presentation, and perhaps indicating a neurodevelopmental component to disease phenotype [201].

FTDP-17 associated with GRN mutations (OMIM#607485) also shows phenotypic variability. Carriers tend to be older than MAPT mutation carriers at age of clinical onset, less likely to have a positive family history, more likely to manifest parietal lobe features and have asymmetric brain atrophy, and have shorter disease duration. The clinical phenotype is variable, including bvFTD, language impairment typical of PNFA or dynamic aphasia, and the corticobasal syndrome, and intrafamilial heterogeneity has been described [202–205]. In one series, patients with aphasic presentations had mean onset three years later than bvFTD presentations [203]. A distinct progranulin-associated phenotype of PPA has been reported, characterized by impoverished propositional speech, anomia, prolonged word-finding pauses, impaired speech repetition for sentences, and impaired verbal short-term memory [206]. In a cohort of patients with progressive language and speech disorders, agrammatic progressive aphasia was reported to be predictive for FTLD-TDP pathology with two-thirds of these patients having GRN mutations [207].

2.2.5.2 Inclusion body myopathy associated with Paget's disease of bone and frontotemporal dementia (IBMPFD): valosin-containing protein (VCP) mutations

This rare autosomal dominant disorder results from mutations in the gene encoding valosin-containing protein (VCP) on chromosome 9p13.3 (OMIM#167320), a member of the AAA-ATPase superfamily that has many roles in cellular metabolism including the ubiquitin-proteasome pathway [208–211]. Around 20 sequence variations are reported to date [85]. The clinical findings are heterogeneous with 90% of cases having myopathy, 40% Paget's disease of bone (Section 7.2.4), and 30% dementia of frontotemporal type. Intrafamilial heterogeneity has been noted. Mutations in the same gene may also cause familial ALS (Section 2.3.5). The neuropathology of the dementia is characterized by the presence of neuronal inclusions containing both ubiquitin and VCP [210]. Allelic heterogeneity has also been noted, one mutation (I27V) causing both bvFTD and an isolated progressive dysarthria [212]. In addition, presentation with fluent aphasia and language difficulties is reported [213].

2.2.5.3 Chromosome 3-linked FTD (FTD3): CHMP2B mutations

This disorder, described in a large Danish kindred, was eventually shown to result from mutations in the charged multivesicular body protein 2B (CHMP2B) on chromosome 3p11.2 (OMIM#600795) [214]. The cognitive phenotype is predominantly a frontal lobe syndrome, although temporal and dominant parietal lobe dysfunction is also recorded, along with late motor signs, both pyramidal and extrapyramidal [215].

2.2.5.4 FTD/ALS: C9ORF72 hexanucleotide repeat

A hexanucleotide repeat (GGGGCC) in the noncoding region of the C9ORF72 gene on chromosome 9p21.2 (OMIM#105550) has been found to be a common cause of FTD, FTDALS, and ALS [216–218]. It is found in around 5% of sporadic FTD cases, around 25% of familial FTD cases, and even higher frequencies in families with both FTD and ALS. The cognitive phenotype is variable, encompassing bvFTD and PNFA, but with only occasional cases of SD. There may also be an association with behavioral features and psychosis [219–221].

2.3 Motor neuron disorders

Traditionally it was taught that motor neuron disease (MND) or amyotrophic lateral sclerosis (ALS) was a disorder confined to the motor system, in which the intellect was preserved and, hence, patients were all too horribly aware of their progressive neurological predicament. Certainly, the earliest description, by Charcot and Joffroy in 1869, made no mention of cognitive changes [222]. Alzheimer may have reported a case of MND with dementia in 1891 [223], but it was not until the later part of the twentieth century that definitive cases of MND with concurrent dementia of frontal type were presented [224–226]. Dementia and cognitive impairment in MND is now a subject of significant research interest, with evident clinical, neuropsychological, pathological, and genetic overlap with FTLD [227,228]. Other conditions potentially relevant to the cognitive disorder of MND/ALS include the ALS/parkinsonism–dementia complex of Guam (Section 2.4.7).

Table 2.5. Typical neuropsychological deficits in motor neuron disease/amyotrophic lateral sclerosis

Attention	↓ Sustained attention; economy of effort, impulsiveness, distractibility
General intelligence	FSIQ may be normal or ↓ due to executive dysfunction
Memory	Not amnesic, but scores may be down due to executive dysfunction
Language	+/– aphasia (may be masked by dysarthria); anomia, ↓ verbal fluency
Perception	Essentially intact
Praxis	Impaired temporal sequencing secondary to executive dysfunction
Executive function	Impaired; ↓ verbal fluency, card sorting

2.3.1 Motor neuron disease (MND), amyotrophic lateral sclerosis (ALS)

The view of MND/ALS as an exclusively motor disorder has been increasingly eroded. Occasional clinical reports of cognitive impairment in MND/ALS patients and of frontotemporal dementia (FTD) complicated by the development of MND/ALS have been followed by more systematic studies, which have suggested that significant numbers of MND/ALS patients, up to 50%, have cognitive deficits when tested, sometimes sufficient to meet diagnostic criteria for FTD [229–231], while neurophysiological investigation of FTD patients has found evidence for subclinical anterior horn cell disease in some cases [232]. FTD and MND/ALS are now thought to represent a spectrum condition, with pure cognitive and pure motor cases at the boundaries but with extensive overlap [227].

Neuropsychological profile (Table 2.5)

Attention

As in bvFTD, economy of effort, impulsiveness, and distractibility may characterize test performance, with poor sustained attention compromising test results [226].

Neurophysiological evidence of impaired selective attention in MND/ALS has been presented, suggesting a reduced focus of attention [233]. Mild dysfunction of the central executive component of working memory, manifested as impairments in semantic and letter verbal fluency, modified Wisconsin Card Sorting Test, trail making test, digit span, Corsi blocks tapping test, and prose memory, has been observed in some patients [234].

General intelligence (IQ)

Performance may be impaired on the WAIS-R, sometimes in all areas, due to underlying executive dysfunction.

Memory

Formal tests of memory, both verbal and visual, may show impaired scores but patients are generally not amnesic, as reflected in their knowledge of autobiographical events and orientation in time and place, as commonly observed in FTD. Occasional cases with amnesia or episodic memory impairment similar to that in AD have been reported, perhaps related to degeneration of the perforant pathway [235].

Language

The frequency of language disorder in MND/ALS is uncertain, as concurrent dysarthria (due to bulbar or pseudobulbar palsy) may mask language dysfunction unless appropriate tests are used. Bulbar MND/ALS with rapidly progressive aphasia has been reported [236,237]. Marked anomia on picture naming and naming from verbal descriptions and impaired letter and category verbal fluency may be observed, indicating a disorder of language production, but with additional impairments on syntactically based tasks of language comprehension (Token Test, Test for the Reception of Grammar) and picture–word matching tests of semantic comprehension [237]. A subgroup of MND/ALS patients with language dysfunction characterized by word-finding difficulties and decreased verbal fluency has been described [238], as has greater difficulty in confrontation naming of verbs than nouns [239].

Perception

As in FTD, there is no evidence for visual perceptual disorder in MND, with preserved spatial navigational skills, spatial localization and orientation, which may be confirmed on tests such as dot counting and maze tracking. Poor performance on tests of drawing may result from lack of planning or strategy or motor deficits rather than visual perceptual impairment.

Praxis

Impaired temporal sequencing of motor skills may be apparent, reflecting executive dysfunction, although this may be difficult to test in the context of motor deficits.

Executive function

Pervasive deficits on frontal executive tests are evident on neuropsychological testing in between one-fifth and one-third of nondemented MND patients [230,231,240,241]. There are impairments on the Wisconsin Card Sorting Test with perseverations, Weigl's Block Test, verbal and design fluency, and WAIS-R Picture Arrangement. These deficits may be more common in patients with predominantly upper motor neuron signs, including primary lateral

sclerosis (Section 2.3.2), and in patients with predominantly bulbar involvement [242].

2.3.2 Primary lateral sclerosis (PLS); progressive symmetric spinobulbar spasticity

Primary lateral sclerosis (PLS) is a rare variant of MND/ALS characterized by progressive spinobulbar spasticity. PLS is thought to result from isolated involvement of upper motor neurons in the precentral gyrus with secondary pyramidal tract degeneration, without either clinical or neurophysiological evidence of lower motor neuron involvement [243,244]. Suggested diagnostic criteria require such isolated upper motor neuron involvement to persist over a period of at least three years [243], PLS tending to pursue a more benign course than typical MND/ALS.

An early study of PLS in which cognitive testing was not undertaken concluded that the intellect was preserved [243]. However, more systematic, albeit retrospective studies in small cohorts have suggested that mild cognitive dysfunction of frontotemporal lobar type is present in PLS, with deficits in executive function, psychomotor speed, and memory, but with normal orientation, spatial skills and language [245–247]. A prospective study of neuropsychological function using a broad battery of tests in 18 PLS patients found heterogeneity, but cognitive impairment according to the definitions of the study was present in 11 patients (61%). Verbal fluency was the most sensitive test, but impairment was also noted on tests of auditory verbal learning, visual (but not verbal) recognition memory, and the Wisconsin Card Sorting Test. Language testing showed impaired category verbal fluency, specifically for nonliving as opposed to living items. These findings overlap with those documented in MND/ALS whereas others do not, such as the finding that confrontation naming of nouns and verbs was relatively intact [244]. A comparison with MND/ALS patients suggested worse performance in the PLS group on verbal fluency tests, possibly related to longer disease duration [248].

2.3.3 Progressive muscular atrophy (PMA)

Variants of MND/ALS with a clinical phenotype of exclusively lower motor neuron involvement, progressive muscular atrophy (PMA), are rare, and may be even rarer if neuropathological findings are taken into account. One study of 12 PMA patients found no significant difference between subjects and healthy controls on any measure of cognitive, behavioral, or emotional function [249]. Further support for the contention that exclusively or predominantly lower motor neuron involvement is not associated with cognitive decline came from a patient with the flail arm syndrome (symmetrical wasting and weakness of the arms with minimal leg or bulbar involvement at clinical presentation), also known as the Vulpian–Bernhardt syndrome [250]. Another 73-year-old man with flail arm syndrome had no complaints of memory problems four years after diagnosis of his illness, and scored 79 on the Addenbrooke's Cognitive Examination-Revised out of a possible 88 (90%), omitting those sections dependent on upper limb function, above the test cutoff excluding dementia (Larner, unpublished observations). However, a more recent study of PMA patients found them to be worse than controls on attention and working memory, category fluency, and the MMSE, but with preserved visuospatial function. Cognitive impairment (>2SD from the mean of normative data on at least three neuropsychological tests) was found in 17% of this group of PMA patients [251].

2.3.4 Mills' syndrome

A syndrome of progressive ascending or descending hemiplegia without significant sensory involvement was first reported by Mills in 1900 [252]. The nosological status of Mills' syndrome has been uncertain, but some cases may be hemiplegic forms of motor neuron disease with exclusively upper motor neuron signs [253,254], although this clinical picture falls outside of proposed diagnostic criteria for PLS [243]. If Mills' syndrome is indeed a localized variant of MND, then the possibility of cognitive

impairment as part of the phenotype might be expected [255].

A case of progressive spastic hemiplegia conforming to the description of Mills' syndrome with concurrent dementia of frontotemporal type has been reported. Pathological examination showed tau-negative, ubiquitin-positive, MND-type inclusions in layer II cortical neurons, hippocampal dentate granule cells, and hypoglossal nerve nucleus neurons [256].

2.3.5 Familial ALS

To date, mutations deterministic for familial ALS have been discovered in several genes, encoding:

- superoxide dismutase-1 (SOD1) gene on chromosome 21q22.1 (OMIM#105400), also known as ALS1;
- fused in sarcoma protein (FUS) on chromosome 16p11.2 (OMIM#608030), also known as ALS6;
- VAPB gene on chromosome 20q13.3 (OMIM#608627), also known as ALS8;
- angiogenin (ANG) gene on chromosome 14q11.2 (OMIM#611895), also known as ALS9;
- TAR-DNA binding protein 43 (TDP-43) on chromosome 1p36.22 (OMIM#612069), also known as ALS10;
- FIG4 gene on chromosome 6q21 (OMIM#612577), also known as ALS11;
- optineurin (OPTN) gene on chromosome 10p13 (OMIM#613435), also known as ALS12;
- valosin-containing protein (VCP) on chromosome 9p13.3 (OMIM#613954), also known as ALS14, allelic with one form of familial FTLD (Section 2.2.5.2);
- ubiquilin 2 (UBQLN2) gene on chromosome Xp11.21 (OMIM#300857), also known as ALS15;
- CHMP2B gene on chromosome 3p11.2 (OMIM#614696), also known as ALS17, allelic with one form of familial FTLD (Section 2.2.5.3);
- C9ORF72 noncoding region hexanucleotide repeat on chromosome 9p21.2 (OMIM#105550), also known as FTDALS.

The overlap with genetic mutations deterministic for familial FTLD (Section 2.2.5) is evident.

Cognitive phenotypes in familial ALS are little described to date. It is reported that in SOD1 mutations significant cognitive changes are less likely compared to non-SOD1 FALS patients [257]. It has been suggested that ALS patients with the C9ORF72 hexanucleotide repeat are characterized by the presence of cognitive and behavioral impairment [258]. Although ALS is the most common phenotype with TDP-43 mutations, FTD in other individuals of the same family or in those with ALS has been reported, usually manifesting with behavioral changes but also with semantic dementia [259].

2.4 Parkinsonian syndromes

In his 1817 account of the disease which later, courtesy of Jean-Martin Charcot, would bear his name, James Parkinson stated that intellect was uninjured (see [260] for a facsimile of Parkinson's book on the shaking palsy). Charcot pointed out that this was not in fact the case and that "psychic faculties are definitely impaired" and "the mind becomes clouded and the memory is lost" [261]; Benjamin Ball also published on this subject in 1882 [262]. It is now generally recognized that Parkinson's disease (PD) is more than simply a motor disorder and that cognitive impairments are common, progressing in some patients to dementia [263,264]. Although this was not reflected in the staging scale for PD developed by Hoehn and Yahr [265], which referred to motor symptoms only, the broader Unified Parkinson's Disease Rating Scale (UPDRS) does encompass intellectual function. The motor stages of PD do not correlate well with cognitive symptoms [266]. Rapid eye movement sleep behavior disorder (REMBD) is one of the nonmotor features of PD (also seen in DLB and MSA; sections 2.4.2 and 2.4.5, respectively), which may predate other disease manifestations by many years [267], and hence be confused with idiopathic REMBD (Section 11.4.1). The pathological hallmark of PD is the finding of Lewy bodies, intracytoplasmic rounded eosinophilic inclusions, in brainstem monoaminergic and cholinergic neurons, which stain for the protein α-synuclein.

Disorders that clinically may superficially resemble idiopathic PD but that, in fact, have different clinical features, course, and pathogenesis have sometimes been labeled as "atypical" parkinsonian syndromes, or sometimes as "parkinsonism plus." The most common of these disorders are PSP, CBD and MSA. The terminology begs the question as to what is "atypical" for PD, but features that should dissuade one from a diagnosis of idiopathic PD include early freezing and falls, rapid disease progression, early dysautonomia, early speech or swallowing problems, levodopa unresponsiveness, and early dementia [268]. It is reported that simple bedside cognitive screening tests such as the Dementia Rating Scale and the Addenbrooke's Cognitive Examination can differentiate the most common "atypical" parkinsonian disorders [269].

The parkinsonian disorders other than PD considered here include PSP and CBD, which are both tauopathies and which are regarded by some authorities as falling within the rubric of FTLD [117]; MSA, a synucleinopathy; dementia pugilistica; and the parkinsonism–dementia complex of Guam. Other disorders with clinical features that might cause them to be regarded as "atypical" parkinsonian syndromes, but which are covered elsewhere, include FTD with parkinsonism linked to chromosome 17 (FTDP-17; Section 2.2.5.1), Huntington's disease (Section 5.1.1), Wilson's disease (Section 5.4.2), neurodegeneration with brain iron accumulation (Section 5.4.3), neuroacanthocytosis (Section 5.4.4), neuroferritinopathy (Section 5.4.5), Kufor–Rakeb syndrome (PARK9; Section 5.4.7), Fahr's disease (Section 5.4.8), Gaucher's disease (Section 5.5.3.4), normal pressure hydrocephalus (Section 7.2.1), postencephalitic parkinsonism (encephalitis lethargica; Section 9.1.11), and some cases of Creutzfeldt–Jakob disease (CJD) (Section 2.5).

2.4.1 Parkinson's disease dementia (PDD)

The frequency of cognitive disorders in PD has been recognized increasingly over the past 20 years [264].

Diagnostic criteria have been developed for Parkinson's disease dementia (PDD) [270,271]. A category of mild cognitive impairment in PD, PD-MCI, has also been recognized [272] and diagnostic criteria developed [273].

Longitudinal cohort studies suggest that the majority (>80%) of patients surviving PD for 20 years will have dementia, which correlates with increasing age [274], evolving around the age of 70 years irrespective of the time of PD onset [275].

However, cognitive deficits may also be evident in newly diagnosed PD patients: around one-third of patients in an incident cohort were impaired on MMSE, pattern recognition task, and the Tower of London Task [276]. At three- to five-year follow-up, 10% of cases had developed dementia and a further 57% had evidence of cognitive impairment, with deficits of frontostriatal function being the most common [277]. REMBD and insomnia may be associated with lower cognitive test scores in de novo PD [278].

Significant predictors of dementia risk in PD are age $\geq$72 years, semantic fluency less than 20 words in 90 seconds, and inability to copy intersecting pentagons [279]. Patients with earlier-onset PD have a preserved linguistic ability prior to dementia onset [274]. PDD seems to be heralded by postural and gait dysfunction and cognitive deficits with a posterior cortical basis, features which are thought to reflect nondopaminergic cortical Lewy body pathology. The cognitive profile in PDD encompasses visuospatial dysfunction, memory problems, and attentional and executive dysfunction. Compared to AD, PDD has worse attentional, executive, and visuospatial functions but memory is better preserved [280].

2.4.2 Dementia with Lewy bodies (DLB)

The finding of Lewy bodies, the pathological hallmark of PD, in the neocortex of patients with dementia and parkinsonism, often with concurrent AD-type pathology, led to the delineation of a syndrome under a variety of names, such as cortical Lewy body disease, senile dementia of the Lewy body type, and the Lewy body variant of AD. All these entities are now subsumed under the rubric of DLB [281]. A distinction has sometimes been drawn between cases with pathological evidence of concurrent AD and Lewy body pathology, labeled Lewy body variant (LBV), and those without significant concomitant AD pathology, labeled diffuse Lewy body disease (DLBD) [282]. The positive immunostaining of Lewy bodies in both PD and DLB with α-synuclein indicates that both disorders fall into the category of synucleinopathies. Lewy body pathology is also common, if sought, in AD caused by mutations in the presenilin-1 gene (Section 2.1.1), suggesting other possible genetic influences on the development of synuclein-related pathology [283].

Clinical and pathological diagnostic criteria for DLB have been developed [284–286] and validated [287]. The central clinical feature is progressive cognitive decline with prominent deficits in attention, visuospatial abilities, and executive function, along with a number of other core features that are essential for diagnosis of probable (two features) or possible (one feature) DLB, namely fluctuating cognition with pronounced variations in attention (the "unstable platform of attention"), recurrent visual hallucinations, and spontaneous motor features of parkinsonism. DLB has been characterized as a visual-perceptual and attentional-executive dementia [288], with greater impairment of attentional and visuospatial function and relative preservation of memory function as compared to AD [289–292]. A number of other clinical features may support the diagnosis, including marked neuroleptic sensitivity [293] and syncopal episodes. Autonomic dysfunction, when sought, is reported to be common [294], and cases of DLB "evolving" from pure autonomic failure have been reported [295,296]. The sensitivity of clinical diagnosis of DLB is low [297]. Inclusion of REMBD as a core clinical feature improves DLB diagnostic accuracy [298].

The relationship between DLB and PDD (Section 2.4.1) has been much discussed. Examination of many PD cases has demonstrated a characteristic pattern of topographical progression of Lewy body changes extending from brainstem to cortex [299], which may support the notion of a

Table 2.6. Typical neuropsychological deficits in Parkinson's disease dementia and in dementia with Lewy bodies

Attention	Prominent deficits: "unstable platform of attention;" difficulty establishing attentional focus, easy disengagement; bradyphrenia; impaired spatial working memory; fluctuating consciousness
General intelligence	FSIQ ↓, PIQ worse than VIQ, possibly related to executive dysfunction
Memory	Subcortical pattern of impairment, recognition better than recall
Language	Relatively intact; verbal fluency may be impaired (?phonemic > category)
Perception	Prominent deficits of visuoperceptual and visuospatial function
Praxis	Possible ideomotor apraxia
Executive function	Prominent deficits: impaired; ↓ verbal fluency, card sorting

spectrum disorder. An arbitrary one-year rule is sometimes used to distinguish PDD from DLB; that is, onset of dementia within one-year of parkinsonism is labeled DLB, while more than one year of parkinsonism before dementia develops is termed PDD. Because there is no clear neuropathological distinction between PDD and DLB, and the clinical boundaries may be blurred, they may reflect similar biological processes, both being neurodegenerative disorders with diffuse cortical Lewy bodies. Cognitive status seems to correlate with neuropathological staging [300].

Although usually a sporadic condition, occasional cases fulfilling diagnostic criteria for DLB have been reported in patients carrying genetic mutations, for example point mutations (E46K) [301] in the α-synuclein gene (SNCA), and in cases associated with triplication of SNCA [302], dementia is said to be a much more common feature [303]. DLB has also been reported with mutations of the presenilin-1 gene (ΔT440) [304], and the prion protein gene (M232R) [305], although the latter may be an uncommon polymorphism rather than a pathogenic mutation. Other disorders that may mimic or be confused with DLB, and hence lead to confounding in defining the neuropsychological profile, include CJD and vascular dementia [306,307].

Neuropsychological profile of PDD and DLB (Table 2.6)

Attention

The basal ganglia are implicated in the regulation of attention [308]. There is evidence that PD patients disengage from attended locations more readily, have less effective mechanisms for resisting interference, and have difficulties establishing a new target of attention [309]. Tests of working memory in PD have shown deficits, with spatial working memory apparently more vulnerable than verbal or visual working memory, which are affected later in the disease course [310]. Bradyphrenia, a slowness of thought or prolonged information processing time, is said to be a cardinal feature of subcortical dementias, in PD perhaps paralleling the motor slowing (bradykinesia). However, if motor slowing is controlled for, cognitive slowing does not seem to be a feature of PD [311,312]. Concurrent depression or mild dementia may also, perhaps in part, account for bradyphrenia. An overview of studies in which PDD was diagnosed by explicit criteria found attention to be more severely affected than in AD [280]. The attentional deficits in PDD are the most important cognitive predictors of impact on activities of daily living [313].

Fluctuating consciousness, clinically distinguishable from delirium, is one of the core features of DLB [284,285]. This may lead to marked variability in performance on cognitive testing both within and between testing sessions. The clinical diagnosis of fluctuating consciousness correlates with psychophysiological measures of variable attentional performance [314]. This "unstable platform of attention" may account for the observed impairments in attentional, mnemonic, and executive functions in DLB. Impairments of attention may be demonstrated using the WAIS-R Digit Span subtest [282] and on complex set-shifting tasks examining shifts of attention [315]. Subtypes of fluctuating cognition that differentiate DLB from AD include daytime drowsiness and lethargy, daytime sleep of more than two hours, staring into space for long periods of time, and episodes of disorganized speech [316], features that form the basis of the Fluctuations Composite Score, which has proved useful in diagnosis of DLB [317].

General intelligence (IQ)

Performance may be impaired on the WAIS-R, for example in Digit Span and Similarities subtests. There may be better VIQ than PIQ.

Memory

There is relatively less impairment of memory in PDD than of visuospatial and executive functions. Memory impairment is not a prerequisite in PDD diagnostic criteria [270]. Nonetheless, memory is not necessarily normal. It is deficient compared to normal controls but better in the verbal domain than in AD although visual memory is poorer [280]. There is impairment of both recent and remote memory, with recognition better than recall consistent with a retrieval deficit typical of impaired subcortical processes. Nevertheless, a meta-analysis indicated that recognition memory is impaired in PDD [318]. Retrieval difficulties may reflect the prominent executive dysfunction, with impaired allocation of attentional resources for effortful free recall tasks and the formulation of retrieval strategies [319]. Registration, storage, and consolidation of memory may be intact [320]. Semantic memory is also impaired [321].

Memory impairment is not essential in DLB consensus clinical diagnostic criteria [286]. Episodic memory deficits are less severe than those of AD patients with an equal degree of dementia [289–292] due to better retention and recognition memory, although learning and delayed recall in the free recall paradigm showed similarly severe impairment. The differences are even more apparent when patients with DLBD (i.e., without concomitant AD pathology) are compared to LBV and AD patients

[322]. Semantic memory is impaired [323]. Memory deficits are more severe in DLB than in PDD [280].

Language

There is relatively less impairment of language in PDD and DLB than visuospatial and executive functions. There is no aphasia, and naming remains intact until late stages, but hypophonia, monotonia, and aprosodia may be evident. Some groups have found reduced information content of spontaneous speech, impaired comprehension of complex commands, and impaired verbal reasoning skills [324,325]. Poor verbal fluency is evident, perhaps more so for phonemic than category fluency [326], and this may be an early indicator of executive dysfunction and developing dementia.

Perception

Visuoperceptual and visuospatial deficits are reported in PDD, and are more pronounced than in AD but less than in DLB [280]. In PD, recorded deficits include prism adaptation [327], facial recognition [328], and complex figure drawing.

In DLB, visuoperceptual and visuospatial impairments are greater than those in PDD and AD [280]. They are evident in tests of fragmented letter identification and overlapping figures [292,323], the Judgment of Line Orientation [329], drawing simple and complex figures [282,289,330,331], and in tests of visual search [332]. These deficits may reflect the underlying attentional problems and/or executive dysfunction, affecting planning and strategy formation, and/or may be related to occipital cortical hypoperfusion observed in functional imaging studies [333]. Pentagon drawing in DLB is worse than in AD or PD, apparently related to deficits in perception and praxis in DLB [331].

Praxis

Praxis may be difficult to evaluate meaningfully in the context of the motor disorder of PD.

However, ideomotor apraxia for transitive movements has been documented in some PD patients, correlating with deficits in tests sensitive to frontal lobe function (verbal fluency, Trail Making, Tower of Hanoi) and suggesting corticostriatal dysfunction [334,335].

Executive function

As with attention, executive function impairments are more severe in PDD than in AD and PD, but less so than in DLB [280].

Executive dysfunction in PD may be manifested as psychomotor slowing, impairments in abstract reasoning on WAIS-R Similarities subtest and Raven's Progressive Matrices, and impaired performance on the Stroop Test and Wisconsin Card Sorting Test [336,337]. Pathological gambling, an executive dysfunction or impulse control disorder, has been reported in some PD patients following treatment with dopamine agonist drugs [338,339].

Treatment of neuropsychological deficits

Because the cholinergic deficit in DLB is greater than that observed in AD, a possible role for cholinesterase inhibitors (ChEI) was anticipated in DLB. A randomized double-blind placebo-controlled trial demonstrated efficacy of rivastigmine for both cognitive and psychiatric features of DLB [340], benefits apparently maintained for up to two years [341]. However, a recent systematic review finds the effects of ChEIs in DLB unclear [342], and the treatment is not licensed currently.

There is greater clarity with respect to PDD where the available evidence supports ChEI use with benefits in cognitive function, activities of daily living, and global assessment [342].

Memantine has also been examined in PDD and DLB, a randomized study suggesting some benefits in global clinical status and behavioral symptoms in mild DLB patients, but not in PDD [343].

Cognitive impairment is generally deemed to be a contraindication to the use of deep brain stimulation in PD.

2.4.3 Progressive supranuclear palsy (PSP)

Progressive supranuclear palsy (PSP) is sometimes known as Steele–Richardson–Olszewski (SRO) syndrome, after the first descriptors of the condition in the early 1960s [344,345], although possible earlier cases, even dating to the nineteenth century, have been noted retrospectively [346]. PSP is an akinetic-rigid syndrome in which the typical features are bradykinesia and axial rigidity without tremor, postural instability with early falls, supranuclear gaze palsy, and bulbar symptoms. Clinical diagnostic criteria for PSP have been published [347]. However, the characteristic eye movement disorder from which PSP takes its name is not always present, as cases with the typical pathological findings but without supranuclear gaze palsy are described. It has been suggested that the typical phenotype be called "Richardson's syndrome," and the atypical form that is often confused with idiopathic PD because of asymmetric onset, tremor, and modest response to levodopa, be called "PSP-P" [348]. The neuropathology of PSP is characterized by neurofibrillary tangles and neuropil threads seen using tau immunohistochemistry. White matter astrocytes containing tangles ("tufted astrocytes") may be seen, an appearance that may be unique to PSP. Cases of apparent PSP with or without dementia have occasionally been reported in association with tau gene mutations (i.e., FTDP-17; Section 2.2.5.1) [349,350].

Dementia as a component of PSP was explicit in the first descriptions [344,345]. The term "subcortical dementia" (Section 1.3.3.1) was first used to describe the neuropsychological deficits observed in PSP, namely forgetfulness, slowing of thought processes, emotional or personality change (apathy, depression with outbursts of irritability), and impaired ability to manipulate acquired knowledge [351]. In the NNIPPS Study, the largest prospective study of PSP, around 60% of PSP patients had impairment on the Dementia Rating Scale [352].

Cognitive slowing and executive dysfunction are the key findings, with relative preservation of instrumental functions [353]. This is manifest as slowed responses to questions or problem solving, impaired verbal fluency, more so for phonological than semantic categories [269,354], and perseveration, as in the "applause test" or "clapping test" (when asked to clap three times, the patient often claps more than three times). On the Dementia Rating Scale, PSP patients are more impaired on the Initiation/Perseveration subtest and less impaired on the Memory subtest than AD patients [355]. Nonetheless, memory for long- and short-term material is also impaired, for both immediate and delayed recall, but unlike the situation in AD or other "cortical dementias," memory performance is significantly improved by cueing and recognition, methods believed to facilitate the retrieval process, itself thought to be related to the frontostriatal system [356]. Ideomotor apraxia may occur, which may cause clinical confusion with CBD, but is usually bilateral [334].

A randomized controlled trial of the ChEI donepezil in PSP proved negative [357].

2.4.4 Corticobasal degeneration (CBD)

Corticobasal degeneration (CBD), also known as cortical-basal ganglionic degeneration, was first defined neuropathologically, characterized by nerve cell loss and gliosis in the cortex, especially frontal and anterior parietal lobes, underlying white matter, thalamus, lentiform nucleus, subthalamic nucleus, substantia nigra, and locus ceruleus, with swollen and chromatolyzed residual nerve cells with eccentric nuclei (achromasia) [358]. Neuronal inclusions resembling the globose neurofibrillary tangles of PSP are present in the substantia nigra. There are no cortical neurofibrillary tangles, Pick bodies or Pick cells, senile plaques, Lewy bodies, granulovacuolar change, or amyloid deposits [359]. Neuropathological diagnostic criteria for CBD have been published

[360]. Clinical diagnosis of CBD is associated with tau-positive pathology [145].

The clinical phenotype is variable: initial reports emphasized a movement disorder, namely a chronic progressive akinetic-rigid syndrome with asymmetric onset, limb apraxia sometimes with the alien limb phenomenon, cortical sensory dysfunction, dystonia, and myoclonus, sometimes with eye movement disorder [361]. However, it was increasingly recognized that CBD is also a cognitive disorder [362,363]. Initial clinicopathological diagnostic criteria for CBD did not reflect this fact [364], but in more recently proposed criteria, this omission has been rectified, including variable degrees of focal or lateralized cognitive dysfunction with relative preservation of learning and memory on neuropsychometric testing as a supportive investigation [365]. Brief bedside cognitive screening instruments such as the Addenbrooke's Cognitive Examination, are reported to be able to detect cognitive deficits in CBD [269].

It is of note that CBD phenocopies are relatively common, the "corticobasal degeneration syndrome" (CBDS). The most common neuropathological substrates of CBDS are AD and tau-positive FTLD (Pick's disease) [19,366], but motor neuron disease-inclusion dementia [367] and NIFID (Section 2.2.4.4) [177] have also been described. Hence, studies of "CBD" without neuropathological confirmation remain open to possible confounding with cases of CBDS, a fact of critical significance when attempting to define the cognitive profile of CBD [368].

Neuropsychological studies in CBD have reported deficits of sustained attention and verbal fluency, more so for letter than category fluency, and deficits of praxis, finger tapping, and motor programing [269]. These latter changes are thought to reflect basal ganglia and posterior frontal lobe involvement in CBD [369,370]. Apraxia affecting limb function is one of the most typical features of CBS, which may be ideomotor and limb-kinetic [335]. Early and prominent language impairments have also been noted [371], specifically phonological impairments overlapping with those observed in progressive nonfluent aphasia variant of FTLD (Section 2.2.2) [372]. Learning and episodic memory are mildly impaired, if at all, particularly in the early stages.

Cases presenting with features of FTD without a motor disorder have also been reported [373], as have occasional patients with parieto-occipital, Balint-like, cortical dysfunction [374]. These findings presumably reflect the regional distribution of pathological change. Some authors have categorized CBD as a frontotemporal lobar degeneration with tau inclusions [117], and this phenotype may be seen in patients harboring mutations in the tau gene (Section 2.2.5.1) [199].

2.4.5 Multiple system atrophy (MSA)

Multiple system atrophy (MSA) is a neurodegenerative disorder characterized as a synucleinopathy on the basis of the signature neuropathological finding of glial cytoplasmic inclusions in basal ganglia, substantia nigra, pontine nuclei, medulla, cerebellum, and white matter, composed of fibrils of polymerized α-synuclein. The clinical phenotype is variable: initially three syndromes were defined, namely olivopontocerebellar atrophy (OPCA), striatonigral degeneration (SND), and Shy–Drager syndrome [375], but the current classification, based on the relative predominance of clinical (and pathological) changes, encompasses MSA-C (cerebellar ataxia), roughly equivalent to OPCA, and MSA-P (parkinsonism), roughly equivalent to SND. All cases have autonomic dysfunction, which was the prominent feature of Shy–Drager syndrome. The phenotype of MSA is broad, with many other neurological features sometimes encountered [376]. Clinicopathological diagnostic criteria for MSA have been proposed [377].

Unlike other parkinsonian syndromes, MSA was previously considered to be largely free from cognitive impairments [269]. Although intelligence is generally normal, systematic studies have shown that there may be neuropsychological impairments in MSA. In the NNIPPS Study, around 20% of MSA patients had impairment on the Dementia Rating Scale, with a cognitive profile similar to that in PSP

and PD [352]. Frontal lobe dysfunction has been a fairly consistent finding, with difficulties in attentional mechanisms and set-shifting impinging on working memory and speed of thinking [353,378, 379]. In MSA-P, verbal fluency (phonemic and category) deficits have been noted despite normality on the WAIS, Wisconsin Card Sorting Test, and Stroop test [380], as well as impairments in visuospatial and constructional function and executive function. MSA-C patients show less severe involvement, with relative sparing of frontal function [381]. Apraxia is not a feature of MSA [334]. Mild cognitive impairment in MSA (MSA–MCI) has been reported to comprise deficits in immediate recall, digit span backward, verbal fluency, Wisconsin Card Sorting Test, and Stroop Test, but with unimpaired recognition memory, long-term forgetting, naming, visuospatial abilities, and constructional praxis [382].

2.4.6 Dementia pugilistica; sports-related head injury

A syndrome of cognitive impairment following repeated blunt head trauma has been described, originally in boxers (hence dementia pugilistica, boxer's dementia, or "punch drunk syndrome") [383], although other professions may also be at risk of sports-related head injury (e.g., steeplechase jockeys after repeated falls). In addition to cognitive impairment, there may be a parkinsonian syndrome dominated by akinesia and variably responsive to levodopa, as well as dysarthria. Brain imaging may show ventricular dilation and a cavum septum pellucidum. Pathologically, the condition is reminiscent of AD, with neurofibrillary tangles, deposition of amyloid-β peptide, and diffuse neuronal loss. Brain trauma is known to increase expression of amyloid-β [384], and epidemiological studies have suggested head injury may be a risk factor for AD, particularly in the presence of the ApoE ϵ4 genotype [385].

Dementia pugilistica lies at the severe end of the spectrum of neuropsychological deficits following head injury [386]. Postconcussional symptoms may be somatic, affective, behavioral, and cognitive. In assessing these latter impairments, allowance may need to be made for premorbid intellectual level and for concurrent alcohol misuse. The neuropsychological sequelae of mild traumatic brain injury have been extensively studied, particularly in American football players [387–389], with the conclusion that following a sports-related concussion, cognitive performance recovers over a three- to seven-day period [390]. However, dementia-related syndromes may be initiated by repeated concussions.

2.4.7 Amyotrophic lateral sclerosis/parkinsonism-dementia complex (ALS/PDC) of Guam; lytico-bodig; Marianas dementia

The Chamorro people of the island of Guam have been recognized to suffer a high prevalence of neurodegenerative disorders, known locally as lytico-bodig, encompassing varying degrees of the clinical features of MND/ALS, PD, and AD. The ALS and parkinsonism-dementia complex (PDC) were initially described separately, but few pure cases of either condition exist, and both have severe neurofibrillary (tau- and TDP-43-positive) pathology with little amyloid, suggesting that there may be shared pathogenetic mechanisms, for which various etiological concepts have been suggested [391,392].

The neuropsychological impairments of PDC encompass recent memory loss, disorientation, and impairments of language, visuospatial and executive function [393], a global pattern similar to that seen in AD. Very occasionally, Chamorros may present with a pure dementing illness without extrapyramidal symptoms or signs, referred to as "Marianas dementia" [394].

2.5 Prion diseases

The etiological agents for the prion group of disorders are conformationally altered proteins, or "prions," which autocatalytically convert normal cellular prion protein (PrP), encoded by the PRNP gene on chromosome 20, to an abnormal form that is highly resistant to degradation [395–397]. Prion diseases (or prionoses) may afflict both humans and animals [398,399]. Human prion disease takes a number of clinicopathological forms, namely sporadic, genetic, or iatrogenic. Because of their unique biology, prion diseases enjoy a high public profile, but in clinical practice they are rare, only a handful of cases being seen each year in regional neuroscience centers [400].

The pathogenesis of neurodegeneration in the various prion disorders is thought to be common to the different etiologies [401]. Polymorphism at codon 129 of the PRNP gene, which may encode either valine or methionine, may have a dramatic effect on disease phenotype, including susceptibility to disease, the incubation period of disease, and the duration of illness [402,403]. No treatment, curative, symptomatic or palliative, is yet described but research into possible therapeutic interventions continues [404,405].

Progressive dementia, often rapid, is common to many prion disorders. Brain tissue (biopsy, autopsy) typically shows spongiform vacuolation affecting any part of the cerebral gray matter, hence the designation of these disorders as "spongiform encephalopathies," with astrocytic proliferation, gliosis, neuronal loss, synaptic degeneration, and variable frequencies of PrP-immunopositive amyloid plaques [406]. Prion disease cases without spongiform change have also been described [407].

2.5.1 Sporadic prion disease: sporadic Creutzfeldt–Jakob disease (sCJD)

Sporadic human prion diseases may be separated into three phenotypes: sporadic Creutzfeldt–Jakob disease (sCJD), sporadic fatal insomnia, and variably protease-sensitive prionopathy [408]. Of these, sCJD is by far (>90%) the most common, occurring with an incidence of around one case per million of the population throughout the world. The older literature defined a number of clinical variants of sCJD, presenting with prominent cerebellar syndrome (Brownell–Oppenheimer or ataxic variant), cortical blindness (Heidenhain variant), or encephalopathy (Nevin–Jones syndrome), but these terms are now seldom used, classification being based on PRNP codon 129 genotype and PrP isotype as detected by Western blotting, resulting in six variants [403]. Diagnostic criteria for sCJD are based on clinical phenotype and investigation findings, including electroencephalographic (EEG) periodic sharp wave complexes (PSWC) at a frequency of around 2–3 Hz in a markedly abnormal background, CSF biomarkers (14-3-3 protein), and MR imaging findings (especially on diffusion-weighted imaging) [409]. Other disorders that may mimic or be clinically confused with CJD, and hence may lead to confounding in defining the neuropsychological profile, include AD [33,410] (Section 2.1), DLB [306,307,410] (Section 2.4.2), progressive subcortical gliosis of Neumann [184] (Section 2.2.4.5), Wernicke–Korsakoff syndrome [411,412] (Section 8.3.1.1), nonconvulsive status epilepticus [413,414], intravascular lymphoma (angioendotheliomatosis) [415] (Section 3.5.7), Hashimoto's encephalopathy [416] (Section 6.13), pellagra encephalopathy [417] (Section 8.2.1.4), and gliomatosis cerebri [418] (Section 7.1.3).

Because rapid progression of sCJD is common, profound cognitive deficits amounting to dementia may be present before clinical presentation. When neuropsychological assessment has been possible, the changes reported have included episodic unresponsiveness, interference effects, and verbal and motor perseverations, perhaps reflecting thalamic involvement [419]. Presentation with isolated aphasia has been reported [420,421]. In a patient undergoing neuropsychological testing in a predementia stage, deficits resembling PSP were reported [422]. A patient with the Heidenhain variant has been reported, in whom the initial symptom was agraphia, followed by hemianopsia and visual hallucinations, and evolving to dementia over a three-month period [423]. Visual symptoms are common in sCJD, which may explain the confusion with DLB, although the visual hallucinations in the latter are generally well formed (animals, people) compared with the rather elemental visual hallucinations (colors, shapes) that may occur in CJD [307,424].

The sporadic form of fatal insomnia is rare, even more so than the familial form (Section 2.5.3).

2.5.2 Iatrogenic prion disease

Acquired, iatrogenic, or transmissible forms of prion disease account for <1% of the total. These include kuru and variant CJD. Iatrogenic disease may also result from exposure to contaminated instrumentation (depth EEG electrodes), grafts (cornea, dura mater), exogenous human pituitary hormones (growth hormone, gonadotrophins), and blood transfusion.

2.5.2.1 Kuru

Kuru, a disorder of the Fore people of the eastern highlands of New Guinea transmitted by ritual endocannibalism of brain tissue, was the first human prion disease to be described extensively [425,426]. It has become less common since the cessation of endocannibalism although some new cases are still reported, reflecting extremely long disease incubation periods of 40–50 years [427]. The profile of cognitive deficits is not reported, because common neuropsychological testing methods are not culturally appropriate.

2.5.2.2 Variant Creutzfeldt–Jakob disease (vCJD)

Variant CJD (vCJD) is caused by the same prion strain responsible for the epidemic of bovine spongiform encephalopathy (BSE) in cattle, presumably reaching man through the food chain (consumption of infected meat products), and thus is sometimes known as "human BSE" [428]. Transmission by blood transfusion is also a possibility [429,430]. Unlike sCJD, vCJD tends to affect younger individuals, and the presentation is often with nonspecific sensory and psychiatric features [431]. Magnetic resonance imaging (MRI) may show high signal intensity in the posterior thalamus, the pulvinar sign [432], although this is not unique to vCJD [410]. EEG PSWC are absent in vCJD. PrP-immunopositive staining may be present in lymphoreticular tissues, even presymptomatically [433,434]. In the appropriate clinical setting, tonsil biopsy may be helpful in the diagnosis of vCJD [435].

In a series of vCJD patients, Hawkins *et al.* found impaired verbal fluency and digit–symbol substitution in all patients, memory and visuoperceptual deficits in most, but with relative preservation of verbal knowledge, immediate memory, and elementary visual processing [436]. A study of ten vCJD patients, in which comparison was made with sCJD and inherited prion disease patients, found evidence for generalized cognitive decline in vCJD but with the suggestion that visual perception might be spared [437].

2.5.2.3 Human growth hormone-related iatrogenic CJD

In a series of five patients with iatrogenic prion disease resulting from exposure to cadaveric human growth hormone, only one had a complaint of mild memory problems but four had evidence for mild intellectual decline on the WAIS-R, and one had selective visual memory and frontal executive impairments [438].

2.5.3 Inherited prion disease: familial CJD; Gerstmann–Straussler–Scheinker disease (GSS); fatal familial insomnia (FFI)

Inherited or familial prion disorders account for approximately 10%–15% of the total. Mutations deterministic for familial prion disorders are located in the PRNP gene on chromosome 20p13, which encodes PrP [439]. These have a broad phenotype, including:

- familial CJD (fCJD) (OMIM#123400);
- Gerstmann–Straussler–Scheinker disease (GSS) (OMIM#137440);
- fatal familial insomnia (FFI) (OMIM#600072);
- Huntington's disease-like 1 (HDL1), due to eight extra octapeptide repeats in the PRNP gene (OMIM#603218) (Section 5.1.1).

A subcortical pattern of cognitive decline has been reported in fCJD, along with episodic unresponsiveness, interference effects, and verbal and motor perseverations, also reported in sporadic prion disease [419]. Another study found generalized cognitive decline in inherited prion disease with relative preservation of nominal function in some cases [437]. In a single case study of fCJD, verbal memory, word finding, and dominant hand tactual performance were impaired with other functions relatively intact [440]. A family with a novel PRNP gene mutation, T183A, has been reported with clinical features that resemble frontotemporal dementia and parkinsonism linked to chromosome 17 (FTDP-17) (Section 2.2.5.1) [441]. In a comparison of two fCJD families, one with the PRNP point mutation (P102L) and one with an insertion of six additional octapeptide repeats (6-OPRI), the latter were found to have lower premorbid function, more executive dysfunction, and more impairment on tests of perception and nominal function [442].

Gerstmann–Straussler–Scheinker disease (GSS) is an autosomal dominant disorder with cerebellar ataxia as an early feature, along with dysarthria and eye movement disorders. Extrapyramidal signs may evolve. Progressive dementia with behavioral disturbance (depression, psychosis) is also reported. Deficits seem to vary among the different reports, including focal abnormalities suggestive of cortical involvement (acalculia, agnosia, apraxia), and more global impairment including attention and executive functions, suggesting possible subcortical involvement [443,444]. This would be in keeping with the multifocal nature of brain involvement in prion disorders. A patient with a FTD phenotype has been described in a family with the P102L PRNP mutation, and in which other affected family members had the typical ataxic GSS presentation [445].

Fatal familial insomnia (FFI), a rare inherited prion disorder linked to mutations of the PRNP gene and a particular polymorphism at codon 129, is characterized clinically by sleep, autonomic, and motor disturbances and pathologically by marked atrophy of the anterior and dorsomedial nuclei of the thalamus. Neuropsychological studies have shown early impairments of attention and vigilance, working memory deficits with a particular difficulty in the ordering of events, and a progressive confusional state [446,447]. The pattern seems to be distinct from that of cortical and subcortical dementias and reflective of a thalamic dementia (Section 1.3.3.2).

REFERENCES

[1] Larner AJ. Alzheimer's disease. In: Cappa SF, Abutalebi J, Démonet JF, Fletcher PC, Garrard P (eds.). *Cognitive Neurology: A Clinical Textbook.* Oxford: Oxford University Press, 2008: 199–227.

[2] Hodges JR. Alzheimer's centennial legacy: origins, landmarks and the current status of knowledge concerning cognitive aspects. *Brain* 2006; 129: 2811–22.

[3] Larner AJ. Alzheimer 100. *Adv Clin Neurosci Rehabil* 2006; 6(5): 24.

[4] Blessed G, Tomlinson BE, Roth M. The association between quantitative measures of dementia and of senile change in the cerebral grey matter of elderly subjects. *Br J Psychiatry* 1968; 114: 797–811.

[5] Tomlinson BE, Blessed G, Roth M. Observations on the brains of non-demented old people. *J Neurol Sci* 1968; 7: 331–56.

[6] Tomlinson BE, Blessed G, Roth M. Observations on the brains of demented old people. *J Neurol Sci* 1970; 11: 205–42.

[7] McKhann G, Drachman D, Folstein M, *et al.* Clinical diagnosis of Alzheimer's disease. Report of the NINCDS–ADRDA work group under the auspices of the Department of Health and Human Service Task forces on Alzheimer's disease. *Neurology* 1984; 34: 939–44.

[8] Cruts M, van Duijn CM, Backhovens H, *et al.* Estimation of the genetic contribution of presenilin-1 and -2 mutations in a population-based study of presenile Alzheimer disease. *Hum Mol Genet* 1998; 7: 43–51.

[9] Caselli RJ, Tariot PN. *Alzheimer's Disease and its Variants: A Diagnostic and Therapeutic Guide.* Oxford: Oxford University Press, 2010.

[10] Jorm AF. Subtypes of Alzheimer's disease: a conceptual analysis. *Psychol Med* 1985; 15: 543–53.

[11] Pogacar S, Williams RS. Alzheimer's disease presenting as slowly progressive aphasia. *R I Med J* 1984; 67: 181–5.

[12] Mendez MF, Zander BA. Dementia presenting with aphasia: clinical characteristics. *J Neurol Neurosurg Psychiatry* 1991; 54: 542–5.

[13] Alladi S, Xuereb J, Bak T, *et al.* Focal cortical presentations of Alzheimer's disease. *Brain* 2007; 130: 2636–45.

[14] Benson DF, Davis RJ, Snyder BD. Posterior cortical atrophy. *Arch Neurol* 1988; 45: 789–93.

[15] Levine DN, Lee JM, Fisher CM. The visual variant of Alzheimer's disease: a clinicopathologic case study. *Neurology* 1993; 43: 305–13.

[16] Crutch SJ, Lehmann M, Schott JM, *et al.* Posterior cortical atrophy. *Lancet Neurol* 2012; 11: 170–8.

[17] Mackenzie Ross SJ, Graham N, Stuart-Green L, *et al.* Progressive biparietal atrophy: an atypical presentation of Alzheimer's disease. *J Neurol Neurosurg Psychiatry* 1996; 61: 388–95.

[18] Crystal HA, Horoupian DS, Katzman R, Jotkowicz S. Biopsy-proved Alzheimer disease presenting as a right parietal lobe syndrome. *Ann Neurol* 1982; 12: 186–8.

[19] Doran M, du Plessis DG, Enevoldson TP, *et al.* Pathological heterogeneity of clinically diagnosed corticobasal degeneration. *J Neurol Sci* 2003; 216: 127–34.

[20] Ball JA, Lantos PL, Jackson M, *et al.* Alien hand sign in association with Alzheimer's histopathology. *J Neurol Neurosurg Psychiatry* 1993; 56: 1020–3.

[21] Johnson JK, Head E, Kim R, Starr A, Cotman CW. Clinical and pathological evidence for a frontal variant of Alzheimer disease. *Arch Neurol* 1999; 56: 1233–9.

[22] Taylor KI, Probst A, Miserez AR, Monsch AU, Tolnay M. Clinical course of neuropathologically confirmed frontal variant Alzheimer's disease. *Nat Clin Pract Neurol* 2008; 4: 226–32.

[23] Larner AJ. Frequency of agnosic, apraxic and aphasic presentations of Alzheimer's disease. *Eur J Neurol* 2006; 13: S193 (abstract P2098).

[24] Larner AJ. Epileptic seizures in AD patients. *Neuromolecular Med* 2010; 12: 71–7.

[25] Friedman D, Honig LS, Scarmeas N. Seizures and epilepsy in Alzheimer's disease. *CNS Neurosci Ther* 2012; 18: 285–94.

[26] Kurlan R, Richard IH, Papka M, Marshall F. Movement disorders in Alzheimer's disease: more rigidity of definitions is needed. *Mov Disord* 2000; 15: 24–9.

[27] Scarmeas N, Hadjigeorgiou GM, Papadimitriou Λ, *et al.* Motor signs during the course of Alzheimer disease. *Neurology* 2004; 63: 975–82.

[28] Rothman SM, Mattson MP. Sleep disturbances in Alzheimer's and Parkinson's diseases. *Neuromolecular Med* 2012; 14: 194–204.

[29] Ballard CG, O'Brien J, James I, Swann A. *Dementia: Management of Behavioural and Psychological Symptoms.* Oxford: Oxford University Press, 2001.

[30] Savva GM, Zaccai J, Matthews FM, *et al.* Prevalence, correlates and course of behavioural and psychological symptoms of dementia in the population. *Br J Psychiatry* 2009; 194: 212–19.

[31] Mendiondo MS, Ashford JW, Kryscio RJ, Schmitt FA. Modelling mini mental state examination changes in Alzheimer's disease. *Stat Med* 2000; 19: 1607–16.

[32] Holmes C, Lovestone S. Long-term cognitive and functional decline in late onset Alzheimer's disease: therapeutic implications. *Age Ageing* 2003; 32: 200–4.

[33] Jayaratnam S, Khoo AK, Basic D. Rapidly progressive Alzheimer's disease and elevated 14-3-3 proteins in cerebrospinal fluid. *Age Ageing* 2008; 37: 467–9.

[34] Larner AJ. "Dementia unmasked": atypical, acute aphasic, presentations of neurodegenerative dementing disease. *Clin Neurol Neurosurg* 2005; 108: 8–10.

[35] Knopman DS, DeKosky ST, Cummings JL, *et al.* Practice parameter: diagnosis of dementia (an evidence-based review). Report of the Quality Standards Subcommittee of the American Academy of Neurology. *Neurology* 2001; 56: 1143–53.

[36] Waldemar G, Dubois B, Emre M, *et al.* Recommendations for the diagnosis and management of Alzheimer's disease and other disorders associated with dementia. *Eur J Neurol* 2007; 14: e1–26.

[37] Hort J, O'Brien JT, Gainotti G, *et al.* EFNS guidelines for the diagnosis and management of Alzheimer's disease. *Eur J Neurol* 2010; 17: 1236–48.

[38] Mirra SS, Heyman A, McKeel D, *et al.* The Consortium to Establish a Registry for Alzheimer's Disease (CERAD). Part II. Standardization of the neuropathologic assessment of Alzheimer's disease. *Neurology* 1991; 41: 479–86.

[39] Braak H, Braak E. Neuropathological stageing [*sic*] of Alzheimer-related changes. *Acta Neuropathol (Berl)* 1991; 82: 239–59.

[40] National Institute on Aging and Reagan Institute Working Group on Diagnostic Criteria for the Neuropathological Assessment of Alzheimer Disease. Consensus recommendations for the post-mortem diagnosis of Alzheimer's disease. *Neurobiol Aging* 1997; 18: S1–2.

[41] Dubois B, Feldman HH, Jacova C, *et al.* Research criteria for the diagnosis of Alzheimer's disease: revising the NINCDS–ADRDA criteria. *Lancet Neurol* 2007; 6: 734–46.

[42] McKhann GM, Knopman DS, Chertkow H, *et al.* The diagnosis of dementia due to Alzheimer's disease: recommendations from the National Institute on Aging–Alzheimer's Association workgroups on diagnostic guidelines for Alzheimer's disease. *Alzheimers Dement* 2011; 7: 263–9.

[43] Albert MS, DeKosky ST, Dickson D, *et al.* The diagnosis of mild cognitive impairment due to Alzheimer's disease: recommendations from the National Institute on Aging–Alzheimer's Association workgroups on diagnostic guidelines for Alzheimer's disease. *Alzheimers Dement* 2011; 7: 270–9.

[44] Sperling RA, Aisen PS, Beckett LA, *et al.* Toward defining the preclinical stages of Alzheimer's disease: recommendations from the National Institute on Aging–Alzheimer's Association workgroups on diagnostic guidelines for Alzheimer's disease. *Alzheimers Dement* 2011; 7: 280–92.

[45] Morris RG, Becker JT (eds.). *Cognitive Neuropsychology of Alzheimer's Disease* (2nd edn.). Oxford: Oxford University Press, 2004.

[46] Perry RJ, Hodges JR. Attention and executive deficits in Alzheimer's disease: a critical review. *Brain* 1999; 122: 383–404.

[47] Parasuraman R. Attentional functioning in Alzheimer's disease. In: Morris RG, Becker JT (eds.). *Cognitive Neuropsychology of Alzheimer's Disease* (2nd edn.). Oxford: Oxford University Press, 2004; 81–102.

[48] McGuinness B, Barrett SL, Criag D, Lawson J, Passmore AP. Attention deficits in Alzheimer's disease and vascular dementia. *J Neurol Neurosurg Psychiatry* 2010; 81: 157–9.

[49] Lawrence AD, Sahakian BJ. Alzheimer's disease, attention, and the cholinergic system. *Alz Dis Assoc Disord* 1995; 9: 43–9.

[50] Baddeley AD, Baddeley HA, Bucks RS, Wilcock GK. Attentional control in Alzheimer's disease. *Brain* 2001; 124: 1492–508.

[51] Huntley JD, Howard RJ. Working memory in early Alzheimer's disease: a neuropsychological review. *Int J Geriatr Psychiatry* 2010; 25: 121–32.

[52] Stopford CL, Thompson JC, Neary D, Richardson AM, Snowden JS. Working memory, attention, and executive function in Alzheimer's disease and frontotemporal dementia. *Cortex* 2012; 48: 429–46.

[53] Overman AA, Becker JT. Information processing defects in episodic memory in Alzheimer's disease. In: Morris RG, Becker JT (eds.). *Cognitive Neuropsychology of Alzheimer's Disease* (2nd edn.). Oxford: Oxford University Press, 2004: 121–40.

[54] Christensen H, Kopelman MD, Stanhope N, Lorentz I, Owen P. Rates of forgetting in Alzheimer dementia. *Neuropsychologia* 1998; 36: 547–57.

[55] Dubois B, Touchon J, Portet F, *et al*. "The 5 words": a simple and sensitive test for the diagnosis of Alzheimer's disease [in French]. *Presse Med* 2002; 31: 1696–9.

[56] Bright P, Kopelman MD. Remote memory in Alzheimer's disease. In: Morris RG, Becker JT (eds.). *Cognitive Neuropsychology of Alzheimer's Disease* (2nd edn.). Oxford: Oxford University Press, 2004; 141–51.

[57] Fox NC, Warrington EK, Seiffer AL, Agnew SK, Rossor MN. Presymptomatic cognitive deficits in individuals at risk of familial Alzheimer's disease: a longitudinal prospective study. *Brain* 1998; 121: 1631–9.

[58] Delacourte A, David JP, Sergeant N, *et al*. The biochemical pathway of neurofibrillary degeneration in aging and Alzheimer's disease. *Neurology* 1999; 52: 1158–65.

[59] Garrard P, Patterson K, Hodges JR. Semantic processing in Alzheimer's disease. In: Morris RG, Becker JT (eds.). *Cognitive Neuropsychology of Alzheimer's Disease* (2nd edn.). Oxford: Oxford University Press, 2004; 179–96.

[60] Henry JD, Crawford JR, Phillips LH. Verbal fluency performance in dementia of the Alzheimer type: a meta-analysis. *Neuropsychologia* 2004; 42: 1212–22.

[61] Verma M, Howard RJ. Semantic memory and language dysfunction in early Alzheimer's disease: a review. *Int J Geriatr Psychiatry* 2012; 27: 1209–15.

[62] Salmon DP, Fennema-Notestine C. Implicit memory in Alzheimer's disease: priming and skill learning. In: Morris RG, Becker JT (eds.). *Cognitive Neuropsychology of Alzheimer's Disease* (2nd edn.). Oxford: Oxford University Press, 2004; 153–78.

[63] Kertesz A. Language in Alzheimer's disease. In: Morris RG, Becker JT (eds.). *Cognitive Neuropsychology of Alzheimer's Disease* (2nd edn.). Oxford: Oxford University Press, 2004; 197–218.

[64] Garrard P, Maloney LM, Hodges JR, Patterson K. The effects of very early Alzheimer's disease on the characteristics of writing by a renowned author. *Brain* 2005; 128: 250–60.

[65] Gorno-Tempini ML, Dronkers NF, Rankin KP, *et al*. Cognition and anatomy in three variants of primary progressive aphasia. *Ann Neurol* 2004; 55: 335–46.

[66] Gorno-Tempini ML, Hillis AE, Weintraub S, *et al*. Classification of primary progressive aphasia and its variants. *Neurology* 2011; 76: 1006–14.

[67] Cronin-Golomb A, Hof PR (eds.). *Vision in Alzheimer's Disease*. Basel: Karger, 2004.

[68] Nestor PJ, Caine D, Fryer TD, Clarke J, Hodges JR. The topography of metabolic deficits in posterior cortical atrophy (the visual variant of Alzheimer's disease) with FDG-PET. *J Neurol Neurosurg Psychiatry* 2003; 74: 1521–9.

[69] Derouesne C, Lagha-Pierucci S, Thibault S, Baudouin-Madec V, Lacomblez L. Apraxic disturbances in patients with mild to moderate Alzheimer's disease. *Neuropsychologia* 2000; 38: 1760–9.

[70] Green RC, Goldstein FC, Mirra SS, *et al*. Slowly progressive apraxia in Alzheimer's disease. *J Neurol Neurosurg Psychiatry* 1995; 59: 312–15.

[71] Ochipa C, Rothi LJG, Heilman KM. Conceptual apraxia in Alzheimer's disease. *Brain* 1992; 115: 1061–71.

[72] Lafleche G, Albert MS. Executive function deficits in mild Alzheimer's disease. *Neuropsychology* 1995; 9: 313–20.

[73] Swanberg MM, Tractenberg RE, Mohs R, Thal LJ, Cummings JL. Executive dysfunction in Alzheimer disease. *Arch Neurol* 2004; 61: 556–60.

[74] Martyr A, Clare L. Executive function and activities of daily living in Alzheimer's disease: a correlational meta-analysis. *Dement Geriatr Cogn Disord* 2012; 33: 189–203.

[75] Birks J. Cholinesterase inhibitors for Alzheimer's disease. *Cochrane Database Syst Rev* 2006; 1:CD005593.

[76] Takeda A, Loveman E, Clegg A, *et al*. A systematic review of the clinical effectiveness of donepezil, rivastigmine and galanatamine on cognition, quality of life and adverse events in Alzheimer's disease. *Int J Geriatr Psychiatry* 2006; 21: 17–28.

[77] Raina P, Santaguida P, Ismaila A, *et al*. Effectiveness of cholinesterase inhibitors and memantine for treating dementia: evidence review for a clinical practice guideline. *Ann Intern Med* 2008; 148: 379–97.

[78] Lopez OL, Becker JT, Wisniewski S, *et al*. Cholinesterase inhibitor treatment alters the natural history of Alzheimer's disease. *J Neurol Neurosurg Psychiatry* 2002; 72: 310–14.

[79] Lopez OL, Becker JT, Saxton J, *et al*. Alteration of a clinically meaningful outcome in the natural history of Alzheimer's disease by cholinesterase inhibition. *J Am Geriatr Soc* 2005; 53: 83–7.

[80] Larner AJ. Do cholinesterase inhibitors alter the course of dementia? *Prog Neurol Psych* 2007; 11(5): 26–8.

[81] McShane R, Areosa Sastre A, Minakaran N. Memantine for dementia. *Cochrane Database Syst Rev* 2006; 2:CD003154.

[82] Tariot PN, Farlow MR, Grossberg GT, *et al*. Memantine treatment in patients with moderate to severe Alzheimer disease already receiving donepezil: a randomized controlled trial. *JAMA* 2004; 291: 317–24.

[83] Atri A, Shaughnessy LW, Locascio JJ, Growdon JH. Long-term course and effectiveness of combination therapy in Alzheimer disease. *Alzheimer Dis Assoc Disord* 2008; 22: 209–21.

[84] Lopez OL, Becker JT, Wahed AS, *et al*. Long-term effects of the concomitant use of memantine with cholinesterase inhibition in Alzheimer disease. *J Neurol Neurosurg Psychiatry* 2009; 80: 600–7.

[85] Alzheimer Disease and Frontotemporal Dementia Mutation Database, www.molgen.ua.ac.be/Admutations (accessed 01/10/12).

[86] Bateman RJ, Xiong C, Benzinger TL, *et al*. Clinical and biomarker changes in dominantly inherited Alzheimer's disease. *N Engl J Med* 2012; 367: 795–804.

[87] Mangialasche F, Solomon A, Winblad B, Mecocci P, Kivipelto M. Alzheimer's disease: clinical trials and drug development. *Lancet Neurol* 2010; 9: 702–16.

[88] Larner AJ, Doran M. Clinical phenotypic heterogeneity of Alzheimer's disease associated with mutations of the presenilin-1 gene. *J Neurol* 2006; 253: 139–58.

[89] Larner AJ, Doran M. Genotype–phenotype relationships of presenilin-1 mutations in Alzheimer's disease: an update. *J Alzheimers Dis* 2009; 17: 259–65.

[90] Larner AJ. Presenilin 1 mutation Alzheimer's disease: a genetic epilepsy syndrome? *Epilepsy Behav* 2011; 21: 20–2.

[91] Godbolt AK, Beck JA, Collinge J, *et al*. A presenilin 1 R278I mutation presenting with language impairment. *Neurology* 2004; 63: 1702–4.

[92] Fox NC, Kennedy AM, Harvey RJ, *et al*. Clinicopathological features of familial Alzheimer's disease associated with the M139V mutation in the presenilin 1 gene. Pedigree but not mutation specific age at onset provides evidence for a further genetic factor. *Brain* 1997; 120: 491–501.

[93] Larner AJ, du Plessis DG. Early-onset Alzheimer's disease with presenilin-1 M139V mutation: clinical, neuropsychological and neuropathological study. *Eur J Neurol* 2003; 10: 319–23.

[94] Mendez MF, McMurtray. Frontotemporal dementia-like phenotypes associated with presenilin-1 mutations. *Am J Alzheimers Dis Other Demen* 2006; 21: 281–6.

[95] Dubois B, Feldman HH, Jacova C, *et al*. Revising the definition of Alzheimer's disease: a new lexicon. *Lancet Neurol* 2010; 9: 1118–27.

[96] Mitchell AJ, Shiri-Feshki M. Rate of progression of mild cognitive impairment to dementia – meta-analysis of 41 robust inception cohort studies. *Acta Psychiatr Scand* 2009; 119: 252–65.

[97] Petersen RC, Smith GE, Waring SC, *et al*. Mild cognitive impairment: clinical characterization and outcome. *Arch Neurol* 1999; 56: 303–8.

[98] Winblad B, Palmer K, Kivipelto M, *et al*. Mild cognitive impairment – beyond controversies, towards a consensus: report of the International Working Group on Mild Cognitive Impairment. *J Int Med* 2004; 256: 240–6.

[99] Petersen RC, Thomas RG, Grundman M, *et al*. Vitamin E and donepezil for the treatment of mild cognitive impairment. *N Engl J Med* 2005; 352: 2379–88.

[100] Feldman HH, Ferris S, Winblad B, *et al*. Effect of rivastigmine on delay to diagnosis of Alzheimer's disease from mild cognitive impairment: the InDDEx study. *Lancet Neurol* 2007; 6: 501–12.

[101] Winblad B, Gauthier S, Scinto L, *et al*. Safety and efficacy of galantamine in subjects with mild cognitive impairment. *Neurology* 2008; 70: 2024–35.

[102] Chen P, Ratcliff G, Belle SH, *et al*. Patterns of cognitive decline in presymptomatic Alzheimer disease: a prospective community study. *Arch Gen Psychiatry* 2001; 58: 853–8.

[103] Bäckman L, Small BJ, Fratiglioni L. Stability of the preclinical episodic memory deficit in Alzheimer's disease. *Brain* 2001; 124: 96–102.

[104] Amieva H, Jacqmin-Gadda H, Orgogozo JM, *et al.* The 9-year cognitive decline before dementia of the Alzheimer type: a prospective population-based study. *Brain* 2005; 128: 1093–101.

[105] Newman SK, Warrington EK, Kennedy AM, Rossor MN. The earliest cognitive change in a person with familial Alzheimer's disease: presymptomatic neuropsychological features in a pedigree with familial Alzheimer's disease confirmed at necropsy. *J Neurol Neurosurg Psychiatry* 1994; 57: 967–72.

[106] Godbolt AK, Cipolotti L, Watt H, *et al.* The natural history of Alzheimer disease: a longitudinal presymptomatic and symptomatic study of a familial cohort. *Arch Neurol* 2004; 61: 1743–8.

[107] Graham A, Hodges J. Pick's disease: its relationship to progressive aphasia, semantic dementia and frontotemporal dementia. In: Burns A, O'Brien J, Ames D (eds.). *Dementia* (3rd edn). London: Hodder Arnold, 2005; 678–88.

[108] Ratnavalli E, Brayne C, Dawson K, Hodges JR. The prevalence of frontotemporal dementia. *Neurology* 2002; 58: 1615–21.

[109] Rosso SM, Donker KL, Baks T, *et al.* Frontotemporal dementia in The Netherlands: patient characteristics and prevalence estimates from a population-based study. *Brain* 2003; 126: 2016–22.

[110] Snowden JS, Neary D, Mann DMA. *Fronto-Temporal Lobar Degeneration: Fronto-Temporal Dementia, Progressive Aphasia, Semantic Dementia*. New York, NY: Churchill Livingstone, 1996.

[111] Hodges JR (ed.). *Frontotemporal Dementia Syndromes*. Cambridge: Cambridge University Press, 2007.

[112] Mendez MF, Lauterbach EC, Sampson SM, ANPA Committee on Research. An evidence-based review of the psychopathology of frontotemporal dementia: a report of the ANPA Committee on Research. *J Neuropsychiatry Clin Neurosci* 2008; 20: 130–49.

[113] Mendez MF, Shapira JS, Woods RJ, Licht EA, Saul RE. Psychotic symptoms in frontotemporal dementia: prevalence and review. *Dement Geriatr Cogn Disord* 2008; 25: 206–11.

[114] Omar R, Sampson EL, Loy CT, *et al.* Delusions in frontotemporal lobar degeneration. *J Neurol* 2009; 256: 600–7.

[115] Miller BL, Cummings J, Mishkin F, *et al.* Emergence of artistic talent in frontotemporal dementia. *Neurology* 1998; 51: 978–82.

[116] Seeley WW, Matthews BR, Crawford RK, *et al.* Unravelling Bolero: progressive aphasia, transmodal creativity and the right posterior neocortex. *Brain* 2008; 131: 39–49.

[117] Kertesz A, Munoz DG (eds.). *Pick's Disease and Pick Complex*. New York, NY: Wiley-Liss, 1998.

[118] Neary D, Snowden JS, Gustafson L, *et al.* Frontotemporal lobar degeneration: a consensus on clinical diagnostic criteria. *Neurology* 1998; 51: 1546–54.

[119] McKhann GM, Albert MS, Grossman M, *et al.* Clinical and pathological diagnosis of frontotemporal dementia. Report of the Work Group on Frontotemporal Dementia and Pick's disease. *Arch Neurol* 2001; 58: 1803–9.

[120] Rascovsky K, Hodges JR, Knopman D, *et al.* Sensitivity of revised diagnostic criteria for the behavioural variant of frontotemporal dementia. *Brain* 2011; 134: 2456–77.

[121] Mackenzie IR, Neumann M, Bigio EH, *et al.* Nomenclature and nosology for neuropathologic subtypes of frontotemporal lobar degeneration: an update. *Acta Neuropathol* 2010; 119: 1–4.

[122] Rosness TA, Haugen PK, Passant U, Engedal K. Frontotemporal dementia – a clinically complex diagnosis. *Int J Geriatr Psychiatry* 2008; 23: 837–42.

[123] Larner AJ. Neurologists still have a role in the dementia care pathway. *Clin Med* 2007; 7: 528–9.

[124] Davies M, Larner AJ. Frontotemporal dementias: development of an integrated care pathway through an experiential survey of patients and carers. *Int J Care Pathways* 2010; 14: 65–9.

[125] Caine D, Patterson K, Hodges JR, Heard R, Halliday G. Severe anterograde amnesia with extensive hippocampal degeneration in a case of rapidly progressive frontotemporal dementia. *Neurocase* 2001; 7: 57–64.

[126] Hodges JR, Davies RR, Xuereb JH, *et al.* Clinicopathological correlates in frontotemporal dementia. *Ann Neurol* 2004; 56: 399–406.

[127] Graham A, Davies R, Xuereb J, *et al.* Pathologically proven frontotemporal dementia presenting with severe amnesia. *Brain* 2005; 128: 597–605.

[128] Baborie A, Griffiths TD, Jaros E, *et al.* Frontotemporal dementia in elderly individuals. *Arch Neurol* 2012; 69: 1052–60.

[129] Irish M, Hornberger M, Lah S, *et al.* Profiles of recent autobiographical memory retrieval in semantic dementia, behavioural-variant frontotemporal dementia, and Alzheimer's disease. *Neuropsychologia* 2011; 49: 2694–702.

[130] Rogers TT, Ivanoiu A, Patterson K, Hodges JR. Semantic memory in Alzheimer's disease and the frontotemporal dementias: a longitudinal study of 236 patients. *Neuropsychology* 2006; 20: 319–35

[131] Rossor M, Warrington EK, Cipolotti L. The isolation of calculation skills. *J Neurol* 1995; 242: 78–81.

[132] Rahman S, Sahakian BJ, Hodges JR, Rogers RD, Robbins TW. Specific cognitive deficits in mild frontal variant frontotemporal dementia. *Brain* 1999; 122: 1469–93.

[133] Lo Coco D, Nacci P. Frontotemporal dementia presenting with pathological gambling. *J Neuropsychiatry Clin Neurosci* 2004; 16: 117–18.

[134] Larner AJ. Cholinesterase inhibitors – beyond Alzheimer's disease. *Expert Rev Neurother* 2010; 10: 1699–705.

[135] Deakin JB, Rahman S, Nestor PJ, Hodges JR, Sahakian BJ. Paroxetine does not improve symptoms and impairs cognition in frontotemporal dementia: a double-blind randomized controlled trial. *Psychopharmacol* 2004; 172: 400–8.

[136] Mesulam MM. Slowly progressive aphasia without generalized dementia. *Ann Neurol* 1982; 11: 592–8.

[137] Mesulam MM. Primary progressive aphasia. *Ann Neurol* 2001; 49: 425–32.

[138] Krefft TA, Graff-Radford NR, Dickson DW, Baker M, Castellani RJ. Familial primary progressive aphasia. *Alzheimer Dis Assoc Disord* 2003; 17: 106–12.

[139] Doran M, Larner AJ. Monozygotic twins discordant for primary progressive aphasia. *Alzheimer Dis Assoc Disord* 2004; 18: 48–9.

[140] Mimura M, Oda T, Tsuchiya K, *et al.* Corticobasal degeneration presenting with nonfluent primary progressive aphasia: a clinicopathological study. *J Neurol Sci* 2001; 183: 19–26.

[141] Ferrer I, Hernandez I, Boada M, *et al.* Primary progressive aphasia as the initial manifestation of corticobasal degeneration and unusual tauopathies. *Acta Neuropathol* 2003; 106: 419–35.

[142] Le Rhun E, Richard F, Pasquier F. Natural history of primary progressive aphasia. *Neurology* 2005; 65: 887–91.

[143] Boeve BF, Dickson D, Duffy J, *et al.* Progressive nonfluent aphasia and subsequent aphasic dementia associated with atypical progressive supranuclear palsy pathology. *Eur Neurol* 2003; 49: 72–8.

[144] Mochizuki A, Ueda Y, Komatsuzaki Y, *et al.* Progressive supranuclear palsy presenting with primary progressive aphasia – clinicopathological report of an autopsy case. *Acta Neuropathol* 2003; 105: 610–4.

[145] Llado A, Sanchez-Valle R, Rey MJ, *et al.* Clinicopathological and genetic correlates of frontotemporal lobar degeneration and corticobasal degeneration. *J Neurol* 2008; 255: 488–94.

[146] Hodges JR, Davies R, Xuereb J, Kril J, Halliday G. Survival in frontotemporal dementia. *Neurology* 2003; 61: 349–54.

[147] Dronkers NF. A new brain region for coordinating speech articulation. *Nature* 1996; 384: 159–61.

[148] Rohrer JD, Rossor MN, Warren JD. Apraxia in progressive nonfluent aphasia. *J Neurol* 2010; 257: 569–74.

[149] Warrington EK. The selective impairment of semantic memory. *Quart J Exp Psychol* 1975; 27: 635–57.

[150] Hodges JR, Patterson K, Oxbury S, Funnell E. Semantic dementia. Progressive fluent aphasia with temporal lobe atrophy. *Brain* 1992; 115: 1783–806.

[151] Chan D, Fox NC, Scahill RI, *et al.* Patterns of temporal lobe atrophy in semantic dementia and Alzheimer's disease. *Ann Neurol* 2001: 49: 433–42.

[152] Thompson SA, Patterson K, Hodges JR. Left/right asymmetry of atrophy in semantic dementia: behavioural-cognitive implications. *Neurology* 2003; 61: 1196–203.

[153] Davies RR, Hodges JR, Kril JJ, *et al.* The pathological basis of semantic dementia. *Brain* 2005; 128: 1984–95.

[154] Godbolt AK, Josephs KA, Revesz T, *et al.* Sporadic and familial dementia with ubiquitin-positive tau-negative inclusions: clinical features of one histopathological abnormality underlying frontotemporal lobar degeneration. *Arch Neurol* 2005; 62: 1097–101.

[155] Evans JJ, Heggs AJ, Antoun N, Hodges JR. Progressive prosopagnosia associated with selective right temporal lobe atrophy. A new syndrome? *Brain* 1995; 118: 1–13.

[156] Larner AJ. Gambling. *Adv Clin Neurosci Rehabil* 2007; 7(1): 26.

[157] Davies RR, Kipps CM, Mitchell J, *et al.* Progression in frontotemporal dementia: identifying a benign

behavioural variant by magnetic resonance imaging. *Arch Neurol* 2006; 63: 1627–31.

[158] Braak H, Braak E. Argyrophilic grain disease: frequency of occurrence in different age categories and neuropathological diagnostic criteria. *J Neural Transm* 1998; 105: 801–19.

[159] Ferrer I, Santpere G, van Leeuwen FW. Argyrophilic grain disease. *Brain* 2008; 131: 1416–32.

[160] Kovacs GG, Pitman A, Revesz T, *et al.* MAPT S305I mutation: implications for argyrophilic grain disease. *Acta Neuropathol* 2008; 116: 103–18.

[161] Steuerwald GM, Baumann TP, Taylor KI, *et al.* Clinical characteristics of dementia associated with argyrophilic grain disease. *Dement Geriatr Cogn Disord* 2007; 24: 229–34.

[162] Thal DR, Schultz C, Botez G, *et al.* The impact of argyrophilic grain disease on the development of dementia and its relationship to concurrent Alzheimer's disease-related pathology. *Neuropath Appl Neurobiol* 2005; 31: 270–9.

[163] Munoz DG, Neumann M, Kusaka H, *et al.* FUS pathology in basophilic inclusion body disease. *Acta Neuropathol* 2009; 118: 617–27.

[164] Ulrich J, Spillantini MG, Goedert M, *et al.* Abundant neurofibrillary tangles without senile plaques in a subset of patients with senile dementia. *Neurodegeneration* 1992; 1: 257–84.

[165] Jellinger KA, Attems J. Neurofibrillary tangle-predominant dementia: comparison with classical Alzheimer disease. *Acta Neuropathol* 2007; 113: 107–17.

[166] Kosaka K. Diffuse neurofibrillary tangles with calcification: a new pre-senile dementia. *J Neurol Neurosurg Psychiatry* 1994; 57: 594–6.

[167] Habuchi C, Iritani S, Sekiguchi H, *et al.* Clinicopathological study of diffuse neurofibrillary tangles with calcification. With special reference to TDP-43 proteinopathy and alpha-synucleinopathy. *J Neurol Sci* 2011; 301: 77–85.

[168] Ito Y, Kato T, Suzuki T, *et al.* Neuroradiologic and clinical abnormalities in dementia of diffuse neurofibrillary tangles with calcification (Kosaka-Shibayama disease). *J Neurol Sci* 2003; 209: 105–9.

[169] Nanda S, Bhatt SP, Pamula J, *et al.* Diffuse neurofibrillary tangles with calcification (DNTC): Kosaka-Shibayama disease in America. *Am J Alzheimers Dis Other Demen* 2007; 22: 535–7.

[170] Langlois NEI, Grieve JHK, Best PV. Changes of diffuse neurofibrillary tangles with calcification (DNTC) in a woman without evidence of dementia. *J Neurol Neurosurg Psychiatry* 1995; 59: 103.

[171] Modrego PJ, Mojonero J, Serrano M, Fayed N. Fahr's syndrome presenting with pure and progressive presenile dementia. *Neurol Sci* 2005; 26: 367–9.

[172] Cairns NJ, Perry RH, Jaros E, *et al.* Patients with a novel neurofilamentopathy: dementia with neurofilament inclusions. *Neurosci Lett* 2003; 341: 177–80.

[173] Bigio EH, Lipton AM, White CL 3rd, Dickson DW, Hirano A. Frontotemporal and motor neurone degeneration with neurofilament inclusion bodies: additional evidence for overlap between FTD and ALS. *Neuropathol Appl Neurobiol* 2003; 29: 239–53.

[174] Josephs KA, Holton JL, Rossor MN, *et al.* Neurofilament inclusion body disease: a new proteinopathy? *Brain* 2003; 126: 2291–303.

[175] Cairns NJ, Grossman M, Arnold SE, *et al.* Clinical and neuropathologic variation in neuronal intermediate filament inclusion disease. *Neurology* 2004; 63: 1376–84.

[176] Mackenzie IRA, Neumann M, Bigio EH, *et al.* Nomenclature for neuropathologic subtypes of frontotemporal lobar degeneration: consensus recommendations. *Acta Neuropathol* 2009; 117: 15–18.

[177] Menon R, Barborie A, Jaros E, *et al.* What's in a name? Neuronal intermediate filament inclusion disease (NIFID), frontotemporal lobar degeneration-intermediate filament (FTLD-IF) or frontotemporal lobar degeneration-fused in sarcoma (FTLD-FUS)? *J Neurol Neurosurg Psychiatry* 2011; 82: 1412–14.

[178] Neumann M, Roeber S, Kretzschmar HA, *et al.* Abundant FUS pathology in neuronal intermediate filament inclusion disease. *Acta Neuropathol* 2009; 118: 605–16.

[179] Neumann MA, Cohn R. Progressive subcortical gliosis, a rare form of presenile dementia. *Brain* 1967; 90: 405–18.

[180] Vermersch P, Daems-Monpeurt C, Parent M, *et al.* Démence sous-corticale type Neumann. Apport de l'imagerie morphologique et fonctionnelle. *Rev Neurol (Paris)* 1994; 150: 354–8.

[181] Larner AJ, Smith ETS, Doran M. Does MRI/MRS permit ante mortem diagnosis of progressive

subcortical gliosis of Neumann? *J Neurol Neurosurg Psychiatry* 2003; 74: 404 (abstract 29).

[182] Goedert M, Spillantini MG, Crowther RA, *et al.* Tau gene mutation in familial progressive subcortical gliosis. *Nat Med* 1999; 5: 454–7.

[183] Lanska DJ, Markesbery WR, Cochran E, *et al.* Late-onset sporadic progressive subcortical gliosis. *J Neurol Sci* 1998; 157: 143–7.

[184] Bergmann M, Gullotta F, Weitbrecht WU. Progressive subkortikale Gliose. *Fortschr Neurol Psychiatr* 1991; 59: 328–34.

[185] Will RG, Lees AJ, Gibb W, Barnard RO. A case of progressive subcortical gliosis presenting clinically as Steele–Richardson–Olszewski syndrome. *J Neurol Neurosurg Psychiatry* 1988; 51:1224–7.

[186] Corey-Bloom J, Sabbagh MN, Bondi MW, *et al.* Hippocampal sclerosis contributes to dementia in the elderly. *Neurology* 1997; 48: 154–60.

[187] Ala T, Beh GO, Frey WM II. Pure hippocampal sclerosis: a rare cause of dementia mimicking Alzheimer's disease. *Neurology* 2000; 54: 843–8.

[188] Leverenz JB, Agustin CM, Tsuang D, *et al.* Clinical and neuropathological characteristics of hippocampal sclerosis: a community-based study. *Arch Neurol* 2002; 59: 1099–106.

[189] Blass DM, Hatanpaa KJ, Brandt J, *et al.* Dementia in hippocampal sclerosis resembles frontotemporal dementia more than Alzheimer disease. *Neurology* 2004; 63: 492–7.

[190] Hatanpaa KJ, Blass DM, Pletnikova O, *et al.* Most cases of dementia with hippocampal sclerosis may represent frontotemporal dementia. *Neurology* 2004; 63: 538–42.

[191] McKeel DW Jr, Burns JM, Meuser TM, Morris JC. *An Atlas of Investigation and Diagnosis: Dementia.* Oxford: Clinical Publishing, 2007: 172.

[192] Probst A, Taylor KI, Tolnay M. Hippocampal sclerosis dementia: a reappraisal. *Acta Neuropathol* 2007; 114: 335–45.

[193] Foster NL, Wilhelmsen K, Sima AAF, *et al.* Frontotemporal dementia and parkinsonism linked to chromosome 17: a consensus conference. *Ann Neurol* 1997; 41: 706–15.

[194] Hutton M, Lendon CL, Rizzu P, *et al.* Association of missense and 5' splice site mutations in tau with the inherited dementia FTDP-17. *Nature* 1998; 393: 702–5.

[195] Poorkaj P, Bird T, Wijsman E, *et al.* Tau is a candidate gene for chromosome 17 frontotemporal dementia. *Ann Neurol* 1998; 43: 815–25.

[196] Spillantini MG, Murrell JR, Goedert M, *et al.* Mutation in the tau gene in familial multiple system tauopathy with presenile dementia. *Proc Natl Acad Sci USA* 1998; 95: 7737–41.

[197] Baker M, Mackenzie IR, Pickering-Brown SM, *et al.* Mutations in progranulin cause tau-negative frontotemporal dementia linked to chromosome 17. *Nature* 2006; 442: 916–19.

[198] Cruts M, Gijselinck I, van der Zee J, *et al.* Null mutations in progranulin cause ubiquitin-positive frontotemporal dementia linked to chromosome 17q21. *Nature* 2006; 442: 920–4.

[199] Larner AJ, Doran M. Clinical heterogeneity associated with tau gene mutations. *Eur Neurol Rev* 2009; 3(2): 31–2.

[200] Larner AJ. Intrafamilial clinical phenotypic heterogeneity with *MAPT* gene splice site IVS10+16C>T mutation. *J Neurol Sci* 2009; 287: 253–6.

[201] Geschwind DH, Robidoux J, Alarcón M, *et al.* Dementia and neurodevelopmental predisposition: cognitive dysfunction in presymptomatic subjects precedes dementia by decades in frontotemporal dementia. *Ann Neurol* 2001; 50: 741–6.

[202] Beck J, Rohrer JD, Campbell T, *et al.* A distinct clinical, neuropsychological and radiological phenotype is associated with progranulin gene mutations in a large UK series. *Brain* 2008; 131: 706–20.

[203] Pickering-Brown SM, Rollinson S, Du Plessis D, *et al.* Frequency and clinical characteristics of progranulin mutation carriers in the Manchester frontotemporal lobar degeneration cohort: comparison with patients with MAPT and no known mutations. *Brain* 2008; 131: 721–31.

[204] Le Ber I, Camuzat A, Hannequin D, *et al.* Phenotype variability in progranulin mutation carriers; a clinical, neuropsychological, imaging and genetic study. *Brain* 2008; 131: 732–46.

[205] Larner AJ. Intrafamilial clinical phenotypic heterogeneity with progranulin gene p.Glu498fs mutation. *J Neurol Sci* 2012; 316: 189–90.

[206] Rohrer JD, Crutch SJ, Warrington EK, Warren JD. Progranulin-associated primary progressive aphasia: a distinct phenotype? *Neuropsychologia* 2010; 48: 288–97.

[207] Deramecourt V, Lebert F, Debachy B, *et al.* Prediction of pathology in primary progressive language and speech disorders. *Neurology* 2010; 74: 42–9.

[208] Watts GDJ, Wymer J, Kovach MJ, *et al.* Inclusion body myopathy associated with Paget disease of bone and frontotemporal dementia is caused by mutant valosin-containing protein. *Nat Genet* 2004; 36: 377–81.

[209] Haubenberger D, Bittner RE, Rauch SS, *et al.* Inclusion body myopathy and Paget disease is linked to a novel mutation in the VCP gene. *Neurology* 2005; 65: 1304–5.

[210] Kimonis VE, Watts GDJ. Autosomal dominant inclusion body myopathy, Paget disease of bone, and frontotemporal dementia. *Alzheimer Dis Assoc Disord* 2005; 19: S44–7.

[211] Schröder R, Watts GDJ, Mehta SG, *et al.* Mutant valosin-containing protein causes a novel type of frontotemporal dementia. *Ann Neurol* 2005; 57: 457–61.

[212] Rohrer JD, Warren JD, Reiman D, *et al.* A novel exon 2 I27V VCP variant is associated with dissimilar clinical syndromes. *J Neurol* 2011; 258: 1494–6.

[213] Kim EJ, Park YE, Kim DS, *et al.* Inclusion body myopathy with Paget disease of bone and frontotemporal dementia linked to VCP p.Arg155Cys in a Korean family. *Arch Neurol* 2011; 68: 787–96.

[214] Skibinski G, Parkinson NJ, Brown J, *et al.* Mutations in the endosomal ESCRTIII complex subunit CHMP2B in frontotemporal dementia. *Nat Genet* 2005; 37: 806–8.

[215] Gydesen S, Brown JM, Brun A, *et al.* Chromosome 3 linked frontotemporal dementia (FTD-3). *Neurology* 2002; 59: 1585–94.

[216] DeJesus-Hernandez M, Mackenzie IR, Boeve BF, *et al.* Expanded GGGGCC hexanucleotide repeat in non-coding region of C9ORF72 causes chromosome 9p-linked FTD and ALS. *Neuron* 2011; 72: 245–56.

[217] Renton AE, Majounie E, Waite A, *et al.* A hexanucleotide repeat expansion in C9ORF72 is the cause of chromosome 9p21-linked ALS-FTD. *Neuron* 2011; 72: 257–68.

[218] Majounie E, Renton AE, Mok K, *et al.* Frequency of the C9orf72 hexanucleotide repeat expansion in patients with amyotrophic lateral sclerosis and frontotemporal dementia: a cross-sectional study. *Lancet Neurol* 2012; 11: 323–30.

[219] Snowden JS, Rollinson S, Thompson JC, *et al.* Distinct clinical and pathological characteristics of frontotemporal dementia associated with C9ORF72 mutations. *Brain* 2012; 135: 693–708.

[220] Hsiung GY, DeJesus-Henrandez M, Feldman HH, *et al.* Clinical and pathological features of familial frontotemporal dementia caused by C9ORF72 mutation on chromosome 9p. *Brain* 2012; 135: 709–22.

[221] Mahoney CJ, Beck J, Rohrer JD, *et al.* Frontotemporal dementia with the C9ORF72 hexanucleotide repeat expansion: clinical, neuroanatomical and neuropathological features. *Brain* 2012; 135: 736–50.

[222] Charcot JM, Joffroy A. Deux cas d'atrophie musculaire progressive avec lésions de la substance grise et des faisceaux antérolatéraux de la moelle épinière. *Archives de Physiologie Normale* 1869; 2: 354–67.

[223] Alzheimer A. On a case of spinal progressive muscle atrophy with accessory disease of bulbar nuclei and the cortex [in German]. *Archiv fur Psychiatrie* 1891; 23: 459–85.

[224] Hudson AJ. Amyotrophic lateral sclerosis and its association with dementia, parkinsonism and other neurological disorders: a review. *Brain* 1981; 104: 217–47.

[225] Mitsuyama Y. Presenile dementia with motor neuron disease in Japan: a clinico-pathological review of 26 cases. *J Neurol Neurosurg Psychiatry* 1984; 47: 953–9.

[226] Neary D, Snowden JS, Mann DMA, *et al.* Frontal lobe dementia and motor neuron disease. *J Neurol Neurosurg Psychiatry* 1990; 53: 23–32.

[227] Strong MJ (ed.). *Dementia and Motor Neuron Disease.* Abingdon: Informa Healthcare, 2006.

[228] Phukan J, Pender NP, Hardiman O. Cognitive impairment in amyotrophic lateral sclerosis. *Lancet Neurol* 2007; 6: 994–1003.

[229] Strong MJ, Grace GM, Orange JB, *et al.* A prospective study of cognitive impairment in ALS. *Neurology* 1999; 53: 1665–70.

[230] Lomen-Hoerth C, Murphy J, Langmore S, *et al.* Are amyotrophic lateral sclerosis patients cognitively normal? *Neurology* 2003; 60: 1094–7.

[231] Ringholz GM, Appel SH, Bradshaw M, *et al.* Prevalence and patterns of cognitive impairment in sporadic ALS. *Neurology* 2005; 65: 586–90.

[232] Lomen-Hoerth C, Anderson T, Miller B. The overlap of amyotrophic lateral sclerosis and frontotemporal dementia. *Neurology* 2002; 59: 1077–9.

[233] Pinkhardt EH, Jurgens R, Becker W, *et al.* Signs of impaired selective attention in patients with amyotrophic lateral sclerosis. *J Neurol* 2008; 255: 532–8.

[234] Volpato C, Piccione F, Silvoni S, *et al.* Working memory in amyotrophic lateral sclerosis: auditory event-related potentials and neuropsychological evidence. *J Clin Neurophysiol* 2010; 27: 198–206.

[235] Takeda T, Uchihara T, Mochizuki Y, Mizutani T, Iwata M. Memory deficits in amyotrophic lateral sclerosis patients with dementia and degeneration of the perforant pathway. A clinicopathological study. *J Neurol Sci* 2007; 260: 225–30.

[236] Caselli RJ, Windebank AJ, Petersen RC, *et al.* Rapidly progressive aphasic dementia and motor neuron disease. *Ann Neurol* 1993; 33: 200–7.

[237] Doran M, Xuereb J, Hodges JR. Rapidly progressive aphasia with bulbar motor neurone disease: a clinical and neuropsychological study. *Behav Neurol* 1995; 9: 169–80.

[238] Rakowicz WP, Hodges JR. Dementia and aphasia in motor neuron disease: an underrecognised association? *J Neurol Neurosurg Psychiatry* 1998; 65: 881–9.

[239] Bak T, Hodges JR. Noun-verb dissociation in three patients with motor neurone disease and aphasia. *Brain Lang* 1997; 60: 38–41.

[240] Massman PJ, Sims J, Cooke N, *et al.* Prevalence and correlates of neuropsychological deficits in amyotrophic lateral sclerosis. *J Neurol Neurosurg Psychiatry* 1996; 61: 450–5.

[241] Evdokimidis I, Constantinidis TS, Gourtzelidis P, *et al.* Frontal lobe dysfunction in amyotrophic lateral sclerosis. *J Neurol Sci* 2002; 195: 25–33.

[242] Schreiber H, Gaigalat T, Wiedemuth-Catrinescu U, *et al.* Cognitive function in bulbar- and spinal-onset amyotrophic lateral sclerosis. A longitudinal study in 52 patients. *J Neurol* 2005; 252: 772–81.

[243] Pringle CE, Hudson AJ, Munoz DG, *et al.* Primary lateral sclerosis: clinical features, neuropathology and diagnostic criteria. *Brain* 1992; 115: 495–520.

[244] Grace GM, Orange JB, Murphy MJ, *et al.* Primary lateral sclerosis: cognitive, language, and cerebral hemodynamic findings. In: Strong MJ (ed.). *Dementia and Motor Neuron Disease.* Abingdon: Informa Healthcare, 2006; 87–97.

[245] Caselli RJ, Smith BE, Osborne D. Primary lateral sclerosis: a neuropsychological study. *Neurology* 1995; 45: 2005–9.

[246] Le Forestier N, Maisonobe T, Piquard A, *et al.* Does primary lateral sclerosis exist? A study of 20 patients and a review of the literature. *Brain* 2001; 124: 1989–99.

[247] Piquard A, Le Forestier N, Baudoin-Madec V, *et al.* Neuropsychological changes in patients with primary lateral sclerosis. *Amyotroph Lateral Scler* 2006; 7: 150–60.

[248] Canu E, Agosta F, Riva N, *et al.* Neuropsychological profiles of patients with primary lateral sclerosis and amyotrophic lateral sclerosis. *J Neurol* 2012; 259: S136 (abstract P545).

[249] Wicks P, Abrahams S, Leigh PN, Williams T, Goldstein LH. Absence of cognitive, behavioural, or emotional dysfunction in progressive muscular atrophy. *Neurology* 2006; 67: 1718–19.

[250] Hu MTM, Ellis CM, Al-Chalabi A, Leigh PN, Shaw CE. Flail arm syndrome: a distinctive variant of amyotrophic lateral sclerosis. *J Neurol Neurosurg Psychiatry* 1998; 65: 950–1.

[251] Raaphorst J, de Visser M, van Tol MJ, *et al.* Cognitive dysfunction in lower motor neuron disease: executive and memory deficits in progressive muscular atrophy. *J Neurol Neurosurg Psychiatry* 2011; 82: 170–5.

[252] Mills CK. A case of unilateral progressive ascending paralysis probably presenting a new form of degenerative disease. *J Nerv Ment Dis* 1900; 27: 195–200.

[253] Malin JP, Poburski R, Reusche E. Clinical variants of amyotrophic lateral sclerosis: hemiplegic type of ALS and Mills syndrome. A critical review [in German]. *Fortschr Neurol Psychiatr* 1986; 54: 101–5.

[254] Gastaut J-L, Bartolomei F. Mills' syndrome: ascending (or descending) progressive hemiplegia: a hemiplegic form of primary lateral sclerosis? *J Neurol Neurosurg Psychiatry* 1994; 57: 1280–1.

[255] Larner AJ, Gardner-Thorpe C. Mills syndrome with dementia. *Eur Neurol J* 2012; 4(2): 29–32.

[256] Doran M, Enevoldson TP, Ghadiali EJ, Larner AJ. Mills syndrome with dementia: broadening the phenotype of FTD/MND. *J Neurol* 2005; 252: 846–7.

[257] Wicks P, Abrahams S, Papps B, *et al.* SOD1 and cognitive dysfunction in familial amyotrophic lateral sclerosis. *J Neurol* 2009; 256: 234–41.

[258] Byrne S, Elamin M, Bede P, *et al.* Cognitive and clinical characteristics of patients with amyotrophic lateral sclerosis carrying a C9orf72 repeat expansion: a population-based cohort study. *Lancet Neurol* 2012; 11: 232–40 [Erratum *Lancet Neurol* 2012; 11: 388].

[259] Al-Chalabi A, Jones A, Troakes C, *et al.* The genetics and neuropathology of amyotrophic lateral sclerosis. *Acta Neuropathol* 2012; 124: 339–52.

[260] Gardner-Thorpe C. *James Parkinson 1755–1824.* Exeter: A Wheaton & Co. Ltd, 1987.

[261] Charcot JM. *Leçons sur les maladies du système nerveux.* Paris: Delahaye, 1985 [1875]; 179.

[262] Ball B. De l'insanité dans la paralysie agitante. *Encéphale* 1882; 2: 22–32.

[263] Starkstein SE, Merello M. *Psychiatric and Cognitive Disorders in Parkinson's Disease.* Cambridge: Cambridge University Press, 2002; 55–87, 100–3.

[264] Emre M (ed.). *Cognitive Impairment and Dementia in Parkinson's Disease.* Oxford: Oxford University Press, 2010.

[265] Hoehn MM, Yahr MD. Parkinsonism: onset, progression, and mortality. *Neurology* 1967; 17: 427–42.

[266] Mortimer JA, Pirozzola FJ, Hansch EC, Webster DD. Relationship of motor symptoms to intellectual deficits in Parkinson's disease. *Neurology* 1982; 32: 133–7.

[267] Boeve BF, Silber MH, Saper CB, *et al.* Pathophysiology of REM sleep behaviour disorder and relevance to neurodegenerative disease. *Brain* 2007; 130: 2770–88.

[268] Quinn N. Other atypical parkinsonian disorders and their differentiation from dementia with Lewy bodies. In: O'Brien J, McKeith I, Ames D, Chiu E (eds.). *Dementia with Lewy Bodies and Parkinson's Disease Dementia.* London: Taylor & Francis, 2006; 241–53.

[269] Bak TH, Crawford LM, Hearn VC, Mathuranath PS, Hodges JR. Subcortical dementia revisited: similarities and differences in cognitive function between progressive supranuclear palsy (PSP), corticobasal degeneration (CBD) and multiple system atrophy (MSA). *Neurocase* 2005; 11: 268–73.

[270] Emre M, Aarsland D, Brown R, *et al.* Clinical diagnostic criteria for dementia associated with Parkinson's disease. *Mov Disord* 2007; 22: 1689–707.

[271] Dubois B, Burn D, Goetz C, *et al.* Diagnostic procedures for Parkinson's disease dementia: recommendations from the Movement Disorder Society task force. *Mov Disord* 2007; 22: 2314–24.

[272] Litvan I, Aarsland D, Adler CH, *et al.* MDS Task Force on mild cognitive impairment in Parkinson's disease: critical review of PD-MCI. *Mov Disord* 2011; 26: 1814–24.

[273] Litvan I, Goldman JG, Troster AI, *et al.* Diagnostic criteria for mild cognitive impairment in Parkinson's disease: Movement Disorder Society Task Force guidelines. *Mov Disord* 2012; 27: 349–56.

[274] Hely MA, Reid WG, Adena MA, Halliday GM, Morris JG. The Sydney multicenter study of Parkinson's disease: the inevitability of dementia at 20 years. *Mov Disord* 2008; 23: 837–44.

[275] Reid WG, Hely MA, Morris JG, Loy C, Halliday GM. Dementia in Parkinson's disease: a 20-year neuropsychological study (Sydney Multicentre Study). *J Neurol Neurosurg Psychiatry* 2011; 82: 1033–7.

[276] Foltynie T, Brayne CE, Robbins TW, Barker RA. The cognitive ability of an incident cohort of Parkinson's patients in the UK. The CamPaIGN study. *Brain* 2004; 127: 550–60.

[277] Williams-Gray CH, Foltyine T, Brayne CE, Robbins TW, Barker RA. Evolution of cognitive dysfunction in an incident Parkinson's disease cohort. *Brain* 2007; 130: 1787–98.

[278] Erro R, Santangelo G, Picillo M, *et al.* Link between non-motor symptoms and cognitive dysfunctions in de novo, drug-naive PD patients. *J Neurol* 2012; 259: 1808–13.

[279] Williams-Gray CH, Evans JR, Goris A, *et al.* The distinct cognitive syndromes of Parkinson's disease: 5-year follow-up of the CamPaIGN cohort. *Brain* 2009; 132; 2958–69.

[280] Brønnick K. Cognitive profile in Parkinson's disease dementia. In: Emre M (ed.). *Cognitive Impairment and Dementia in Parkinson's Disease.* Oxford: Oxford University Press, 2010: 27–43.

[281] O'Brien J, McKeith I, Ames D, Chiu E (eds.). *Dementia with Lewy Bodies and Parkinson's Disease Dementia.* London: Taylor & Francis, 2006.

[282] Hansen L, Salmon D, Galasko D, *et al.* The Lewy body variant of Alzheimer's disease: a clinical and pathologic entity. *Neurology* 1990; 40: 1–8.

[283] Leverenz JB, Fishel MA, Peskind ER, *et al.* Lewy body pathology in familial Alzheimer disease: evidence for disease- and mutation-specific pathologic phenotype. *Arch Neurol* 2006; 63: 370–6.

[284] McKeith IG, Galasko D, Kosaka K, *et al.* Consensus guidelines for the clinical and pathologic diagnosis of dementia with Lewy bodies (DLB): report of the consortium on DLB international workshop. *Neurology* 1996; 47: 1113–24.

[285] McKeith IG, Perry EK, Perry RH for the Consortium on Dementia with Lewy Bodies. Report of the second

Dementia with Lewy body international workshop. *Neurology* 1999; 53: 902–5.

[286] McKeith IG, Dickson DW, Lowe J, *et al.* Diagnosis and management of dementia with Lewy bodies: third report of the DLB Consortium. *Neurology* 2005; 65: 1863–72.

[287] McKeith IG, Ballard CG, Perry RH, *et al.* Prospective validation of consensus criteria for the diagnosis of dementia with Lewy bodies. *Neurology* 2000; 54: 1050–8.

[288] Collerton D, Burn D, McKeith I, O'Brien J. Systematic review and meta-analysis show that dementia with Lewy bodies is a visual-perceptual and attentional-executive dementia. *Dement Geriatr Cogn Disord* 2003; 16: 229–37.

[289] Salmon DP, Galasko D, Hansen LA, *et al.* Neuropsychological deficits associated with diffuse Lewy body disease. *Brain Cogn* 1996; 31: 148–65.

[290] Downes JJ, Priestley NM, Doran M, *et al.* Intellectual, mnemonic and frontal functions in dementia with Lewy bodies: a comparison with early and advanced Parkinson's disease. *Behav Neurol* 1998; 11: 173–83.

[291] Ballard CG, Ayre G, O'Brien J, *et al.* Simple standardised neuropsychological assessments aid in the differential diagnosis of dementia with Lewy bodies from Alzheimer's disease and vascular dementia. *Dement Geriatr Cogn Disord* 1999; 10: 104–8.

[292] Calderon J, Perry R, Erzinclioglu S, *et al.* Perception, attention and working memory are disproportionately impaired in dementia with Lewy bodies compared with Alzheimer's disease. *J Neurol Neurosurg Psychiatry* 2001; 70: 157–64.

[293] McKeith I, Fairbairn A, Perry R, Thompson P, Perry E. Neuroleptic sensitivity in patients with senile dementia of Lewy body type. *BMJ* 1992; 305: 673–8.

[294] Horimoto Y, Matsumoto M, Akatsu H, *et al.* Autonomic dysfunctions in dementia with Lewy bodies. *J Neurol* 2003; 250: 530–3.

[295] Larner AJ, Mathias CJ, Rossor MN. Autonomic failure preceding dementia with Lewy bodies. *J Neurol* 2000; 247: 229–31.

[296] Kaufmann H, Nahm K, Purohit D, Wolfe D. Autonomic failure as the initial presentation of Parkinson disease and dementia with Lewy bodies. *Neurology* 2004; 63: 1093–5.

[297] Nelson PT, Jicha GA, Kryscio RJ, *et al.* Low sensitivity in clinical diagnoses of dementia with Lewy bodies. *J Neurol* 2010; 257: 359–66.

[298] Ferman TJ, Boeve BF, Smith GE, *et al.* Inclusion of RBD improves the diagnostic classification of dementia with Lewy bodies. *Neurology* 2011; 77: 875–82.

[299] Braak H, Del Tredici K, Rüb U, *et al.* Staging of brain pathology related to sporadic Parkinson's disease. *Neurobiol Aging* 2003; 24: 197–211.

[300] Braak H, Rüb U, Jansen-Steur ENH, Del Tredici K, de Vos RAI. Cognitive status correlates with neuropathologic stage in Parkinson disease. *Neurology* 2005; 64: 1404–10.

[301] Zarranz JJ, Alegre J, Gomez-Esteban JC, *et al.* The new mutation, E46K, of alpha-synuclein causes Parkinson and Lewy body dementia. *Ann Neurol* 2004; 55: 164–73.

[302] Singleton AB, Farrer M, Johnson J, *et al.* Alpha-synuclein locus triplication causes Parkinson's disease. *Science* 2003; 302: 841.

[303] Houlden H, Singleton AB. The genetics and neuropathology of Parkinson's disease. *Acta Neuropathol* 2012; 124: 325–38 [at 327].

[304] Ishikawa A, Piao YS, Miyashita A, *et al.* A mutant PSEN1 causes dementia with Lewy bodies and variant Alzheimer's disease. *Ann Neurol* 2005; 57: 429–34.

[305] Koide T, Ohtake H, Nakajima T, *et al.* A patient with dementia with Lewy bodies and codon 232 mutation of PRNP. *Neurology* 2002; 59: 1619–21.

[306] Doran M, Larner AJ. EEG findings in dementia with Lewy bodies causing diagnostic confusion with sporadic Creutzfeldt–Jakob disease. *Eur J Neurol* 2004; 11: 838–41.

[307] Du Plessis DG, Larner AJ. Phenotypic similarities causing clinical misdiagnosis of pathologically-confirmed sporadic Creutzfeldt–Jakob disease as dementia with Lewy bodies. *Clin Neurol Neurosurg* 2008; 110: 194–7.

[308] Brown P, Marsden CD. What do the basal ganglia do? *Lancet* 1998; 351: 1801–4.

[309] Dujardin K, Degreef JF, Rogelet P, Defebvre L, Destee A. Impairment of the supervisory attentional system in early untreated patients with Parkinson's disease. *J Neurol* 1999; 246: 783–8.

[310] Owen AM, Iddon JL, Hodges JR, Summers BA, Robbins TW. Spatial and non-spatial working memory at different stages of Parkinson's disease. *Neuropsychologia* 1997; 35: 519–32.

[311] Rafal RD, Posner MJ, Walker JA, Friedrich FJ. Cognition and the basal ganglia: separating mental and

motor components of performance in Parkinson's disease. *Brain* 1984; 107: 1083–94.

[312] Smith MC, Goldman WP, Janer KW, Baty JD, Morris JC. Cognitive speed in nondemented Parkinson's disease. *J Int Neuropsychol Soc* 1998; 4: 584–92.

[313] Brønnick K, Ehrt U, Emre M, *et al.* Attentional deficits affect activities of daily living in dementia associated with Parkinson's disease. *J Neurol Neurosurg Psychiatry* 2006; 77: 1136–42.

[314] Walker MP, Ayre GA, Cummings JL, *et al.* The clinical assessment of fluctuation and the one day fluctuation assessment scale. Two methods to assess fluctuating confusion in dementia. *Br J Psychiatry* 2000; 177: 252–6.

[315] Saghal A, Galloway PH, McKeith IG, *et al.* A comparative study of attentional deficits in senile dementias of Alzheimer and Lewy body types. *Dementia* 1992; 3: 350–4.

[316] Ferman TJ, Smith GE, Boeve BF, *et al.* DLB fluctuations: specific features that reliably differentiate DLB from AD and normal aging. *Neurology* 2004; 62: 181–7.

[317] Larner AJ. Can the informant Fluctuation Composite Score help in the diagnosis of synucleinopathies? A pragmatic study. *Int J Geriatr Psychiatry* 2012; 27: 1094–5.

[318] Whittington CJ, Podd J, Kan MM. Recognition memory impairment in Parkinson's disease: power and meta-analyses. *Neuropsychology* 2000; 14: 233–46.

[319] Ivory SJ, Knight RG, Longmore BE, Caradoc-Davies T. Verbal memory in non-demented patients with idiopathic Parkinson's disease. *Neuropsychologia* 1999; 37: 817–28.

[320] Pillon B, Deweer B, Agid Y, Dubois B. Explicit memory in Alzheimer's, Huntington's, and Parkinson's diseases. *Arch Neurol* 1993; 50: 374–9.

[321] Portin R, Laatu S, Revonsuo A, Rinne UK. Impairment of semantic knowledge in Parkinson disease. *Arch Neurol* 2000; 57: 1338–43.

[322] Hamilton JM, Salmon DP, Galasko D, *et al.* A comparison of episodic memory deficits in neuropathologically-confirmed dementia with Lewy bodies and Alzheimer's disease. *J Int Neuropsychol Soc* 2004; 10: 689–97.

[323] Lambon Ralph MA, Powell J, Howard D, *et al.* Semantic memory is impaired in both dementia with Lewy bodies and dementia of Alzheimer's type: a comparative neuropsychological study and literature review. *J Neurol Neurosurg Psychiatry* 2001; 70: 149–56.

[324] Cummings JL, Darkins A, Mendez M, Hill MA, Benson DF. Alzheimer's disease and Parkinson's disease: comparison of speech and language alterations. *Neurology* 1988; 38: 680–4.

[325] Lewis FM, Lapointe L, Murdoch BE, Chenery HJ. Language impairment in Parkinson's disease. *Aphasiology* 1998; 12: 193–206.

[326] Troyer AK, Moscovitch M, Winocur G, Leach L, Freedman M. Clustering and switching on verbal fluency tests in Alzheimer's and Parkinson's disease. *J Int Neuropsychol Soc* 1998; 4: 137–43.

[327] Canavan AGM, Passingham RE, Marsden CD. Prism adaptation and other tasks involving spatial abilities in patients with Parkinson's disease, patients with frontal lobe lesions and patients with unilateral temporal lobectomies. *Neuropsychologia* 1990; 28: 969–84.

[328] Levin BE, Llabre MM, Reisman S, *et al.* Visuospatial impairment in Parkinson's disease. *Neurology* 1991; 41: 365–9.

[329] Simard M, van Reekum R, Myran D. Visuospatial impairment in dementia with Lewy bodies and Alzheimer's disease: a process analysis approach. *Int J Geriatr Psychiatry* 2003; 18: 387–91.

[330] Gnanalingham KK, Byrne EJ, Thornton A. Clock-face drawing to differentiate Lewy body and Alzheimer type dementia syndromes. *Lancet* 1996; 347: 696–7.

[331] Cormack F, Aarsland D, Ballard C, Tovée MJ. Pentagon drawing and neuropsychological performance in dementia with Lewy bodies, Alzheimer's disease, Parkinson's disease and Parkinson's disease with dementia. *Int J Geriatr Psychiatry* 2004; 19: 371–7.

[332] Cormack F, Gray A, Ballard C, Tovée MJ. A failure of "pop-out" in visual search tasks in dementia with Lewy bodies as compared to Alzheimer's and Parkinson's disease. *Int J Geriatr Psychiatry* 2004; 19: 763–72.

[333] Lobotesis K, Fenwick JD, Phipps A, *et al.* Occipital hypoperfusion on SPECT in dementia with Lewy bodies but not AD. *Neurology* 2001; 56: 643–9.

[334] Leiguarda RC, Pramstaller PP, Merello M, *et al.* Apraxia in Parkinson's disease, progressive supranuclear palsy, multiple system atrophy and neuroleptic-induced parkinsonism. *Brain* 1997; 120: 75–90.

[335] Zadikoff C, Lang AE. Apraxia in movement disorders. *Brain* 2005; 128: 1480–97.

[336] Lees AJ, Smith E. Cognitive deficits in the early stages of Parkinson's disease. *Brain* 1983; 106: 257–70.

[337] Brown RG, Marsden CD. Dual task performance and processing resources in normal subjects and patients with Parkinson's disease. *Brain* 1991; 114: 215–31.

[338] Larner AJ. Medical hazards of the internet: gambling in Parkinson's disease. *Mov Disord* 2006; 21: 1789.

[339] Djamshidian A, Cardoso F, Grosset D, Bowden-Jones H, Lees AJ. Pathological gambling in Parkinson's disease – a review of the literature. *Mov Disord* 2011; 26: 1976–84.

[340] McKeith I, Del Ser T, Spano P, *et al.* Efficacy of rivastigmine in dementia with Lewy bodies: a randomised, double-blind, placebo-controlled international study. *Lancet* 2000; 356: 2031–6.

[341] Grace J, Daniel S, Stevens T, *et al.* Long-term use of rivastigmine in patients with dementia with Lewy bodies: an open-label trial. *Int Psychogeriatr* 2001; 13: 199–205.

[342] Rolinksi M, Fox C, Maidment I, McShane R. Cholinesterase inhibitors for dementia with Lewy bodies, Parkinson's disease dementia and cognitive impairment in Parkinson's disease. *Cochrane Database Syst Rev* 2012; 3: CD006504.

[343] Emre M, Tsolaki M, Bonuccelli U, *et al.* Memantine for patients with Parkinson's disease dementia or dementia with Lewy bodies: a randomised, double-blind, placebo-controlled trial. *Lancet Neurol* 2010; 9: 969–77.

[344] Richardson JC, Steele J, Olszewski J. Supranuclear ophthalmoplegia, pseudobulbar palsy, nuchal dystonia and dementia. A clinical report on eight cases of heterogeneous system degeneration. *Trans Am Neurol Assoc* 1963; 88: 25–9.

[345] Steele JC, Richardson JC, Olszewski J. Progressive supranuclear palsy: a heterogeneous degeneration involving the brainstem, basal ganglia and cerebellum with vertical gaze and pseudobulbar palsy, nuchal dystonia and dementia. *Arch Neurol* 1964; 10: 333–58.

[346] Larner AJ. Did Charles Dickens describe progressive supranuclear palsy in 1857? *Mov Disord* 2002; 17: 832–3.

[347] Litvan I, Agid Y, Calne D, *et al.* Clinical research criteria for the diagnosis of progressive supranuclear palsy (Steele–Richardson–Olszewski syndrome): report of the NINDS–SPSP International Workshop. *Neurology* 1996; 47: 1–9.

[348] Williams DR, de Silva R, Paviour DC, *et al.* Characteristics of two distinct clinical phenotypes in pathologically proven progressive supranuclear palsy: Richardson's syndrome and PSP-parkinsonism. *Brain* 2005; 128: 1247–58.

[349] Morris HR, Osaki Y, Holton J, *et al.* Tau exon 10 +16 mutation FTDP-17 presenting clinically as sporadic young onset PSP. *Neurology* 2003; 61: 102–4.

[350] Larner AJ. A 50-year old man with deteriorating cognitive function and impaired movement. *PLoS Med* 2009; 6: e1000019.

[351] Albert ML, Feldman RG, Willis AL. The "subcortical dementia" of progressive supranuclear palsy. *J Neurol Neurosurg Psychiatry* 1974; 37: 121–30.

[352] Brown RG, Lacomblez L, Landwehrmeyer BG, *et al.* Cognitive impairment in patients with multiple system atrophy and progressive supranuclear palsy. *Brain* 2010; 133: 2382–93.

[353] Robbins TW, James M, Lange KW, *et al.* Cognitive deficits in progressive supranuclear palsy, Parkinson's disease, and multiple system atrophy in tests sensitive to frontal lobe dysfunction. *J Neurol Neurosurg Psychiatry* 1994; 57: 79–88.

[354] Rosser AE, Hodges JR. Initial letter and semantic category fluency in Alzheimer's disease, Huntington's disease and progressive supranuclear palsy. *J Neurol Neurosurg Psychiatry* 1994; 57: 1389–94.

[355] Rosser AE, Hodges JR. The Dementia Rating Scale in Alzheimer's disease, Huntington's disease and progressive supranuclear palsy. *J Neurol* 1994; 241: 531–6.

[356] Pillon B, Deweer B, Michon A, *et al.* Are explicit memory disorders of progressive supranuclear palsy related to damage to striatofrontal circuits? Comparison with Alzheimer's, Parkinson's and Huntington's diseases. *Neurology* 1994; 44: 1264–70.

[357] Litvan I, Phipps M, Pharr VL, *et al.* Randomized placebo-controlled trial of donepezil in patients with progressive supranuclear palsy. *Neurology* 2001; 57: 467–73.

[358] Rebeiz JJ, Kolodny EH, Richardson EP. Corticodentatonigral degeneration with neuronal achromasia: a progressive disorder of late adult life. *Trans Am Neurol Assoc* 1967; 92: 23–6.

[359] Mahapatra RK, Edwards MJ, Schott JM, Bhatia KP. Corticobasal degeneration. *Lancet Neurol* 2004; 3: 736–43.

[360] Dickson DW, Bergeron C, Chin SS, *et al.* Office of Rare Diseases neuropathologic criteria for corticobasal degeneration. *J Neuropathol Exp Neurol* 2002; 61: 935–46.

[361] Thompson PD, Marsden CD. Corticobasal degeneration. In: Rossor MN (ed.). *Unusual Dementias.* London: Bailliere Tindall, 1992; 677–86.

[362] Grimes DA, Lang AE, Bergeron CB. Dementia as the most common presentation of cortical-basal ganglionic degeneration. *Neurology* 1999; 53: 1969–74.

[363] Graham NL, Bak TH, Hodges JR. Corticobasal degeneration as a cognitive disorder. *Mov Disord* 2003; 18: 1224–32.

[364] Lang AE, Riley DE, Bergeron C. Cortical-basal ganglionic degeneration. In: Calne DB (ed.). *Neurodegenerative Diseases.* Philadelphia, PA: WB Saunders, 1994; 877–94.

[365] Boeve BF, Lang AE, Litvan I. Corticobasal degeneration and its relationship to progressive supranuclear palsy and frontotemporal dementia. *Ann Neurol* 2003; 54: S15–19.

[366] Boeve BF, Maraganore MD, Parisi JE, *et al.* Pathologic heterogeneity in clinically diagnosed corticobasal degeneration. *Neurology* 1999; 53: 795–800.

[367] Grimes DA, Bergeron CB, Lang AE. Motor neuron disease-inclusion dementia presenting as cortical-basal ganglionic degeneration. *Mov Disord* 1999; 14: 674–80.

[368] Larner AJ, Doran M. Language function and dysfunction in corticobasal degeneration. *Neurology* 2004; 62: 1238.

[369] Pillon B, Blin J, Vidailhet M, *et al.* The neuropsychological pattern of corticobasal degeneration: comparison with progressive supranuclear palsy and Alzheimer's disease. *Neurology* 1995; 45: 1477–83.

[370] Massman PJ, Kreiter KT, Jankovic J, Doody RS. Neuropsychological functioning in cortical-basal ganglionic degeneration: differentiation from Alzheimer's disease. *Neurology* 1996; 46: 720–6.

[371] Lippa CF, Cohen R, Smith TW, Drachman DA. Primary progressive aphasia with focal neuronal achromasia. *Neurology* 1991; 41: 882–6.

[372] Graham NL, Bak T, Patterson K, Hodges JR. Language function and dysfunction in corticobasal degeneration. *Neurology* 2003; 61: 493–9.

[373] Mathuranath PS, Xuereb JH, Bak T, Hodges JR. Corticobasal ganglionic degeneration and/or frontotemporal dementia? A report of two overlap cases and review of literature. *J Neurol Neurosurg Psychiatry* 2000; 68: 304–12.

[374] Tang-Wai DF, Josephs KA, Boeve BF, *et al.* Pathologically confirmed corticobasal degeneration presenting with visuospatial dysfunction. *Neurology* 2003; 61: 1134–5.

[375] Graham JG, Oppenheimer DR. Orthostatic hypotension and nicotine sensitivity in a case of multiple system atrophy. *J Neurol Neurosurg Psychiatry* 1969; 32: 28–34.

[376] Stefanova N, Bücke P, Duerr S, Wenning GK. Multiple system atrophy: an update. *Lancet Neurol* 2009; 8: 1172–8.

[377] Gilman S, Wenning GK, Low PA, *et al.* Second consensus statement on the diagnosis of multiple system atrophy. *Neurology* 2008; 71: 670–6.

[378] Robbins TW, James M, Lange KW, *et al.* Cognitive performance in multiple system atrophy. *Brain* 1992; 115: 271–91.

[379] Meco G, Gasparini M, Doricchi F. Attentional functions in multiple system atrophy and Parkinson's disease. *J Neurol Neurosurg Psychiatry* 1996; 60: 393–8.

[380] Pillon B, Gouider-Khouja N, Deweer B, *et al.* Neuropsychological pattern of striatonigral degeneration: comparison with Parkinson's disease and progressive supranuclear palsy. *J Neurol Neurosurg Psychiatry* 1995; 58: 174–9.

[381] Kawai Y, Suenaga M, Takeda A, *et al.* Cognitive impairments in multiple system atrophy: MSA-C vs MSA-P. *Neurology* 2008; 70: 1390–6.

[382] Skelina S, Pavlova R, Petrova M, *et al.* Mild cognitive impairment in patients with multiple system atrophy. *J Neurol* 2012; 259: S25 (abstract O228).

[383] Corsellis JAN, Bruton CJ, Freeman-Browne D. The aftermath of boxing. *Psychol Med* 1973; 3: 270–303.

[384] Roberts GW, Gentleman SM, Lynch A, *et al.* β-amyloid protein deposition in the brain following severe head injury: implications for the pathogenesis of Alzheimer's disease. *J Neurol Neurosurg Psychiatry* 1994; 57: 419–25.

[385] Nicoll JAR, Roberts GW, Graham DI. Apolipoprotein E epsilon-4 allele is associated with deposition of

amyloid beta-protein following head injury. *Nat Med* 1995; 1: 135–7.

[386] Erlanger DM, Kutner KC, Barth JT, Barnes R. Neuropsychology of sports-related head injury: dementia pugilistica to post concussion syndrome. *Clin Neuropsychol* 1999; 13: 193–209.

[387] Echemendia RJ, Julian LJ. Mild traumatic brain injury in sports: neuropsychology's contribution to a developing field. *Neuropsychol Rev* 2001; 11: 69–88.

[388] Guskiewicz KM, Marshall SW, Bailes J, *et al.* Association between recurrent concussion and late-life cognitive impairment in retired professional football players. *Neurosurgery* 2005; 57: 719–26.

[389] McCrea MA. *Mild Traumatic Brain Injury and Post-concussion Syndrome. The New Evidence Base for Diagnosis and Treatment.* Oxford: Oxford University Press, 2008.

[390] Bleiberg J, Cernich AN, Cameron K, *et al.* Duration of cognitive impairment after sports concussion. *Neurosurgery* 2004; 54: 1073–8.

[391] Perl DP. Amyotrophic lateral sclerosis/parkinsonism-dementia complex of Guam. In: Strong MJ (ed.). *Dementia and Motor Neuron Disease.* Abingdon: Informa Healthcare, 2006; 177–91.

[392] Miklossy J, Steele JC, Yu S, *et al.* Enduring involvement of tau, beta-amyloid, alpha-synuclein, ubiquitin and TDP-43 pathology in the amyotrophic lateral sclerosis/parkinsonism dementia complex of Guam (ALS/PDC). *Acta Neuropathol* 2008; 116: 625–37.

[393] Galasko D, Salmon DP, Craig UK, *et al.* Clinical features and changing patterns of neurodegenerative disorders on Guam, 1997–2000. *Neurology* 2002; 58: 90–7.

[394] Perl DP, Hof PR, Steele JC, *et al.* Neuropathologic studies of a pure dementing syndrome (Marianas dementia) among the inhabitants of Guam, a form of ALS/parkinsonism dementia complex. *Brain Pathol* 1994; 4: 529 (abstract P31–13).

[395] Prusiner SB. Novel proteinaceous particles cause scrapie. *Science* 1982; 216: 136–44.

[396] Prusiner SB. Shattuck lecture – neurodegenerative diseases and prions. *N Engl J Med* 2001; 344: 1516–26.

[397] Collinge J. Prion diseases of humans and animals: their causes and molecular basis. *Annu Rev Neurosci* 2001; 24: 519–50.

[398] Collinge J, Palmer MS (eds.). *Prion Diseases.* Oxford: Oxford University Press, 1997.

[399] Prusiner SB (ed.). *Prion Biology and Diseases.* Cold Spring Harbor, NY: Cold Spring Harbor Laboratory Press, 1999.

[400] Larner AJ, Doran M. Prion disease at a regional neuroscience centre: retrospective audit. *J Neurol Neurosurg Psychiatry* 2004; 75: 1789–90.

[401] Hegde RS, Tremblay P, Groth D, *et al.* Transmissible and genetic prion diseases share a common pathway of neurodegeneration. *Nature* 1999; 402: 822–6.

[402] Palmer MS, Dryden AJ, Hughes JT, Collinge J. Homozygous prion protein genotype predisposes to sporadic Creutzfeldt–Jakob disease. *Nature* 1991; 352: 340–2.

[403] Parchi P, Giese A, Capellari S, *et al.* Classification of sporadic Creutzfeldt–Jakob disease based on molecular and phenotypic analysis of 300 subjects. *Ann Neurol* 1999; 46: 224–33.

[404] Larner AJ, Doran M. Prion diseases: update on therapeutic patents, 1999–2002. *Exp Opin Ther Patents* 2003; 13: 67–78.

[405] Trevitt CR, Collinge J. A systematic review of prion therapeutics in experimental models. *Brain* 2006; 129: 2241–65.

[406] Ironside JW, Head MW. Human prion diseases. In: Esiri MM, Lee VM-Y, Trojanowski JQ (eds.). *The Neuropathology of Dementia* (2nd edn.). Cambridge: Cambridge University Press, 2004; 402–26.

[407] Collinge J, Owen F, Poulter M, *et al.* Prion dementia without characteristic pathology. *Lancet* 1990; 336: 7–9.

[408] Puoti G, Bizzi A, Forloni G, *et al.* Sporadic human prion diseases: molecular insights and diagnosis. *Lancet Neurol* 2012; 11: 618–28.

[409] Zerr I, Kallenberg K, Summers DM, *et al.* Updated clinical diagnostic criteria for sporadic Creutzfeldt–Jakob disease. *Brain* 2009; 132: 2659–68 [Erratum *Brain* 2012; 135: 1335].

[410] Tschampa HJ, Neumann M, Zerr I, *et al.* Patients with Alzheimer's disease and dementia with Lewy bodies mistaken for Creutzfeldt–Jakob disease. *J Neurol Neurosurg Psychiatry* 2001; 71: 33–9.

[411] Pietrini V. Creutzfeldt–Jakob disease presenting as Wernicke-Korsakoff syndrome. *J Neurol Sci* 1992; 108: 149–53.

[412] Monaghan TS, Murphy DT, Tubridy N, Hutchinson M. The woman who mistook the past for the present. *Adv Clin Neurosci Rehabil* 2006; 6(3): 27–8.

[413] Cohen D, Kutluay E, Edwards J, Peltier A, Beydoun A. Sporadic Creutzfeldt–Jakob disease

presenting with nonconvulsive status epilepticus. *Epilepsy Behav* 2004; 5: 792–6.

[414] Vaz J, Sierazdan K, Kane N. Non convulsive status epilepticus in Creutzfeldt–Jakob disease – a short report. *J Neurol Neurosurg Psychiatry* 2005; 76: 1318 (abstract 030).

[415] Drlicek M, Grisold W, Liszka U, Hitzenberger P, Machacek E. Angiotropic lymphoma (malignant angioendotheliomatosis) presenting with rapidly progressive dementia. *Acta Neuropathol* 1991; 82: 533–5.

[416] Schott JM, Warren JD, Rossor MN. The uncertain nosology of Hashimoto encephalopathy. *Arch Neurol* 2003; 60: 1812.

[417] Pellisé A, Navarro O, Rey M, Cardozo A, Ferrer I. Protein 14-3-3 in pellagra encephalopathy. *Neurologia* 2002; 17: 655–6.

[418] Slee M, Pretorius P, Ansorge O, Stacey R, Butterworth R. Parkinsonism and dementia due to gliomatosis cerebri mimicking sporadic Creutzfeldt–Jakob disease (CJD). *J Neurol Neurosurg Psychiatry* 2006; 77: 283–4

[419] Snowden JA, Mann DMA, Neary D. Distinct neuropsychological characteristics in Creutzfeldt-Jakob disease. *J Neurol Neurosurg Psychiatry* 2002; 73: 686–94.

[420] Mandell AM, Alexander MP, Carpenter S. Creutzfeldt–Jakob disease presenting as isolated aphasia. *Neurology* 1989; 39: 55–8.

[421] Greene JDW, Hodges JR, Ironside JW, Warlow CP. Progressive aphasia with rapidly progressive dementia in a 49 year old woman. *J Neurol Neurosurg Psychiatry* 1999; 66: 238–43.

[422] Zarei M, Nouraei SA, Caine D, Hodges JR, Carpenter RH. Neuropsychological and quantitative oculometric study of a case of sporadic Creutzfeldt–Jakob disease at predementia stage. *J Neurol Neurosurg Psychiatry* 2002; 73: 56–8.

[423] Pachalska M, Kurzbauer H, MacQueen BD, Forminska-Kapuscik M, Herman-Sucharska I. Neuropsychological features of rapidly progressive dementia in a patient with an atypical presentation of Creutzfeldt–Jakob disease. *Med Sci Monit* 2001; 7: 1307–15.

[424] Armstrong RA. Creutzfeldt–Jakob disease and vision. *Clin Exp Optom* 2006; 89: 3–9.

[425] Gajdusek DC. Unconventional viruses and the origin and disappearance of kuru. *Science* 1977; 197: 943–60.

[426] Zigas V. *Laughing Death: the Untold Story of Kuru.* Clifton, NJ: Humana, 1990.

[427] Collinge J, Whitfield J, McKintosh E, *et al.* Kuru in the 21st century – an acquired human prion disease with very long incubation periods. *Lancet* 2006; 367: 2068–74.

[428] Collinge J. Variant Creutzfeldt–Jakob disease. *Lancet* 1999; 354: 317–23.

[429] Peden AH, Head MW, Ritchie DL, Bell JE, Ironside JW. Preclinical vCJD after blood transfusion in a PRNP codon 129 heterozygous patient. *Lancet* 2004; 364: 527–9.

[430] Wroe SJ, Pal S, Siddique D, *et al.* Clinical presentation and pre-mortem diagnosis of variant Creutzfeldt–Jakob disease associated with blood transfusion: a case report. *Lancet* 2006; 368: 2061–7.

[431] Spencer MS, Knight RSG, Will RG. First hundred cases of variant Creutzfeldt–Jakob disease: retrospective case note review of early psychiatric and neurological features. *BMJ* 2002; 324: 1479–82.

[432] Zeidler M, Sellar RJ, Collie DA, *et al.* The pulvinar sign on magnetic resonance imaging in variant Creutzfeldt–Jakob disease. *Lancet* 2000; 355: 1412–8.

[433] Hilton DA, Fathers E, Edwards P, Ironside JW, Zajicek J. Prion immunoreactivity in appendix before clinical onset of variant Creutzfeldt–Jakob disease. *Lancet* 1998; 352: 703–4.

[434] Hilton D, Ghani AC, Conyers L, *et al.* Accumulation of prion protein in tonsil and appendix: review of tissue samples. *BMJ* 2002; 325: 633–4.

[435] Hill AF, Butterworth RJ, Joiner S, *et al.* Investigation of variant Creutzfeldt–Jakob disease and other human prion diseases with tonsil biopsy samples. *Lancet* 1999; 353: 183–9.

[436] Hawkins K, Chohan G, Kipps C, Will R, Kapur N. Variant Creutzfeldt–Jakob disease: neuropsychological profile in an extended series of cases. *J Int Neuropsychol Soc* 2009; 15: 807–10.

[437] Cordery RJ, Alner K, Cipolotti L, *et al.* The neuropsychology of variant CJD: a comparative study with inherited and sporadic forms of prion disease. *J Neurol Neurosurg Psychiatry* 2005; 76: 330–6.

[438] Cordery RJ, Hall M, Cipolotti L, *et al.* Early cognitive decline in Creutzfeldt–Jakob disease associated with human growth hormone treatment. *J Neurol Neurosurg Psychiatry* 2003; 74: 1412–16.

[439] Kovacs GG, Trabattoni G, Hainfellner JA, *et al*. Mutations of the prion protein gene: phenotypic spectrum. *J Neurol* 2002; 249: 1567–82.

[440] Gass CS, Luis CA, Meyers TL, Kuljis RO. Familial Creutzfeldt-Jakob disease: a neuropsychological case study. *Arch Clin Neuropsychol* 2000; 15: 165–75.

[441] Nitrini R, Teixeira-da-Silva LS, Rosemberg S, *et al*. Prion disease resembling frontotemporal dementia and parkinsonism linked to chromosome 17. *Arq Neuropsiquiatr* 2001; 59: 161–4.

[442] Alner K, Hyare H, Mead S, *et al*. Distinct neuropsychological profiles correspond to distribution of cortical thinning in inherited prion disease caused by insertional mutation. *J Neurol Neurosurg Psychiatry* 2012; 83: 109–14.

[443] Farlow MR, Yee RD, Dlouhy SR, *et al*. Gerstmann–Straussler–Scheinker disease. I. Extending the clinical spectrum. *Neurology* 1989; 39: 1446–52.

[444] Unverzagt FW, Farlow MR, Norton J, *et al*. Neuropsychological function in patients with Gerstmann–Straussler disease from the Indiana kindred (F198S). *J Int Neuropsychol Soc* 1997; 3: 169–78.

[445] Giovagnoli AR, Di Fede G, Aresi A, *et al*. Atypical frontotemporal dementia as a new clinical phenotype of Gerstmann–Straussler–Scheinker disease with the PrP-P102L mutation. Description of a previously unreported Italian family. *Neurol Sci* 2008; 29: 405–10.

[446] Gallassi R, Morreale A, Montagna P, Gambetti P, Lugaresi E. Fatal familial insomnia: neuropsychological study of a disease with thalamic degeneration. *Cortex* 1992; 28: 175–87.

[447] Gallassi R, Morreale A, Montagna P, *et al*. Fatal familial insomnia: behavioral and cognitive features. *Neurology* 1996; 46: 935–9.

Cerebrovascular disease: vascular dementia and vascular cognitive impairment

3.1 Vascular dementia (VaD); vascular cognitive impairment (VCI)

Cognitive impairment and dementia associated with cerebrovascular disease is not a unitary entity, but one typified by clinical, pathological, and etiological heterogeneity. Different variants or subtypes have been noted for over a century, but the classification and categorization of vascular dementia (VaD) and vascular cognitive impairment (VCI) is evolving, current taxonomies incorporating combinations of lesion etiology, pathological features, neuroanatomical location, and clinical syndrome [1–6].

Various consensus diagnostic criteria for VaD have been proposed, including the State of California Alzheimer's Disease Diagnostic and Treatment Centers (ADDTC) criteria [7] and the National Institute of Neurological Disorders and Stroke and the Association Internationale pour la Recherche et l'Enseignement en Neurosciences (NINDS–AIREN) criteria [8,9], as well as the general criteria of *Diagnostic and Statistical Manual* (DSM) and the *International Classification of Diseases* (ICD). NINDS–AIREN recognizes the need to establish a causal relationship between cerebrovascular lesions and cognitive deficit both spatially and temporally, emphasizing the importance of neuroimaging to corroborate clinical findings. However, because memory impairment is the most salient feature in Alzheimer's disease (AD), the most common cause of dementia, it has been noted that many of these diagnostic criteria have been inadvertently "Alzheimerized," with undue emphasis placed on memory loss at the expense of other neuropsychological features. This may account for the low sensitivity but high specificity of these criteria [10].

Perhaps one of the reasons for this poor sensitivity is that cerebrovascular disease is very common in AD. In one community-based study, most patients with dementia coming to autopsy had mixed AD/cerebrovascular disease [11]. Considering the shared vascular risk factors for AD and VaD [12], this observation is perhaps not surprising. Conversely, there have been reports of series of patients clinically diagnosed as VaD who, at postmortem, proved to have either AD alone or mixed disease [13]. Dual pathology may lower the threshold for the clinical manifestation of cognitive deficits [14,15]. An integrative approach to classification envisages a continuum running from pure AD to pure VaD through entities such as "AD with vascular lesions" and "VaD with AD changes." Pure VaD may be a rare cause of dementia, and mixed dementia a frequent one [16]. The delineation of VCI [1] represented a new conceptual approach, stemming in part from the realization that older concepts were unduly influenced by thinking on AD, and in part from the realization that cognitive decline due to vascular disease is amenable to prevention. VCI might be envisaged as one form of mild cognitive impairment (MCI; Section 1.3.2).

Therefore, it is not surprising that clinically the distinction between AD and VaD is not always clear cut. The Hachinski Ischaemic Score (HIS) has been suggested to differentiate patients with VaD from those with AD [17] but is recognized to have shortcomings. In a neuropathologically confirmed series of dementia patients, items from the HIS showing independent correlation with VaD were, stepwise deterioration, fluctuating course, and a history of hypertension, stroke, and focal neurological symptoms [18].

Attempts to define the neuropsychological profile of VaD have often been undertaken in comparison with AD, but this has proved difficult because of diagnostic and methodological inconsistencies, and no reliable profile has emerged. Nonetheless, reviewing such studies and using strict inclusion and exclusion criteria, such as matching for level of overall cognitive decline, Sachdev and Looi [19] found relative preservation of long-term memory and greater deficits in executive function in VaD patients, corroborating previous qualitative reviews [20]. Cognitive domains not permitting discrimination of VaD from AD included digit span, attention, visuoconstructive, and conceptual tasks, while language was thought to be an area in which AD would be predicted to be superior to VaD [19]. Verbal fluency for letter is more affected in VaD [21] while category fluency is equally impaired in VaD and AD [22]. The heterogeneity of the VaD group may mandate subdivision in order to find diagnostically meaningful cognitive profiles. In clinical practice, typically used cognitive screening instruments, such as the Mini-Mental State Examination (MMSE), may not be optimal for the detection of cognitive deficits of vascular origin. This may require new, specifically designed, neuropsychological test instruments, rather than those typically used for AD; for example, the vascular equivalent of the ADAS-Cog and CAM-COG, "VaDAS-Cog" and R-CAMCOG, respectively. Other tests designed specifically to detect VCI are described [23].

Pending the development of empirically derived rather than consensus criteria, which are operationalized and have undergone validation, classification of VaD remains somewhat arbitrary. NINDS–AIREN suggested a pathogenetic classification based on hypoxia–ischemia and infarction (encompassing multi-infarct, small vessel, and strategic infarct dementia), hypoperfusion (incomplete infarctions), and intracerebral hemorrhage dementia [8]. These mechanisms are not necessarily mutually exclusive, and similarly the neuropathological substrates of VaD are heterogeneous and may overlap [24].

For the purposes of this chapter, classification is largely clinical, examining cortical, subcortical, and strategic infarct subtypes. Hemodynamic or hypoperfusion dementia, associated with occlusive carotid artery disease or watershed infarcts (also known as distal field or borderzone infarcts), is included with cortical VaD. The entity of "cardiogenic dementia" discussed in the older literature [25] is also assumed to fall within this rubric. The category of hemorrhagic dementia is broad, and potentially may include any cause of intraparenchymal or subarachnoid hemorrhage (Section 3.3). The hereditary causes of vascular disease are defined increasingly [26], some of which may be associated with dementia, such as CADASIL (Section 3.5.1), MELAS and other mitochondrial disorders (Section 5.5.1), and Fabry's disease (Section 5.5.3.2). Other brain vascular disorders considered here include arteriovenous malformations, certain vasculopathies (cerebral vasculitides are discussed in the chapter on inflammatory and systemic disorders; Section 6.11), concluding with a miscellaneous group of conditions in which vascular mechanisms may be suspected rather than proved.

3.1.1 Cortical vascular dementia; multi-infarct dementia (MID); poststroke dementia

Originally conceived of as multi-infarct dementia (MID) [27], cortical VaD refers to cognitive impairment following large vessel disease, cardiac and carotid embolic events, and hence poststroke dementia [28], resulting in large cortical and corticosubcortical complete infarcts in arterial territory distribution.

Within this category may also be included hemodynamic or hypoperfusion dementia; for example, related to occlusive carotid artery disease or watershed infarction between the territories of anterior, middle, and posterior cerebral arteries (also known as distal field or borderzone infarction), and incomplete infarctions related to global cerebral ischemia following profound and prolonged hypotension, as associated with cardiac arrest, cardiac arrhythmias, or hypovolemic shock. Atrial fibrillation may be associated with cognitive decline even in the absence of overt stroke [29].

The pathological studies of Tomlinson *et al.* [30] suggested that dementia correlated with increasing volume of infarcted tissue, above a threshold of 100 mL. Classically cortical VaD is characterized as having an abrupt onset and stepwise deterioration, and is associated with focal neurological signs (e.g., hemiparesis, hemianopia, gait impairment, pseudobulbar palsy), as expected with stroke [17].

The cognitive profile of cortical VaD is dependent upon the precise arterial territory affected, but is said to include memory impairment, cortical signs such as aphasia, apraxia, or agnosia, visuospatial and/or visuoconstructive difficulties, and executive dysfunction, although the latter is not as marked as in subcortical VaD. The fact that around 10% or more of stroke patients have preexisting dementia ("prestroke dementia") [31,32], which may result from vascular lesions and/or concurrent AD, may potentially confound these observations. MMSE is adequate in screening for moderate cognitive deficits or dementia one month after stroke but has only modest performance in screening for mild cognitive disturbances [33].

3.1.1.1 Carotid artery disease

Occlusive carotid artery disease is a well-recognized risk factor for the development of transient ischemic attacks (TIA) and stroke. Studies have been undertaken to assess whether occlusive carotid artery disease is also associated with cognitive impairment. A systematic review of such studies [34] found marked heterogeneity in terms of study design, neuropsychological assessment procedures, and interpretation, making it difficult to draw meaningful conclusions. Accepting a degree of case selection bias (i.e., those likely to undergo surgery), the majority of studies found evidence of cognitive impairment, generally mild, in both symptomatic and asymptomatic patients. This was associated with either generalized cognitive impairment

or with specific deficits in memory, reasoning, and psychomotor skills. Hence, cognitive impairment may be the sole symptom of carotid artery stenosis [35].

A more recent study of patients with "asymptomatic" carotid artery disease found cognitive deficits in all domains with the exception of executive function for moderate stenosis, severe stenosis, and occluded groups [36].

Data on the effects on cognition of carotid endarterectomy for carotid artery occlusive disease are also difficult to interpret because of methodological issues [37]. Although the majority of studies suggest postoperative improvement, for example in verbal memory, constructive abilities, and visual attention [38], others suggest no change, making it impossible to draw clear conclusions about the efficacy of this procedure for the treatment of cognitive problems [37]. Cognitive improvement in a patient with bilateral carotid artery occlusions who underwent extracranial–intracranial bypass surgery has been reported [39].

3.1.1.2 Postcardiac surgery cognitive impairment ("pumphead")

There is a large amount of literature on cognitive problems appearing after cardiac surgery, most often coronary artery bypass grafting (CABG) [40], deficits sometimes evocatively referred to as "pumphead". Although most patients undergoing CABG do so without cognitive complication, there is undoubtedly a cognitive morbidity to the procedure that cannot be ascribed to depression [41]. These defects are multifactorial, and may in part be a consequence of watershed area injury secondary to hypoperfusion and/or embolic factors related to cardiopulmonary bypass. Occasionally, CABG may "unmask" an underlying neurodegenerative disorder such as AD or frontotemporal dementia (FTD) [42]. Late cognitive decline, one to five years postsurgery, is also observed, possibly related to known vascular risk factors rather than to surgery per se [43].

3.1.2 Subcortical vascular dementia; Binswanger's disease; lacunar state; subcortical ischemic vascular dementia (SIVD)

Diffuse damage to subcortical structures is probably the most common cause of VaD or VCI, due to small vessel disease in individuals with hypertension. Subcortical forms of VaD and VCI encompass both the leukoencephalopathy originally described by Binswanger and the *état lacunaire* originally described by Marie.

In 1894, Otto Binswanger reported subcortical obliteration of small cerebral arteries and arterioles, often in association with systemic hypertension, leading to pathological periventricular demyelination and the clinical correlate of dementia [44] (translation by Blass *et al.* [45]). The condition, subsequently known as Binswanger's disease, Binswanger's encephalopathy, or subcortical arteriosclerotic encephalopathy (SAE) [46], was judged relatively rare until the advent of structural neuroimaging showed radiological evidence of basal ganglia infarcts and periventricular white matter disease, often with sparing of subcortical U fibers, the white matter changes sometimes known as leukoaraiosis [47].

The *état lacunaire* or lacunar state, described by Pierre Marie in 1901, comprised small cavitary lesions in the brain parenchyma, particularly in deep gray matter, internal capsule, basis pontis, and deep hemispheric white matter, reflecting small vessel disease, occurring frequently in patients with hypertension [48]. Lacunar infarcts, also known as small deep infarcts, are readily seen on neuroimaging, and may be associated with a variety of clinical syndromes, originally described by Fisher [49], such as pure motor stroke, pure sensory stroke, sensorimotor stroke, and ataxic hemiparesis. In addition, lacunar strokes may be associated with cognitive impairment which, in contrast to cortical VaD, is often of insidious rather than abrupt onset and has a progressive rather than stepwise course.

Longitudinal studies have shown that white matter changes (leukoaraiosis) and small vessel disease are associated with cognitive impairment and an increase in the risk of transition from autonomy to dependency [50]. Cerebral microbleeds, evident on T2*-weighted gradient-echo magnetic resonance imaging (MRI), may also contribute to executive dysfunction independent of white matter change [51].

The cognitive profile of subcortical VaD is typically that of executive dysfunction, as may be anticipated with lesions affecting subcortical circuits, with slowed information processing and impairments of initiation, planning, sequencing, and abstracting [52]. Episodic memory impairment may or may not be present, and is typically milder than in AD, with impaired recall but better recognition, and with benefit from cueing [53]. There may be additional neuropsychiatric signs (depression, inertia, emotional lability) and neurological signs, although the latter are fewer than in cortical VaD, including gait disorder of frontal type (broad-based, short-stepped), subtle upper motor neuron signs, dysarthria, urinary incontinence, and extrapyramidal signs. Although there is overlap, mild subcortical VaD may be differentiated from AD on the basis of greater impairment in tests of semantic memory, executive function, and visuospatial and perceptual skills [54]. Use of the MMSE is generally insensitive for the detection of the deficits typical in subcortical VaD and VCI, for which other tests have been developed [23,55].

Within the spectrum of subcortical vascular ischemic disorders associated with cognitive impairment and dementia, an entity named subcortical ischemic vascular dementia (SIVD) has been delineated, and research diagnostic criteria for its identification suggested, based on the relationship between clinical and radiological findings, specifically the presence of extensive white matter lesions and multiple lacunar infarcts due to small vessel disease [56,57]. In a series of radiologically (MRI) defined cases of SIVD, executive deficits and subtle delayed memory deficits were found, thought to reflect disruption of frontosubcortical circuits and medial temporal lobe atrophy, respectively [58].

Treatment of neuropsychological deficits

As VaD may be associated with cholinergic deficits, the use of cholinesterase inhibitors (ChEIs) in treatment has been explored in a number of studies. A meta-analysis indicated that ChEIs produce small benefits of uncertain relevance in cognition, likewise memantime, and did not recommend widespread use of these agents in VaD but rather a need to identify subgroups who might benefit [59]. A report of improved aphasia in some patients with chronic poststroke aphasia treated with galantamine has appeared [60]. An open-label trial of donepezil in Binswanger-type subcortical VaD was reported to be beneficial and well tolerated [61]. In CADASIL, another subcortical white matter disorder that may result in dementia (Section 3.5.1), a trial of ChEIs was negative.

3.2 Strategic infarct dementia; strategic strokes

Strategic infarct dementia refers to focal ischemic lesions in regions eloquent for cognitive processes, although they may not cause dementia in the strict sense of the DSM or ICD criteria for dementia, hence strategic strokes may be a better term. The possibility that other subclinical lesions may contribute to the clinical picture cannot be excluded entirely. Nonetheless, a variety of locations have been associated with cognitive deficits [62,63], including exclusively subcortical infarction [64].

3.2.1 Angular gyrus

The angular gyrus is located in the posterior parieto-temporal region of the dominant hemisphere in the territory of the posterior branch of the middle cerebral artery. Infarction of the angular gyrus may be associated with combinations of aphasia, alexia with agraphia, and Gerstmann syndrome (acalculia, right–left disorientation, finger

agnosia), sometimes in the absence of focal sensorimotor deficit and sometimes simulating AD [65,66].

3.2.2 Corpus callosum and fornix

Acute anterograde amnesia following ischemic infarct of the genu of the corpus callosum and both columns and the body of the fornix has been reported [67,68], with subjective improvement in memory on follow-up [67]. Multiple infarctions along the entire length of the corpus callosum, due to bilateral internal carotid artery occlusion, producing a rapidly progressive dementia has been reported [69], whereas an isolated retrosplenial infarct produced a transient global amnesia (Sections 7.1.7 and 3.6.2) [70].

Acute bilateral anterior fornix infarction, presumed to be due to pericallosal artery branch occlusion, has been reported as causing not only amnesia for verbal and visual material but also visuospatial and executive dysfunction amounting to dementia [71]. Selective damage to the fornix is more commonly seen after surgery for third ventricle lesions such as colloid cyst (Section 7.2.3).

3.2.3 Thalamus

Several types of thalamic infarct have been described, involving differing thalamic vascular territories and damaging differing nuclei [72]. Various neuropsychological deficits have been described with thalamic infarctions, including aphasia, hemineglect, amnesia, and dementia, sometimes known as thalamic dementia (Section 1.3.3.2) [73].

A single branch of the posterior cerebral artery, sometimes known as the artery of Percheron, may supply the medial thalamic nuclei bilaterally. Occlusion of this paramedian thalamic artery, therefore, may cause bilateral medial thalamic infarction, with acute onset of confusion followed by a persistent amnesia, so-called diencephalic amnesia. This amnesia may be global, may resemble Wernicke–Korsakoff syndrome (Section 8.3.1.1), or may manifest principally as autobiographical amnesia [74–77]. Anterograde memory impairment for verbal material has been reported after left dorsomedial thalamic infarct, and for visuospatial material after right dorsomedial thalamic infarct [78,79]. Selective verbal memory impairment after a left thalamic infarct involving the mammillothalamic tract has been reported [80]. Although the classical verbal/nonverbal left/right dichotomy was observed for learning, naming, and gnosic difficulties associated with laterothalamic infarcts causing hemisensory disturbance, executive dysfunction was more apparent with right thalamic infarcts, suggesting disruption of frontothalamic subcortical loops [81]. Executive impairment and attentional deficit may contribute to cognitive dysfunction after thalamic infarction [72], and utilization behavior may be seen occasionally [82]. Aphasia, usually of nonfluent type, may occur with left-sided thalamic lesions ("thalamic aphasia"), and hemineglect and anosognosia with right-sided lesions [83]. Apraxia has also been reported with thalamic infarction [84]. Observations of cognitive dysfunction in thalamic infarcts support the idea of a "lateralized cognitive thalamus" [73].

3.2.4 Genu of the internal capsule

Infarction of the inferior genu of the internal capsule may cause an acute confusional state with inattention, memory loss, psychomotor retardation, apathy, and abulia [85]. Persistent deficits associated with dominant hemisphere lesions include verbal memory, naming, and verbal fluency, reflecting damage to the limbic system [86–90]. As with thalamic infarcts, these neuropsychological sequelae may reflect disruption of thalamocortical pathways.

3.2.5 Caudate nucleus and globus pallidus

Cognitive and neurobehavioral problems are common with vascular lesions of the caudate nucleus, which may also extend to involve the anterior limb of the internal capsule and the putamen. Mendez *et al.* [91] found impaired sustained attention and executive function, and poor recall on tests of immediate and delayed recall, in a series of 12 patients with mostly unilateral caudate lesions; some were apathetic or abulic, others disinhibited and impulsive. Similar observations have been made in other series, with additional aphasia with left-sided lesions and neglect with right-sided lesions [92,93]. Executive dysfunction has also been noted [93] as has utilization behavior [94]. A two-year study of subcortical strokes found that patients with caudate lesions had lower scores on the MMSE (although this is not an ideal instrument for the assessment of subcortical deficits) on long-term follow-up than patients with strokes in other locations, with evidence of deterioration despite no new events [95]. These various cognitive changes have been ascribed to interruption of striatal efferents to the cortex.

A role for the globus pallidus in cognitive processing, in addition to its motor functions, has been postulated. Isolated athymhormia (psychic akinesia) has been reported with ischemic pallidal lesions [96], and two patients with left globus pallidus infarction were found to have inattention, reduced verbal fluency, and amnesia [97].

3.2.6 Hippocampus

Stroke limited to the hippocampus is a rare event; first-ever stroke confined to the hippocampus even more so. One patient with possible hippocampal ischemic infarcts causing bilateral hippocampal volume loss has been extensively studied, showing impaired recall but relatively preserved item recognition memory [98]. In a 41-year-old right-handed man with first-ever stroke affecting the left posterior choroidal artery territory and involving the left posterior hippocampus, presentation was with an amnesic syndrome resembling transient global amnesia (Section 3.6.2) but with additional "amnestic aphasia." Improvement over 24–48 hours was followed by a severe deficit of episodic long-term memory, particularly in the verbal modality, with default of encoding and semantic intrusions. This case suggested specialization of the left hippocampus for encoding of verbal material [99]. Another patient with pure left hippocampal stroke has been described with transient global amnesia-like syndrome [100].

3.2.7 Basal forebrain

"Basal forebrain amnesia" has been reported following subarachnoid hemorrhage due to rupture or surgery for anterior communicating artery aneurysm (Section 3.3.1) [101–103], presumably due to disruption of the basal forebrain cholinergic projection to the hippocampus (which is also a key site of pathology in AD). Features may be akin to the amnesia seen in Wernicke–Korsakoff syndrome (Section 8.3.1.1), although this is not invariably so. ChEIs have not proved beneficial in this situation [103].

3.2.8 Brainstem and cerebellum

Can isolated infratentorial ischemic lesions cause cognitive impairment? Transient amnesia has been reported as a herald of brainstem infarction and basilar artery thrombosis [104,105], but these syndromes may conceivably have involved memory eloquent structures in the thalamus (Section 3.2.3). The question may be addressed by examining patients with lesions confined to the brainstem and cerebellum.

In a series of 17 patients with lacunar infarcts in the brainstem, neuropsychological evaluation showed impairments in naming, category fluency, and trailmaking, a profile similar to that seen with supratentorial lacunar infarcts, prompting the conclusion that small white matter infarcts affect cognitive function in a nonspecific way [106]. Occasional cases of cognitive impairment in patients with brainstem vascular events complicated by peduncular hallucinosis have been reported [107]. Patients with locked-in syndrome due to bilateral ventral pontine infarct or hemorrhage have been reported

to show preserved cognitive function in the absence of other supratentorial mesencephalic lesions [108], but another series found difficulties in auditory recognition, oral comprehension, delayed visuospatial memory, and mental calculation, although the more severely impaired patients had additional hemispheric lesions [109]. Cognitive testing in de-efferented patients is obviously difficult, response being largely limited to yes/no answers.

In a series of 15 patients with isolated cerebellar infarcts confirmed by MRI, neuropsychological testing showed changes consistent with a frontal deficit in comparison with controls [110]. A study of 26 patients with exclusively cerebellar infarcts found slow performance on visuospatial tasks with left-sided lesions and in verbal memory with right-sided lesions. The subtle deficits were interpreted as being mediated by the contralateral cortical hemisphere [111]. Patients with chronic cerebellar lesions as a consequence of infarcts were found to have generally preserved cognitive function but impaired verbal fluency, especially with right-sided lesions [112].

Hence, from the limited information currently available, it would seem likely that isolated ischemic infratentorial lesions can result in subtle effects on cognition.

3.3 Subarachnoid hemorrhage (SAH)

Subarachnoid hemorrhage (SAH), bleeding into the space between the arachnoid and pia mater, is the least common form of stroke, accounting for perhaps 5% of the total. Bleeding may originate from structural lesions such as a ruptured intracranial aneurysm or an arteriovenous malformation (Section 3.4.1), but in some cases no specific bleeding source is identified [113]. Unruptured intracranial aneurysms may be discovered as a result of screening in families with a history of SAH [114] or incidentally when neuroimaging is undertaken for other reasons. A careful reckoning of the risk:benefit ratio must be undertaken before deciding on treatment of such asymptomatic lesions.

SAH patients are heterogeneous with respect to bleeding source (aneurysms may be on the internal carotid, anterior communicating, middle cerebral, posterior cerebral, or basilar artery), severity of the initial bleed (which may be graded, for example using the Hunt and Hess classification or the World Federation of Neurological Surgeons scale based on the Glasgow Coma Scale), degree of brain injury, occurrence of complications such as vasospasm or hydrocephalus, and treatment method used. Ruptured aneurysms may be treated by open surgical clipping or by intravascular embolization ("coiling"), both procedures isolating the aneurysm from the circulation. Coiling has become more frequently undertaken in recent times, and has a better outcome according to the International Subarachnoid Aneurysm Trial (ISAT) [115]. When the significant psychological sequelae of SAH, including fatigue and anxiety, are factored into the clinical picture, the difficulty of defining a neuropsychological profile associated with SAH becomes apparent.

3.3.1 Aneurysmal SAH; unruptured aneurysms

Patients who survive the acute phase of SAH may be left with significant neuropsychological deficits despite an apparently excellent neurological outcome, with problems in memory, executive function, and language being common [116,117]. The pattern of cognitive impairments is global in some patients, even amounting to dementia, whereas in others general intelligence as measured by conventional IQ tests remains intact but there may be specific impairments of psychomotor speed, language function, and verbal memory. Working memory and verbal short-term memory seem most affected, with features sometimes reported to resemble the amnesia of Wernicke–Korsakoff syndrome, with or without confabulation. Basal forebrain injury, damaging the septohippocampal system, may be responsible for amnesia [101]. Concurrent frontal lobe injury may be required for the presence of confabulations

[118]. In addition, there may be deficits in perceptual speed and accuracy, visuospatial and visuoconstructive function, and abstraction and cognitive flexibility, for example in the Wisconsin Card Sorting Test, the latter suggesting frontocortical cognitive dysfunction [119]. Executive dysfunction may affect anterograde memory function significantly [120]. The similarity of this profile to that seen following mild traumatic brain injury has been noted. Deficits have a negative impact on functional status and quality of life.

Although older studies suggested that cognitive deficits were greatest with ruptured anterior communicating artery (AcoA) aneurysms, even postulating the existence of an "AcoA syndrome" characterized by severe memory deficit, confabulation, and personality change [121], more systematic studies have found the pattern of deficits to be unrelated to the location of the ruptured aneurysm, and to be persistent over time [122–124]. The cognitive dysfunction may be aggravated by concurrent infarction in the vascular territory of the ruptured aneurysm. Left-sided infarcts and global cerebral edema were reported to be predictors of post-SAH cognitive dysfunction in one study [125].

Comparison of cognitive outcome between aneurysm coiling and clipping showed a poorer outcome in the surgical group in ISAT. Overall, around one-third of survivors who were not otherwise disabled according to the modified Rankin Scale had cognitive impairment, but this was less common in those allocated endovascular treatment (odds ratio = 0.58) [126].

The detection and management of unruptured intracranial aneurysms remains an area of investigation. Cognitive outcome following surgery for unruptured aneurysms seems to be good [127,128].

3.3.2 Perimesencephalic (non-aneurysmal) SAH

In perimesencephalic SAH (pSAH), no underlying aneurysm(s) may be identified with conventional angiography in 15%–20% of cases. Hence, pSAH differs from other types of SAH in its excellent prognosis, as there is a very low risk of rebleeding [129]. Only minor cognitive deficits have been identified on follow-up of pSAH patients, but high scores on a depression scale, suggesting that vigorous reassurance and treatment of depression might improve outcome in this subgroup [130].

3.3.3 Superficial siderosis of the nervous system

Deposition of ferritin in the superficial layers of the CNS as a consequence of repeated or continuous leakage of blood into the cerebrospinal fluid (CSF) is the cause of this unusual condition, with subsequent gliosis and neuronal loss, particularly in the eighth cranial nerve, the cerebellar vermis, and the inferior frontal cerebral cortex. Clinical features include sensorineural hearing loss, cerebellar ataxia, dysarthria, anosmia, and pyramidal signs, with typical appearances of signal void around affected areas of the brain on T_2-weighted MRIs, corresponding to deposition of hemosiderin [131].

In a review of the literature, 14 cases of superficial siderosis of the nervous system with dementia of variable severity were identified, with onset between one and more than 30 years after disease onset [131]. Only one systematic study of the cognitive impairments in superficial siderosis has been reported [132]. In six patients tested, general intellectual function was well preserved, but speech production difficulties, impairment of visual recall, and executive impairments formed the core neuropsychological deficits. Impaired executive function was evident in tests of both initiation (phonemic fluency, Hayling sentence completion part A) and inhibition (Stroop, Hayling sentence completion part B). Functions relatively preserved included naming, literacy, calculation, visual perceptual and visuospatial skills, verbal and visual recognition memory, verbal recall memory, and speed of information processing. All patients also failed a theory of mind test, indicating a mentalizing impairment.

Overall the deficits were akin to the previously described cerebellar cognitive affective syndrome (Section 1.3.3.2) [133].

3.4 Intracranial vascular malformations

The classification of intracranial arteriovenous vascular anomalies has been subject to various approaches, lesions not always having been described in a standardized way. Distinction may be made between hemangiomas, in which endothelial hyperplasia occurs, and nonproliferating vascular anomalies in which there is no hyperplasia. These latter include arterial malformations (angiodysplasia, aneurysms) and lesions in which there is arteriovenous shunting of blood, either through a tangled anastomosis of vessels ("arteriovenous malformation," AVM) or a direct high flow connection between artery and vein ("arteriovenous fistula," AVF). AVMs and AVFs may be within the brain parenchyma or in the dura [134].

3.4.1 Arteriovenous malformations (AVMs)

Whether AVMs cause cognitive deficits, over and above the hemorrhagic and epileptic complications that bring them to clinical attention, is uncertain [135]. Some early studies suggested "mental changes" in 50% of patients with "AVMs" [136] whereas others found normal fullscale IQ and no lateralizing changes comparable with those seen with acute focal lesions [137]. Mahalick *et al.* [138] reported a series of 24 patients, 12 each with right and left AVMs, and found compromised higher cortical function (attention, memory, learning, fluency) both ipsilateral and contralateral to the lesion, more so ipsilateral, prompting them to argue that a vascular "steal" phenomenon accounted for contralateral deficits. However, there were no concomitant vascular imaging studies. To answer the question of the neuropsychological effects of AVMs, ideally one would wish to study asymptomatic individuals, perhaps discovered by chance on brain imaging for other reasons.

3.4.2 Intracranial dural arteriovenous fistula (dAVF)

Cases of higher cortical dysfunction have been reported in association with intracranial dural arteriovenous fistuals (dAVFs), sometimes amounting to dementia. Although rare, such cases are important because cognitive impairment may be reversible with definitive treatment, either resection or embolization [139]. For example, in the series of Hurst *et al.* [140], five out of 40 cases had dementia or encephalopathy with remission after embolization. Accounts of the precise neuropsychological deficits in dAVF and serial documentation of cognitive function are few, perhaps due in part to the necessity for prompt therapeutic intervention when there is acute neurological deterioration. Wilson *et al.* [139] reported three cases with pre- and posttreatment cognitive assessment, finding deficits in all domains that improved after embolization, most notably in memory and executive function, although complete reversal was not seen.

The mechanism of cognitive impairment in these patients relates to the high flow through the AV shunt combined with venous outflow obstruction resulting in impaired cerebral venous drainage, slowed cerebral vascular transit time, and hence widespread venous hypertension and diffuse ischemia, which may be manifested neuroradiologically as a leukoencephalopathy [141], sometimes with thalamic involvement [142]. Progressive cognitive dysfunction in intracranial dAVF may thus be analogous to the progressive myelopathy (Foix–Alajouanine syndrome) seen with spinal dural AVFs [140]. Irreversible cognitive changes may be a consequence of complete or partial venous infarction of tissues subject to venous hypertension, especially if prolonged [139].

3.4.3 Cavernous hemangiomas

Cavernous hemangiomas or cavernomas are thin-walled vascular spaces lacking a shunt, hence are not arteriovenous malformations. They may present as space-occupying lesions, with epileptic seizures or relapsing-remitting symptoms related to hemorrhage. Multiple cavernous angiomas (cavernomatosis) that undergo multiple and recurrent hemorrhages may rarely be associated with cognitive decline and dementia [143–146]. Dementia associated with right medial temporal lobe cavernous angioma has been reported, although the cognitive syndrome may have resulted, at least in part, from partial epileptic seizures [147].

3.5 Vasculopathies

Vasculopathy is a relatively nonspecific term for blood vessel abnormalities, which is interpreted here to encompass not only primary abnormalities of blood vessel wall structure predisposing to intraluminal thrombosis, but also rheologic abnormalities promoting a thrombotic tendency. Although there may be overlap at the level of pathophysiology, inflammatory disorders of blood vessels such as the primary and secondary cerebral vasculitides are considered elsewhere (Sections 6.11.1 and 6.11.2, respectively), likewise primary metabolic disorders affecting blood vessels such Fabry's disease (Section 5.5.3.2).

3.5.1 CADASIL

Cerebral autosomal dominant arteriopathy with subcortical infarcts and leukoencephalopathy (CADASIL) is an autosomal dominant vasculopathy resulting from mutations within the gene encoding the notch3 protein on chromosome 19q12 (OMIM#125310) [148]. It is characterized clinically by recurrent subcortical strokes, both symptomatic and silent, migraine, psychiatric disturbances, with late pseudobulbar palsy, occasionally epilepsy, and a reversible encephalopathy. Skin biopsy may show granular osmiophilic material adjacent to the basement membrane of smooth muscle cells of dermal arterioles; similar deposits may be observed in the thickened arterial media in vessels on brain biopsy. MRI of the brain shows confluent high signal in periventricular and deep white matter, basal ganglia lacunar infarcts, and characteristic high signal in the anterior temporal pole and external capsule [149].

A subcortical type, white matter vascular dementia may also occur in CADASIL, with both step-wise and progressive course. Cognitive impairment may occur in the absence of neurological features other than migraine [150], and changes in working memory and executive function prior to stroke have been documented [151,152]. The neuropsychological profile is characterized by a deficit in sustained attention, cognitive slowing, impaired learning with intact recognition, and perseveration, in other words a pattern resembling that in other white matter disorders [153]. In a cross-sectional study of 42 patients, Buffon *et al.* [154] found a heterogeneous cognitive profile at disease onset, most often affecting executive skills leading to impaired memory and attention, evolving to a more homogeneous pattern affecting all domains with increasing age, including language and visuospatial function, although distinct from AD. Retrieval was better with cueing, suggesting that encoding was relatively spared, as were recognition and semantic memory. The authors speculated that this pattern resulted from initial damage to frontosubcortical networks with sparing of the hippocampus, with diffuse cortical dysfunction in later disease reflecting the accumulation of subcortical ischemic insults, although as history of stroke was not associated with dementia, most of these events must be silent. In one series of 64 patients, not selected for the presence or absence of dementia, a significant inverse correlation was noted between overall cognitive performance, as assessed with the MMSE score, and total MRI lesion volume [155]. The NINDS–AIREN criteria for SIVD are the most sensitive VaD critera in CADASIL [156].

Cholinergic denervation was shown in one pathologically examined case of CADASIL, despite this being a pure vascular dementia [157]. A trial of donepezil for the subcortical vascular cognitive impairment in CADASIL has been reported, showing no effect on the primary outcome measure (VADAS-Cog scores) but possibly some improvements in executive function [158].

3.5.2 CARASIL

An autosomal recessive variant of CADASIL, cerebral autosomal recessive arteriopathy with subcortical infarcts and leukoencephalopathy (CARASIL), has also been described [159], often associated with alopecia and degenerative disease in the lumbar spine and knees. This condition is linked to chromosome 10q26.13 and results from mutations in the HTRA1 gene (OMIM#600142). A condition initially described as "familial young-adult onset arteriosclerotic leukoencephalopathy with alopecia and lumbago without arterial hypertension" also falls within this rubric. In this rare syndrome, reported only in Japanese families, progressive subcortical dementia is common, with accompanying pseudobulbar palsy and pyramidal signs. Lacunar strokes occurred in about half of the patients [160]. More recent descriptions of CARASIL with HTRA1 gene mutations noted the presence of progressive dementia in some cases [161].

3.5.3 Cerebral amyloid angiopathies (CAA)

The cerebral amyloid angiopathies (CAA) are so named because of the deposition of amyloidogenic peptides in the walls of small parenchymal and leptomeningeal arteries, known as congophilic angiopathy, which sometimes extends from around vessel walls into the brain parenchyma, known as dyshoric angiopathy. CAA may be one feature of AD brain pathology, but may also occur in relative isolation as either a sporadic or familial condition. Cerebral hemorrhage in a lobar distribution is the most common complication of CAA [162,163], although other transient focal neurological features may occur, including transient ischemic attacks, focal epileptic seizures, and multifocal cortical myoclonus [164,165], as well as a leuko-encephalopathy. Dementia without major lobar hemorrhage is also reported [164]. A variant in which CAA is associated with inflammatory changes, CAA-I, has been described [166], and which may produce prominent cognitive problems (Section 6.11.1).

All sporadic CAA cases are due to deposition of amyloid-β, originating from proteolytic cleavage of the amyloid precursor protein (APP) [163]. Of the familial CAAs, hereditary cerebral hemorrhage with amyloidosis Dutch type (HCHWA-D) results from mutations at codon 693 of the APP gene (OMIM#605714; other mutations within this gene are deterministic for autosomal dominant AD; Section 2.1.1). The phenotype is one of cerebral hemorrhages that may result in cognitive impairment of the cortical type [167], although dementia in the absence of a history of stroke or focal radiological change may occur. Dementia in HCHWA-D is independent of neurofibrillary pathology, plaque density, and age, but related to the CAA load in the frontal cortex, as quantified by computerized morphometry, and vessel-wall thickening, suggesting that CAA per se may cause dementia [168]. Hereditary cerebral hemorrhage with amyloidosis Icelandic type (HCHWA-I), resulting from mutations in the cystatin c gene (OMIM#105150), also causes intracerebral hemorrhages. One family with a late-onset dementia as the only manifestation of HCHWA-I has been reported, with cortical and subcortical infarctions [169]. Familial British dementia and familial Danish dementia are autosomal dominant familial CAAs that cause dementia usually without strokes or hemorrhages. Both result from mutations in the ITM2B gene on chromosome 13q14.2 (OMIM#176500 and #117300, respectively; Section 5.1.3 for further details).

Treatment options are currently limited in CAA, but a favorable response to immunosuppressive treatment has been noted in CAA-I [164], suggesting that a trial of such medication might be considered without brain biopsy in suspected CAA patients.

3.5.3.1 Familial occipital calcifications, hemorrhagic strokes, leukoencephalopathy, dementia, and external carotid dysplasia (FOCHS–LADD)

Described in one family of Spanish descent, with presumed autosomal dominant transmission, this syndrome was characterized by dementia and cerebral hemorrhages with radiological evidence of fine tram-line occipital calcifications. Of the six affected individuals in two generations, neuropsychological testing was only reported in one patient who developed progressive memory decline in the early 1960s with additional evidence of visuoconstructional problems, "ideokinetic" apraxia, calculation and writing errors, and frontal lobe symptoms [170]. A mutation in the APP gene (N694D) was subsequently shown in two members of this pedigree [171], demonstrating that this is a form of CAA (OMIM#605714).

3.5.4 Hereditary endotheliopathy with retinopathy, nephropathy, and stroke (HERNS)

This microangiopathy of the brain and retina, inherited as an autosomal dominant condition linked to chromosome 3p21, is characterized clinically by progressive visual loss, headache, epileptic seizures, focal neurological deficits, and progressive cognitive decline [172,173].

3.5.5 Hereditary multi-infarct dementia of Swedish type

Sourander and Wålinder [174] described a Swedish pedigree with a hereditary disorder characterized by multiple infarcts and cognitive decline in 1977. When CADASIL was described as such in 1993 (Section 3.5.1), it was thought that the Swedish "hereditary multi-infarct dementia" was in fact an example of CADASIL. However, further clinical, neuroradiological, neuropathological, and neurogenetic examination of the Swedish pedigree refutes this suggestion. Patients from this kindred did not have migraine, MRI appearances did not show the typical anterior temporal pole or external capsule hyper-intensities seen in CADASIL, skin biopsy did not show granular osmiophilic deposits, and neuro-genetic testing found no pathogenic mutation in the notch3 gene. Hence, Swedish multi-infarct dementia is a novel small vessel disease [175].

3.5.6 Hughes' syndrome (primary antiphospholipid antibody syndrome)

Antiphospholipid antibodies may occur in association with conditions such as systemic lupus erythematosus (SLE), Sjögren's syndrome, rheumatoid arthritis, and systemic sclerosis (Sections 6.5, 6.6, 6.8, and 6.9, respectively), known as secondary antiphospholipid antibody syndromes; or without evidence of accompanying connective tissue disease, known as primary antiphospholipid antibody syndrome or Hughes' syndrome. There is overlap between Hughes's syndrome and Sneddon's syndrome (Section 3.5.11). Suggested diagnostic criteria for Hughes' syndrome require both clinical (thrombotic) and laboratory features, and there is also a "probable" category in which the antibodies occur without a history of large vessel thromboses [176]. Antiphospholipid antibodies (lupus anticoagulant, or anticardiolipin antibodies) may be associated with various neurological features including epileptic seizures, chorea, transverse myelitis, migraine, depression, psychosis, and cognitive decline. Whether these clinical features are linked to arterial and venous thromboses or to immune-mediated mechanisms, or both, remains uncertain.

Cognitive impairment and dementia have been recorded in primary antiphospholipid antibody syndrome. For example, in a young woman not meeting diagnostic criteria for SLE, decline in intellect and occupational failure were the presenting features, with a MMSE score of 28/30 (5 minute recall = 1/3), poor right–left orientation, right inattention, reduced motor speed, mild impulsivity, and poor concentration. MRI of the brain showed small high signal lesions in the right caudate and fronto-subcortical white matter. The patient improved after treatment with corticosteroids, aspirin, and hydroxychloroquine [177]. Reviewing the literature over the period 1983–2003 and their own experience, Gómez-Puerta et al. [178] identified 30 cases of dementia associated with antiphospholipid syndrome (primary:secondary = 14:16, the latter having SLE or "lupus-like syndrome"). On brain imaging, cortical infarcts were common (in more than half of cases), subcortical and basal ganglia infarcts less so (in less than one-third). Hence, dementia would seem to be an unusual complication of antiphospholipid syndromes. Because pathogenesis is uncertain, optimal treatment (antiplatelet and anticoagulant therapy or immunosuppression or both) is not established.

3.5.7 Intravascular lymphomatosis (angioendotheliomatosis)

Intravascular lymphomatosis, also known as angioendotheliomatosis or neoplastic angio-endotheliomatosis, is a malignant intravascular proliferation of endothelial cells or lymphocytes defined as an angiotropic intravascular large-cell lymphoma of B-cell type (see Section 7.1.6 for cognitive effects of other forms of lymphoma). The most common clinical presentation is with multifocal ischemic events due to vascular occlusion with neoplastic cells, but it may also cause dementia, leading to classification with the vascular dementias. Brain and/or meningeal biopsy is usually required for diagnosis [179–183]. A case associated with a reversible dementia following immunosuppressive treatment in a transplant recipient has been reported [181].

3.5.8 Moyamoya

Moyamoya is an occlusive vasculopathy of uncertain etiology, often presenting in childhood as a syndrome of recurrent cerebral ischemia and infarction. There may be associated headache, epileptic seizures, and cognitive impairment. In adults, moyamoya more usually presents with recurrent intracerebral hemorrhage or subarachnoid hemorrhage. Radiologically there is severe stenosis or occlusion of one or both distal internal carotid arteries, sometimes extending to the circle of Willis, with fine anastomotic (telangiectatic) collateral vessels developing from perforating and pial arteries at the base of the brain, orbital and ethmoidal branches of the external carotid artery, and leptomeningeal vessels. These vessels are the source of hemorrhage in cases presenting in adulthood, and may be visualized on cerebral angiography as a "puff of smoke" or "haze," from the Japanese term for which the syndrome takes its name.

A study of 29 adult patients found cognitive impairment in two-thirds, particularly apparent in tests of processing speed, verbal memory, verbal fluency, and executive function, suggesting involvement of frontal and subcortical regions, presumably as a result of chronic small vessel ischemia due to hypoperfusion [184].

Another series of adult patients noted that executive functioning was most affected with relative sparing of memory and intellect, but not as severely as in pediatric cases [185].

3.5.9 Polycythemia rubra vera

Polycythemia rubra vera is a myeloproliferative disease characterized by increased red cell mass and blood volume, resulting in erythrocytosis (raised hematocrit) and increased blood viscosity. Associated neurological features include transient ischemic attacks and thrombotic strokes, less commonly with cerebral hemorrhage, and chorea. Cases presenting with cognitive impairment [186] or with cognitive decline, which partially reversed on reduction of the hematocrit, have been reported [187].

3.5.10 Sickle cell disease

Dementia may be a feature of sickle cell disease as a consequence of multiple ischemic strokes, although diffuse brain injury, perhaps related to hypoxia, may also contribute [188]. Children with sickle cell disease have been found to have cognitive defects even in the absence of cerebral infarction [189].

3.5.11 Sneddon's syndrome

Sneddon's syndrome is a noninflammatory, thrombo-occlusive, arteriolar vasculopathy affecting skin and brain, which is often but not invariably associated with antiphospholipid antibodies (Section 3.5.6). The disorder occurs primarily in young patients, with a female preponderance. Clinical features include livedo reticularis or livedo racemosa, recurrent strokes in the absence of obvious risk factors, focal neurological signs, epileptic seizures, and sometimes cognitive decline [190,191]. Cases presenting with cognitive decline or dementia without a clinical history of stroke, but with imaging evidence of cortical and subcortical infarcts with brain atrophy, have been reported [192,193]. Of 30 patients with dementia and antiphospholipid antibody syndrome reported in a 20-year literature review, ten had Sneddon's syndrome [178].

3.5.12 Spatz–Lindenberg disease (von Winiwarter–Buerger's disease)

This rarely described condition is characterized pathologically by isolated cerebral noninflammatory occlusive vasculopathy ("thromboangiitis obliterans"), hence Buerger's disease confined to the brain [194]. A vascular dementia with additional upper motor neuron signs (hemiparesis, aphasia) and epileptic seizures may result [195], but no systematic exploration of the neuropsychological deficits has been reported.

3.5.13 Susac syndrome

Susac syndrome, or retinocochleocerebral vasculopathy, is a rare, idiopathic, noninflammatory vasculopathy principally affecting young women. It usually follows a monophasic but fluctuating course, causing small infarcts in the cochlea, retina, and brain. Characteristic clinical features are sensorineural deafness, branch retinal arteriolar occlusions, encephalopathy, acute psychiatric features, upper motor neuron limb signs, cranial nerve palsies, and epileptic seizures.

Cognitive dysfunction, specifically impaired short-term memory, has been reported and dementia is said to be a rare late sequela [196]. A detailed study of three patients showed impaired verbal long-term memory at disease onset with impaired executive functions and reduced speed in attentional tasks in two, but preserved language and short-term memory. There was general cognitive improvement over time, although full recovery was not achieved, especially in executive function and attention [197].

3.5.14 Venous sinus thrombosis

Cortical venous sinus thrombosis is a rare cause of stroke, with many possible causes [198]. Studies examining cognitive outcomes have been few. De Bruijn *et al.* [199] found cognitive impairments in around one-third of survivors at one year, suggesting an unfavorable outcome, whereas Buccino *et al.* [200] found mild nonfluent aphasia in 9% and working memory deficits in 18% of a cohort of 34 patients seen over a 10-year period, suggesting good cognitive long-term outcome. The variable results may relate to case mix and duration of follow-up.

3.6 Other disorders of possible vascular etiology

3.6.1 Migraine, including familial hemiplegic migraine (FHM)

Migraine is the most common cause of primary or idiopathic headache, which may occur with or without aura (MA, MO) [201]. Migraine is occasionally a symptom of a neurological disorder that may also cause cognitive impairment; for example, CADASIL (Section 3.5.1) and mitochondrial disease (Section 5.5.1). The rare entity of migraine stroke, a diagnosis of exclusion, may be associated with focal deficits including cognitive impairments, as with strokes of other etiologies. White matter hyperintensities and infarcts are often seen on MRIs of the brain in MA,

but are not associated with cognitive impairment [202]. Whether migraine is associated with cognitive deficits, either between or within attacks, is a subject of ongoing debate, with research findings being inconsistent [203].

Mental slowness may be a feature of headache prodrome, and amnesia is one of the atypical auras of migraine [204,205]. During migraine attacks, simple reaction time, sustained attention, and visuospatial processing may be adversely affected [206,207]. However, it is difficult to know whether these findings relate to concurrent pain or the neural pathophysiology of the headache syndrome per se. Moreover, information processing speed and memory may be influenced by age, independent of migraine [208]. Migraine postdrome may be attended with impaired concentration.

Interictal deficits have been reported involving certain frontal lobe functions [209], or associated with right-sided pain [210], or with higher frequency of attacks or length of migraine history [211]. Certainly, migraine patients show a disturbance of subcortical sensory modulation systems, which may account for interictal loss of normal cognitive habituation.

Epidemiological studies have not suggested any long-term cognitive implications of a history of migraine. A ten-year study suggested impairments of immediate and delayed memory in MA patients at baseline but less decline over time than in controls [212]. Likewise, no increased risk for cognitive decline from migraine has been found in population-based studies [213–215].

Familial hemiplegic migraine (FHM) due to mutations in the CACNA1A gene at chromosome 19p13.2 (OMIM#T41500) is allelic with episodic ataxia type 2 and spinocerebellar ataxia type 6 (SCA6; Section 5.2.1.4). Cognitive deficits have been detected in this form of FHM, sometimes with minimal headache history [216]. In a study of one family, a distinct neuropsychological profile was recorded with preserved linguistic and verbal memory abilities but deficits in figural memory, executive functions, and some aspects of attention [217]. These findings were associated with cerebellar atrophy and ataxia, and converge with cognitive findings in SCA6, previously considered to be a "pure" cerebellar syndrome (Section 5.2.1.4).

3.6.2 Transient global amnesia (TGA)

The syndrome of transient global amnesia (TGA) consists of an abrupt attack of impaired anterograde memory, often manifest as repeated questioning, without clouding of consciousness or focal neurological signs. Episodes are of brief duration (<24 hr), with no recollection of the amnesic period following resolution [218,219]. TGA subgroups have been suggested on the basis of different precipitating events in men (physical) and women (emotional), with headache being a risk factor in younger individuals [220]. The etiopathogenesis of TGA is imperfectly understood although there is evidence of vascular involvement, specifically from diffusion-weighted MRI techniques [221]. Others have taken the view that "TGA is probably a migraine aura in most cases" [222], or that the neurophysiological process of spreading depression might be causative [223]. Herpes simplex encephalitis (Section 9.1.1) presenting with TGA has been reported [224] and a TGA-like syndrome has been seen in pure hippocampal stroke (Section 3.2.6). The differential diagnosis of TGA includes transient epileptic amnesia (Section 4.3.1) but electroencephalography (EEG) is generally normal during an attack of TGA [225] and recurrence rate much lower. Psychogenic amnesia (Section 12.5.1) also enters the differential diagnosis.

As expected for an acute and transient syndrome, most TGA cases that come to medical attention are seen by primary care physicians in the community or district general hospitals [226], thus neuropsychological assessment during an attack is uncommon. When undertaken, this shows dense anterograde amnesia, with a variably severe retrograde amnesia, but intact working memory and semantic memory. Implicit memory functions (e.g., for driving) are usually intact [227]. A variant in which transient impairment of semantic memory was present has been described [228]. In the recovery phase, retrograde amnesia recovers before anterograde amnesia, but the shrinkage of the former may be heterogeneous, with or without temporal gradient [229].

REFERENCES

[1] Bowler JV, Hachinski V. Vascular cognitive impairment: a new approach to vascular dementia. In: Hachinski V (ed.). *Cerebrovascular Disease*. London: Bailliere Tindall, 1995; 357–76.

[2] Bowler JV, Hachinski V (eds.). *Vascular Cognitive Impairment: Reversible Dementia*. Oxford: Oxford University Press, 2003.

[3] O'Brien J, Ames D, Gustafson L, Folstein MF, Chiu E (eds.). *Cerebrovascular Disease, Cognitive Impairment and Dementia*. London: Martin Dunitz, 2004.

[4] Godefroy O, Bogousslavsky J. *The Behavioral and Cognitive Neurology of Stroke*. Cambridge: Cambridge University Press, 2007.

[5] Moorhouse P, Rockwood K. Vascular cognitive impairment: current concepts and clinical developments. *Lancet Neurol* 2008; 7: 246–55.

[6] Wahlund L-O, Erkinjuntti T, Gauthier S (eds.). *Vascular Cognitive Impairment in Clinical Practice*. Cambridge: Cambridge University Press, 2009.

[7] Chui HC, Victoroff JI, Margolin D, *et al.* Criteria for the diagnosis of ischemic vascular dementia proposed by the State of California Alzheimer's Disease Diagnostic and Treatment Centers. *Neurology* 1992; 42: 473–80.

[8] Román GC, Tatemichi TK, Erkinjuntti T, *et al.* Vascular dementia: diagnostic criteria for research studies. Report of the NINDS–AIREN international workshop. *Neurology* 1993; 43: 250–60.

[9] van Straaten EC, Scheltens P, Knol DL, *et al.* Operational definitions for the NINDS–AIREN criteria for vascular dementia: an interobserver study. *Stroke* 2003; 34: 1907–12.

[10] Holmes C, Cairns N, Lantos P, *et al.* Validity of current clinical criteria for Alzheimer's disease, vascular dementia and dementia with Lewy bodies. *Br J Psychiatry* 1999; 174: 45–50.

[11] MRC CFAS. Pathological correlates of late-onset dementia in a multicentre, community-based population in England and Wales. Neuropathology Group of the Medical Research Council Cognitive Function and Ageing Study. *Lancet* 2001; 357: 169–75.

[12] Stewart R. Vascular factors and Alzheimer's disease. In: Ames D, Burns A, O'Brien J (eds.). *Dementia* (4th edn.). London: Hodder Arnold, 2010; 529–37.

[13] Nolan KA, Lino MM, Seligmann AW, *et al.* Absence of vascular dementia in an autopsy series from a dementia clinic. *J Am Geriatr Soc* 1998; 46: 597–604.

[14] Snowdon DA, Greiner LH, Mortimer JA, *et al.* Brain infarction and the clinical expression of Alzheimer's disease. The Nun Study. *JAMA* 1997; 277: 813–17.

[15] Snowdon D. *Aging with Grace. The Nun Study and the Science of Old Age. How We Can All Live Longer, Healthier and More Vital Lives.* London: Fourth Estate, 2001.

[16] Langa KM, Foster NL, Larson EB. Mixed dementia: emerging concepts and therapeutic implications. *JAMA* 2004; 292: 2901–8.

[17] Hachinski VC, Iliff LD, Zilkha E, *et al.* Cerebral blood flow in dementia. *Arch Neurol* 1975; 32: 632–7.

[18] Moroney JT, Bagiella E, Desmond DW, *et al.* Meta-analysis of the Hachinski Ischemic Score in pathologically verified dementias. *Neurology* 1997; 49: 1096–105.

[19] Sachdev PC, Looi JCL. Neuropsychological differentiation of Alzheimer's disease and vascular dementia. In: Bowler JV, Hachinski V (eds.). *Vascular Cognitive Impairment: Reversible Dementia.* Oxford: Oxford University Press, 2003; 153–75.

[20] Hodges JR, Graham NL. Vascular dementias. In: Hodges JR (ed.). *Early-Onset Dementia: a Multidisciplinary Approach.* Oxford: Oxford University Press, 2001; 319–37.

[21] Duff Canning SJ, Leach L, Stuss D, Ngo L, Black SE. Diagnostic utility of abbreviated fluency measures in Alzheimer disease and vascular dementia. *Neurology* 2004; 62: 556–62.

[22] Bentham PW, Jones S, Hodges JR. A comparison of semantic memory in vascular dementia and dementia of Alzheimer's type. *Int J Geriatr Psychiatry* 1997; 12: 575–80.

[23] Brookes RL, Hannesdottir K, Lawrence R, Morris RG, Markus HS. Brief Memory and Executive Test: evaluation of a new screening test for cognitive impairment due to small vessel disease. *Age Ageing* 2012; 41: 212–18.

[24] Morris JH, Kalimo H, Viitanen M. Vascular dementias. In: Esiri MM, Trojanowski JQ, Lee VMY (eds.). *The Neuropathology of Dementia* (2nd edn.). Cambridge: Cambridge University Press, 2004; 289–329.

[25] Lane RJM. "Cardiogenic dementia" revisited. *J R Soc Med* 1991; 84: 577–9.

[26] Markus HS (ed.). *Stroke Genetics.* Oxford: Oxford University Press, 2003.

[27] Hachinski VC, Lassen NA, Marshall J. Multi-infarct dementia. A cause of mental deterioration in the elderly. *Lancet* 1974; 2: 207–10.

[28] Leys D, Henon H, Mackowiak Cordoliani MA, Pasquier F. Poststroke dementia. *Lancet Neurol* 2005; 4: 752–9.

[29] Marzona I, O'Donnell M, Teo K, *et al.* Increased risk of cognitive and functional decline in patients with atrial fibrillation: results of the ONTARGET and TRANSCEND studies. *CMAJ* 2012; 184: E329–36.

[30] Tomlinson BE, Blessed G, Roth M. Observations on the brains of demented old people. *J Neurol Sci* 1970; 11: 205–42.

[31] Hénon H, Pasquier F, Durieu I, *et al.* Preexisting dementia in stroke patients: baseline frequency, associated factors, and outcome. *Stroke* 1997; 28: 2429–36.

[32] Klimkowicz A, Dziedzic T, Slowik A, *et al.* Incidence of pre- and poststroke dementia: Cracow Stroke Registry. *Dement Geriatr Cogn Disord* 2002; 14: 137–40.

[33] Bour A, Rasquin S, Boreas A, Limburg M, Verhey F. How predictive is the MMSE for cognitive performance after stroke? *J Neurol* 2010; 257: 630–7.

[34] Bakker FC, Klijn CJM, Jennekens-Schinkel A, Kappelle LJ. Cognitive disorder in patients with occlusive disease of the carotid artery: a systematic review of the literature. *J Neurol* 2000; 247: 669–76.

[35] Lehrner J, Willfort A, Mlekusch I, *et al.* Neuropsychological outcome 6 months after unilateral carotid stenting. *J Clin Exp Neuropsychol* 2005; 27: 859–66.

[36] Landgraff NC, Whitney SL, Rubinstein EN, Yonas H. Cognitive and physical performance in patients with asymptomatic carotid artery disease. *J Neurol* 2010; 257: 982–91.

[37] Lunn S, Crawley F, Harrison MJG, Brown MM, Newman SP. Impact of carotid endarterectomy upon cognitive functioning. A systematic review of the literature. *Cerebrovasc Dis* 1999; 9: 74–81.

[38] Antonelli Incalzi R, Gemma A, Landi F, *et al.* Neuropsychologic effects of carotid endarterectomy. *J Clin Exp Neuropsychol* 1997; 19: 785–94.

[39] Tatemichi TK, Desmond DW, Prohovnik I, Eidelberg D. Dementia associated with bilateral carotid occlusions: neuropsychological and haemodynamic course after extracranial to intracranial bypass

surgery. *J Neurol Neurosurg Psychiatry* 1995; 58: 633–6.

[40] Selnes OA, Gottesman RF, Grega MA, *et al.* Cognitive and neurologic outcome after coronary-artery bypass surgery. *N Engl J Med* 2012; 366: 250–7.

[41] McKhann GM, Borowicz LM, Goldsborough MA, Enger C, Selnes OA. Depression and cognitive decline after coronary artery bypass grafting. *Lancet* 1997; 349: 1282–4.

[42] Larner AJ. "Dementia unmasked": atypical, acute aphasic, presentations of neurodegenerative dementing disease. *Clin Neurol Neurosurg* 2005; 108: 8–10.

[43] Selnes OA, Grega MA, Bailey MM, *et al.* Cognition 6 years after surgical or medical therapy for coronary artery disease. *Ann Neurol* 2008; 63: 581–90.

[44] Binswanger O. Die Abgrenzung der allgemeinen progressiven paralyse. *Berliner Klinische Wochenschrift* 1894; 31: 1102–5, 1137–9, 1180–6.

[45] Blass JP, Hoyer S, Nitsch R. A translation of Otto Binswanger's article, "The delineation of the generalized progressive paralyses," 1894. *Arch Neurol* 1991; 48: 961–72.

[46] Caplan LR, Gomes JA. Binswanger disease–an update. *J Neurol Sci* 2010; 299: 9–10.

[47] Hachinski VC. Leukoaraiosis. *Arch Neurol* 1987; 44: 21–3.

[48] Marie P. Des foyers lacunaires de désintégration de différents autres états cavitaires du cerveau. *Rev Méd* 1901; 21: 281–98.

[49] Fisher CM. Lacunar strokes and infarcts: a review. *Neurology* 1982; 32: 871–6.

[50] LADIS Study Group. 2001–2011: a decade of the LADIS (Leukoaraiosis And DISability) Study: what have we learned about white matter changes and small-vessel disease? *Cerebrovasc Dis* 2011; 32: 577–88.

[51] Werring DJ, Frazer DW, Coward LJ, *et al.* Cognitive dysfunction in patients with cerebral microbleeds on T2*-weighted gradient-echo MRI. *Brain* 2004; 127: 2265–75.

[52] Kramer JH, Reed BR, Mungas D, Weiner MW, Chui HC. Executive dysfunction in subcortical ischaemic vascular disease. *J Neurol Neurosurg Psychiatry* 2002; 72: 217–20.

[53] Desmond DW, Erkinjuntti T, Sano M, *et al.* The cognitive syndrome of vascular dementia: implications for clinical trials. *Alzheimer Dis Assoc Disord* 1999; 13: S21–9.

[54] Graham NL, Emery T, Hodges JR. Distinctive cognitive profiles in Alzheimer's disease and subcortical vascular dementia. *J Neurol Neurosurg Psychiatry* 2004; 75: 61–71.

[55] O'Sullivan M, Morris RG, Markus HS. Brief cognitive assessment for patients with cerebral small vessel disease. *J Neurol Neurosurg Psychiatry* 2005; 76: 1140–5.

[56] Román GC, Erkinjuntti T, Pantoni L, Wallin A, Chui HC. Subcortical ischaemic vascular dementia. *Lancet Neurol* 2002; 1: 426–36.

[57] Erkinjuntti T, Inzitari D, Pantoni L, *et al.* Research criteria for subcortical vascular dementia in clinical trials. *J Neural Transm Suppl* 2000; 59: 23–30.

[58] Jokinen H, Kalska H, Mäntylä R, *et al.* Cognitive profile of subcortical ischaemic vascular disease. *J Neurol Neurosurg Psychiatry* 2006; 77: 28–33.

[59] Kavirajan H, Schneider LS. Efficacy and adverse effects of cholinesterase inhibitors and memantine in vascular dementia: a meta-analysis of randomised controlled trials. *Lancet Neurol* 2007; 6: 782–92.

[60] Hong JM, Shin DH, Lim TS, Lee JS, Huh K. Galantamine administration in chronic post-stroke aphasia. *J Neurol Neurosurg Psychiatry* 2012; 83: 675–80.

[61] Kwon JC, Kim EG, Kim JW, *et al.* A multicenter, open-label, 24-week follow-up study for efficacy on cognitive function of donepezil in Binswanger-type subcortical vascular dementia. *Am J Alzheimers Dis Other Demen* 2009; 24: 293–301.

[62] Katz DI, Alexander MP, Mandell AM. Dementia following strokes in the mesencephalon and diencephalon. *Arch Neurol* 1987; 44: 1127–33.

[63] Tatemichi TK, Desmond DW, Prohovnik I. Strategic infarcts in vascular dementia: a clinical and brain imaging experience. *Arzneim-Forsch/Drug Res* 1995; 45: 371–85.

[64] Corbett A, Bennett H, Kos S. Cognitive dysfunction following subcortical infarction. *Arch Neurol* 1994; 51: 999–1007.

[65] Benson DF, Cummings JL, Tsai SY. Angular gyrus syndrome simulating Alzheimer's disease. *Arch Neurol* 1982; 39: 616–20.

[66] Roeltgen DP, Sevush S, Heilman KM. Pure Gerstmann's syndrome from a focal lesion. *Arch Neurol* 1983; 40: 46–7.

[67] Moudgil SS, Azzouz M, Al-Azzaz A, Haut M, Gutmann L. Amnesia due to fornix infarction. *Stroke* 2000; 31: 1418–19.

[68] Saito Y, Matsumura K, Shimizu T. Anterograde amnesia associated with infarction of the anterior fornix and genu of the corpus callosum. *J Stroke Cerebrovasc Dis* 2006; 15: 176–7.

[69] Rabinstein AA, Romano JG, Forteza AM, Koch S. Rapidly progressive dementia due to bilateral internal carotid artery occlusion with infarction of the total length of the corpus callosum. *J Neuroimaging* 2004; 14: 176–9.

[70] Saito K, Kimura K, Minematsu K, Shiraishi A, Nakajima M. Transient global amnesia associated with an acute infarction in the retrosplenium of the corpus callosum. *J Neurol Sci* 2003; 210: 95–7.

[71] Yang KI, Joung JH, Oh HG, *et al.* Strategic infarct dementia after bilateral anterior fornix infarction. *Eur J Neurol* 2009; 16: 414 (abstract P2214).

[72] Schmahmann JD. Vascular syndromes of the thalamus. *Stroke* 2003; 34: 2264–78.

[73] De Witte L, Brouns R, Kavadias D, *et al.* Cognitive, affective and behavioural disturbances following vascular thalamic lesions: a review. *Cortex* 2011; 47: 273–319.

[74] Parkin AJ, Rees JE, Hunkin NM, Rose PE. Impairment of memory following discrete thalamic infarction. *Neuropsychologia* 1994; 32: 39–51.

[75] Graff-Radford NR, Tranel D, Van Hoesen GW, Brandt JP. Diencephalic amnesia. *Brain* 1990; 113: 1–25.

[76] Hodges JR, McCarthy RA. Autobiographical amnesia resulting from bilateral paramedian thalamic infarction. *Brain* 1993; 116: 921–40.

[77] Crews WD, Manning CA, Skalabrin E. Neuropsychological impairments of executive functions and memory in a case of bilateral paramedian thalamic infarction. *Neurocase* 1996; 2: 405–12.

[78] Speedie LJ, Heilman KM. Amnestic disturbance following infarction of the left dorsomedial nucleus of the thalamus. *Neuropsychologia* 1982; 20: 597–604.

[79] Speedie LJ, Heilman KM. Anterograde memory deficits for visuospatial material after infarction of the right thalamus. *Arch Neurol* 1983; 40: 183–6.

[80] Schott JM, Crutch SJ, Fox NC, Warrington EK. Development of selective verbal memory impairment secondary to a left thalamic infarct: a longitudinal case study. *J Neurol Neurosurg Psychiatry* 2003; 74: 255–7.

[81] Annoni JM, Khateb A, Gramigna S, *et al.* Chronic cognitive impairment following laterothalamic infarcts: a study of 9 cases. *Arch Neurol* 2003; 60: 1439–43.

[82] Eslinger PJ, Warner GC, Grattan LM, Easton JD. Frontal lobe utilization behavior associated with

paramedian thalamic infarction. *Neurology* 1991; 41: 450–2.

[83] Karussis D, Leker RR, Abramsky O. Cognitive dysfunction following thalamic stroke: a study of 16 cases and review of the literature. *J Neurol Sci* 2000; 172: 25–9.

[84] Nadeau SE, Roeltgen DP, Sevush S, Ballinger WE, Watson RT. Apraxia due to a pathologically documented thalamic infarction. *Neurology* 1994; 44: 2133–7.

[85] Tatemichi TK, Desmond DW, Prohovnik I, *et al.* Confusion and memory loss from capsular genu infarction: a thalamocortical disconnection syndrome? *Neurology* 1992; 42: 1966–79.

[86] Kooistra CA Heilman KM. Memory loss from a subcortical white matter infarct. *J Neurol Neurosurg Psychiatry* 1988; 51: 866–9.

[87] Schnider A, Gutbrod K, Hess CW, Schroth G. Memory without context: amnesia with confabulations after infarction of the right capsular genu. *J Neurol Neurosurg Psychiatry* 1996; 61: 186–93.

[88] Madureira S, Guerreiro M, Ferro JM. A follow-up study of cognitive impairment due to inferior capsular genu infarction. *J Neurol* 1999; 246: 764–9.

[89] van Zandvoort MJ, Aleman A, Kappelle LJ, De Haan EH. Cognitive functioning before and after a lacunar infarct. *Cerebrovasc Dis* 2000; 10: 478–9.

[90] Pantoni L, Basile AM, Romanelli M, *et al.* Abulia and cognitive impairment in two patients with capsular genu infarct. *Acta Neurol Scand* 2001; 104: 185–90.

[91] Mendez MF, Adams NL, Lewandowski KS. Neurobehavioral changes associated with caudate lesions. *Neurology* 1989; 39: 349–54.

[92] Caplan LR, Schmahmann JD, Kase CS, *et al.* Caudate infarcts. *Arch Neurol* 1990; 47: 133–43.

[93] Kumral E, Evyapan D, Balkir K. Acute caudate vascular lesions. *Stroke* 1999; 30: 100–8.

[94] Rudd R, Maruff P, MacCupsie-Moore C, *et al.* Stimulus relevance in eliciting utilisation behaviour: case study in a patient with a caudate lesion. *Cogn Neuropsychiatry* 1998; 3: 287–98.

[95] Bokura H, Robinson RG. Long-term cognitive impairment associated with caudate stroke. *Stroke* 1997; 28: 970–5.

[96] Mori E, Yamashita H, Takauchi S, Kondo K. Isolated athymhormia following hypoxic bilateral pallidal lesions. *Behav Neurol* 1996; 9: 17–23.

[97] Kim SH, Park KH, Sung YH, *et al.* Dementia mimicking a sudden cognitive and behavioral change

induced by left globus pallidus infarction: review of two cases. *J Neurol Sci* 2008; 272: 178–82.

[98] Mayes AR, Holdstock JS, Isaac CL, Hunkin NM, Roberts N. Relative sparing of item recognition memory in a patient with adult-onset damage limited to the hippocampus. *Hippocampus* 2002; 12: 325–40.

[99] Scacchi F, Carota A, Morier J, Bogousslavsky J. Predominantly verbal deficit of encoding with stroke limited to the left posterior hippocampus. *J Neurol* 2006; 253: II137 (abstract P543).

[100] Carota A, Lysandropoulos AP, Calabrese P. Pure left hippocampal stroke: a transient global amnesia-plus syndrome. *J Neurol* 2012; 259: 989–92.

[101] Damasio AR, Graff-Radford NR, Eslinger PJ, Damasio H, Kassell N. Amnesia following basal forebrain lesions. *Arch Neurol* 1985; 42: 263–71.

[102] Rajaram S. Basal forebrain amnesia. *Neurocase* 1997; 3: 405–15.

[103] Wright RA, Boeve BF, Malec JF. Amnesia after basal forebrain damage due to anterior communicating artery aneurysm rupture. *J Clin Neurosci* 1999; 6: 511–15.

[104] Howard RS, Festenstein R, Mellers J, Kartsounis LD, Ron M. Transient amnesia heralding brain stem infarction. *J Neurol Neurosurg Psychiatry* 1992; 55: 977.

[105] Taylor RA, Wu GF, Hurst RW, Kasner SE, Cucchiara BL. Transient global amnesia heralding basilar artery thrombosis. *Clin Neurol Neurosurg* 2005; 108: 60–2.

[106] van Zandvoort M, de Haan E, van Gijn J, Kappelle LJ. Cognitive functioning in patients with a small infarct in the brainstem. *J Int Neuropsychol Soc* 2003; 9: 490–4.

[107] Benke T. Peduncular hallucinosis. A syndrome of impaired reality monitoring. *J Neurol* 2006; 253: 1561–71.

[108] Schnakers C, Majerus S, Goldman S, *et al.* Cognitive function in the locked-in syndrome. *J Neurol* 2008; 255: 323–30.

[109] Rousseaux M, Castelnot E, Rigaux P, Kozlowski O, Danzé F. Evidence of persisting cognitive impairment in a case series of patients with locked-in syndrome. *J Neurol Neurosurg Psychiatry* 2009; 80: 166–70.

[110] Neau J-P, Arroyo-Anllo E, Bonnaud V, Ingrand P, Gil R. Neuropsychological disturbances in cerebellar infarcts. *Acta Neurol Scand* 2000; 102: 363–70.

[111] Hokkanen LS, Kauranen V, Roine RO, Salonen O, Kotila M. Subtle cognitive deficits after cerebellar infarcts. *Eur J Neurol* 2006; 13: 161–70.

[112] Richter S, Gerwig M, Aslan B, *et al.* Cognitive functions in patients with MR-defined chronic focal cerebellar lesions. *J Neurol* 2007; 254: 1193–203.

[113] Van Gijn J, Rinkel GJE. Sub-arachnoid haemorrhage: diagnosis, causes and management. *Brain* 2001; 124: 249–78.

[114] Teasdale GM, Wardlaw JM, White PM, *et al.* The familial risk of subarachnoid haemorrhage. *Brain* 2005; 128: 1677–85.

[115] Molyneux AJ, Kerr RS, Birks J, *et al.* Risk of recurrent subarachnoid haemorrhage, death, or dependence and standardized mortality ratios after clipping or coiling of an intracranial aneurysm in the International Subarachnoid Aneurysm Trial (ISAT): long-term follow-up. *Lancet Neurol* 2009; 8: 427–33.

[116] Hütter BO. *Neuropsychological Sequelae of Subarachnoid Hemorrhage and its Treatment.* Berlin: Springer, 2000.

[117] Al-Khindi T, Macdonald RL, Schweizer TA. Cognitive and functional outcome after aneurismal subarachnoid hemorrhage. *Stroke* 2010; 41: e519–36.

[118] Downes JJ, Mayes AR. How bad memories can sometimes lead to fantastic beliefs and strange visions. In: Campbell R, Conway MA (eds.). *Broken Memories: Case Studies in Memory Impairment.* Oxford: Blackwell, 1995; 115–23.

[119] Stenhouse LM, Knight RG, Longmore BE, Bishara SN. Long-term cognitive deficits in patients after surgery on aneurysms of the anterior communicating artery. *J Neurol Neurosurg Psychiatry* 1991; 54: 909–14.

[120] Diamond BJ, DeLuca J, Kelley SM. Memory and executive functions in amnesic and non-amnesic patients with aneurysms of the anterior communicating artery. *Brain* 1997; 120: 1015–25.

[121] Talland GA, Sweet WH, Ballantine HT Jr. Amnesic syndrome with anterior communicating artery aneurysm. *J Nerv Ment Dis* 1967; 145: 179–92.

[122] Maurice-Williams RS, Willison JR, Hatfield R. The cognitive and psychological sequelae of uncomplicated aneurysm surgery. *J Neurol Neurosurg Psychiatry* 1991; 54: 335–40.

[123] Ogden JA, Mee EW, Henning M. A prospective study of impairment of cognition and memory and recovery after subarachnoid haemorrhage. *Neurosurgery* 1993; 33: 572–87.

[124] Tidswell P, Dias PS, Sagar HJ, Mayes AR, Battersby RD. Cognitive outcome after aneurysm rupture: relationship to aneurysm site and perioperative complications. *Neurology* 1995; 45: 875–82.

[125] Kreiter KT, Copeland D, Bernardini GL, *et al.* Predictors of cognitive dysfunction after subarachnoid haemorrhage. *Stroke* 2002; 33: 200–8.

[126] Scott RB, Eccles F, Molyneux AJ, *et al.* Improved cognitive outcomes with endovascular coiling of ruptured intracranial aneurysms: neuropsychological outcomes from the International Subarachnoid Aneurysm Trial (ISAT). *Stroke* 2010; 41: 1743–7.

[127] Otawara Y, Ogasawara K, Ogawa A, Yamadate K. Cognitive function before and after surgery in patients with unruptured intracranial aneurysm. *Stroke* 2005; 36: 142–3.

[128] Kubo Y, Ogasawara K, Kashimura H, *et al.* Cognitive function and anxiety before and after surgery for asymptomatic unruptured intracranial aneurysms in elderly patients. *World Neurosurg* 2010; 73: 350–3.

[129] van Gin J, van Dongen KJ, Vermeulen M, Hijdra A. Perimesencephalic hemorrhage: a nonaneurysmal and benign form of subarachnoid hemorrhage. *Neurology* 1985; 35: 493–7.

[130] Madureira S, Canhao P, Guerreiro M, Ferro JM. Cognitive and emotional consequences of perimesencephalic subarachnoid haemorrhage. *J Neurol* 2000; 247: 862–7.

[131] Fearnley JM, Stevens JM, Rudge P. Superficial siderosis of the central nervous system. *Brain* 1995; 118: 1051–66.

[132] van Harskamp NJ, Rudge P, Cipolotti L. Cognitive and social impairments in patients with superficial siderosis. *Brain* 2005; 128: 1082–92.

[133] Schmahmann JD, Sherman JC. The cerebellar cognitive affective syndrome. *Brain* 1998; 121: 561–79.

[134] Choi JH, Mohr JP. Brain arteriovenous malformations in adults. *Lancet Neurol* 2005; 4: 299–308.

[135] Al-Shahi R, Warlow CP. A systematic review of the frequency and prognosis of arteriovenous malformations of the brain in adults. *Brain* 2001; 124: 1900–26.

[136] Olivecrona H, Reeves J. Arteriovenous malformations of the brain. Their diagnosis and treatment. *Arch Neurol Psychiatry Chicago* 1948; 59: 567–602.

[137] Waltimo O, Putkonen A-R. Intellectual performance of patients with intracranial arteriovenous malformations. *Brain* 1974; 97: 511–20.

[138] Mahalick DM, Ruff RM, U HS. Neuropsychological sequelae of arteriovenous malformations. *Neurosurgery* 1991; 29: 351–7.

[139] Wilson M, Doran M, Enevoldson TP, Larner AJ. Cognitive profiles associated with intracranial dural arteriovenous fistula. *Age Ageing* 2010; 39: 389–92.

[140] Hurst RW, Bagley LJ, Galetta S, *et al.* Dementia resulting from dural arteriovenous fistulas: the pathologic findings of venous hypertensive encephalopathy. *AJNR Am J Neuroradiol* 1998; 19: 1267–73.

[141] Waragai M, Takeuchi H, Fukushima T, Haisa T, Yonemitsu T. MRI and SPECT studies of dural arteriovenous fistulas presenting as pure progressive dementia with leukoencephalopathy: a cause of treatable dementia. *Eur J Neurol* 2006; 13: 754–9.

[142] Tanaka K, Morooka Y, Nakagawa Y, Shimizu S. Dural arteriovenous malformation manifesting as dementia due to ischemia in bilateral thalami. A case report. *Surg Neurol* 1999; 51: 489–93.

[143] Hayman L, Evans R, Ferrell R, *et al.* Familial cavernous angiomas: natural history and genetic study over a 5-year period. *Am J Med Genet* 1982; 11: 147–60.

[144] Gil-Nagel A, Wilcox KJ, Stewart JM, *et al.* Familial cerebral cavernous angioma: clinical analysis of a family and phenotypic classification. *Epilepsy Res* 1995; 21: 27–36.

[145] Kageyama Y, Kodama Y, Yamamoto S, *et al.* A case of multiple intracranial cavernous angiomas presented with dementia and parkinsonism – clinical and MRI study for 10 years [in Japanese]. *Rinsho Shinkeigaku* 2000; 40: 1105–9.

[146] Kariya S, Kawahara M, Suzumura A. A case of multiple cavernous angioma with dementia [in Japanese]. *Rinsho Shinkeigaku* 2000; 40: 1003–7.

[147] Balamoutsos G, Karabela O, Kosmidis M, *et al.* Cavernous angioma presenting as dementia: a case report. *Eur J Neurol* 2009; 16 (Suppl 3): 446 (abstract p. 2327).

[148] Joutel A, Corpechot C, Ducros A, *et al.* Notch3 mutations in CADASIL, a hereditary adult-onset condition causing stroke and dementia. *Nature* 1996; 383: 707–10.

[149] Chabriat H, Joutal A, Dichgans M, Tournier-Lasserve E, Bousser MG. CADASIL. *Lancet Neurol* 2009; 8: 643–53.

[150] Mellies JK, Bäumer T, Müller JA, *et al.* SPECT study of a German CADASIL family: a phenotype with

migraine and progressive dementia only. *Neurology* 1998; 50: 1715–21.

[151] Taillia H, Chabriat H, Kurtz A, *et al.* Cognitive alterations in non-demented CADASIL patients. *Cerebrovasc Dis* 1998; 8: 97–101.

[152] Amberla K, Waljas M, Tuominen S, *et al.* Insidious cognitive decline in CADASIL. *Stroke* 2004; 35: 1598–602.

[153] Filley CM, Thompson LL, Sze CI, *et al.* White matter dementia in CADASIL. *J Neurol Sci* 1999; 163: 163–7.

[154] Buffon F, Porcher R, Hernandez K, *et al.* Cognitive profile in CADASIL. *J Neurol Neurosurg Psychiatry* 2006; 77: 175–80.

[155] Dichgans M, Filippi M, Brüning R, *et al.* Quantitative MRI in CADASIL. Correlation with disability and cognitive performance. *Neurology* 1999; 52: 1361–7.

[156] Benisty S, Hernandez K, Viswanathan A, *et al.* Diagnostic criteria of vascular dementia in CADASIL. *Stroke* 2008; 39: 838–44.

[157] Mesulam M, Siddique T, Cohen B. Cholinergic denervation in a pure multi-infarct state. Observations in CADASIL. *Neurology* 2003; 60: 1183–5.

[158] Dichgans M, Markus HS, Salloway S, *et al.* Donepezil in patients with subcortical vascular cognitive impairment: a randomised double-blind trial in CADASIL. *Lancet Neurol* 2008; 7: 310–18.

[159] Bowler JV, Hachinski V. Progress in the genetics of cerebrovascular disease: inherited subcortical arteriopathies. *Stroke* 1994; 25: 1696–8.

[160] Fukutake T, Hirayama K. Familial young-adult-onset arteriosclerotic leukoencephalopathy with alopecia and lumbago without arterial hypertension. *Eur Neurol* 1995; 35: 69–79.

[161] Hara K, Shiga A, Fukutake T, *et al.* Association of HTRA1 mutations and familial ischemic cerebral small-vessel disease. *N Engl J Med* 2009; 360: 1729–39.

[162] Revesz T, Holton JL, Lashley T, *et al.* Genetics and molecular pathogenesis of sporadic and hereditary cerebral amyloid angiopathies. *Acta Neuropathol* 2009; 118: 115–30.

[163] Biffi A, Greenberg SM. Cerebral amyloid angiopathy: a systematic review. *J Clin Neurol* 2011; 7: 1–9.

[164] Greenberg SM, Vonsattel JP, Stekes JW, Gruber M, Finklestein SP. The clinical spectrum of cerebral amyloid angiopathy: presentations without lobar haemorrhage. *Neurology* 1993; 43: 2073–9.

[165] Larner AJ, Elkington P, Mehta H, *et al.* Multifocal cortical myoclonus and cerebral amyloid β-peptide angiopathy. *J Neurol Neurosurg Psychiatry* 1998; 65: 951–2.

[166] Chung KK, Anderson NE, Hutchinson D, Synek B, Barber PA. Cerebral amyloid angiopathy related inflammation: three case reports and a review. *J Neurol Neurosurg Psychiatry* 2011; 82: 20–6.

[167] Haan J, Lanser JB, Zijderveld I, van der Does IG, Roos RA. Dementia in hereditary cerebral haemorrhage with amyloidosis–Dutch type. *Arch Neurol* 1990; 47: 965–7.

[168] Natté R, Maat-Schieman MLC, Haan J, *et al.* Dementia in hereditary cerebral hemorrhage with amyloidosis-Dutch type is associated with cerebral amyloid angiopathy but is independent of plaques and neurofibrillary tangles. *Ann Neurol* 2001; 50: 765–72.

[169] Sveinbjörnsdóttir S, Blöndal H, Gudmundsson G, *et al.* Progressive dementia and leucoencephalopathy as the initial presentation of late onset hereditary cystatin-C amyloidosis. Clinicopathological presentation of two cases. *J Neurol Sci* 1996; 140: 101–8.

[170] Iglesias S, Chapon F, Baron JC. Familial occipital calcifications, haemorrhagic strokes, leukoencephalopathy, dementia and external carotid dysplasia. *Neurology* 2000; 55: 1661–7 [Erratum Neurology 2001; 56: 823].

[171] Greenberg SM, Shin Y, Grabowski TJ, *et al.* Hemorrhagic stroke associated with the Iowa amyloid precursor protein mutation. *Neurology* 2003; 60: 1020–2.

[172] Grand MG, Kaine J, Fulling K, *et al.* Cerebroretinal vasculopathy. A new hereditary syndrome. *Ophthalmology* 1988; 95: 649–59.

[173] Jen J, Cohen AH, Yue Q, *et al.* Hereditary endotheliopathy with retinopathy, nephropathy and stroke (HERNS). *Neurology* 1997; 49: 1322–30.

[174] Sourander P, Wålinder J. Hereditary multi-infarct dementia. Morphological and clinical studies of a new disease. *Acta Neuropathol (Berl)* 1977; 39: 247–54.

[175] Low WC, Junna M, Borjesson-Hanson A, *et al.* Hereditary multi-infarct dementia of the Swedish type is a novel disorder different from *NOTCH3* causing CADASIL. *Brain* 2007; 130: 357–67.

[176] Asherson RA. New subsets of the antiphospholipid syndrome in 2006: PRE-APS (probable APS) and microangiopathic antiphospholipid syndromes (MAPS). *Autoimmun Rev* 2006; 6: 76–80.

[177] Van Horn G, Arnett FC, Dimachkie MM. Reversible dementia and chorea in a young woman with the lupus anticoagulant. *Neurology* 1996; 46: 1599–603.

[178] Gómez-Puerta JA, Cervera R, Calvo LM, *et al.* Dementia associated with the antiphospholipid syndrome: clinical and radiological characteristics of 30 patients. *Rheumatology (Oxford)* 2005; 44: 95–9.

[179] Reinglass JL, Muller J, Wissman S, Wellman H. Central nervous system angioendotheliosis: a treatable multiple infarct dementia. *Stroke* 1977; 8: 218–21.

[180] Drlicek M, Grisold W, Liszka U, Hitzenberger P, Machacek E. Angiotropic lymphoma (malignant angioendotheliomatosis) presenting with rapidly progressive dementia. *Acta Neuropathol* 1991; 82: 533–5.

[181] Heafield MT, Carey M, Williams AC, Cullen M. Neoplastic angioendotheliomatosis: a treatable "vascular dementia" occurring in an immunosuppressed transplant recipient. *Clin Neuropathol* 1993; 12: 102–6.

[182] Treves TA, Gadoth N, Blumen S, Korczyn AD. Intravascular malignant lymphomatosis: a cause of subacute dementia. *Dementia* 1995; 6: 286–93.

[183] Beristain X, Azzarelli B. The neurological masquerade of intravascular lymphomatosis. *Arch Neurol* 2002; 59: 439–43.

[184] Festa JR, Schwarz LR, Pliskin N, *et al.* Neurocognitive dysfunction in adult moyamoya disease. *J Neurol* 2010; 257: 806–15.

[185] Karzmark P, Zeiffert PD, Tan S, *et al.* Effect of moyamoya disease on neuropsychological functioning in adults. *Neurosurgery* 2008; 62: 1048–51.

[186] Alkemade GM, Willems JM. Polycytemia [*sic*] vera presenting as sudden-onset cognitive impairment. *J Am Geriatr Soc* 2008; 56: 2362–3.

[187] Di Pollina L, Mulligan R, Juillerat van der Linden A, Michel JP, Gold G. Cognitive impairment in polycythaemia rubra vera: partial reversibility upon lowering of the hematocrit. *Eur Neurol* 2000; 44: 57–9.

[188] Steen RG, Miles MA, Helton KJ, *et al.* Cognitive impairment in children with hemoglobin SS sickle cell disease: relationship to MR imaging findings and hematocrit. *AJNR Am J Neuroradiol* 2003; 24: 382–9.

[189] Schatz J, Finke RL, Kellett JM, Kramer JH. Cognitive functioning in children with sickle cell disease: a meta-analysis. *J Pediatr Psychol* 2002; 27: 739–48.

[190] Sneddon IB. Cerebrovascular lesions and livedo reticularis. *Br J Dermatol* 1965; 77: 180–5.

[191] Frances C, Papo T, Wechsler B, *et al.* Sneddon syndrome with or without antiphospholipid antibodies: a comparative study in 46 patients. *Medicine (Baltimore)* 1999; 78: 209–19.

[192] Wright RA, Kokmen E. Gradually progressive dementia without discrete cerebrovascular events in a patient with Sneddon's syndrome. *Mayo Clin Proc* 1999; 74: 57–61.

[193] Adair JC, Digre KB, Swanda RM, *et al.* Sneddon's syndrome: a cause of cognitive decline in young adults. *Neuropsychiatry Neuropsychol Behav Neurol* 2001; 14: 197–204.

[194] Zhan S-S, Beyreuther K, Schmitt HP. Vascular dementia in Spatz–Lindenberg disease (SLD): cortical synaptophysin immunoreactivity as compared with dementia of Alzheimer type and nondemented controls. *Acta Neuropathol (Berl)* 1993; 86: 259–64.

[195] Larner AJ, Kidd D, Elkington P, Rudge P, Scaravilli F. Spatz–Lindenberg disease: a rare cause of vascular dementia. *Stroke* 1999; 30: 687–9.

[196] Papo T, Biousse V, Lehoang P, *et al.* Susac syndrome. *Medicine (Baltimore)* 1998; 77: 3–11.

[197] Turconi E, Coyette F, van Meerbeeck P, *et al.* Three cases of Susac syndrome: clinical features, MRI findings and cognitive follow-up. *Eur J Neurol* 2007; 14: 102 (abstract P1272).

[198] Bousser M-G, Ross Russell RW. *Cerebral Venous Thrombosis.* London: Saunders, 1997.

[199] De Bruijn SF, Budde M, Teunisse S, de Haan RJ, Stam J. Long-term outcome of cognition and functional health after cerebral venous sinus thrombosis. *Neurology* 2000; 54: 1687–9.

[200] Buccino G, Scoditti U, Patteri I, Bertolino C, Mancia D. Neurological and cognitive long-term outcome in patients with cerebral venous sinus thrombosis. *Acta Neurol Scand* 2003; 107: 330–5.

[201] International Headache Society Classification Subcommittee. The International Classification of Headache Disorders, second edition. *Cephalalgia* 2004; 24: 1–160.

[202] Kurth T, Mohamed S, Maillard P, *et al.* Headache, migraine, and structural brain lesions and function: population based epidemiology of vascular ageing–MRI study. *BMJ* 2011; 342: c7357.

[203] O'Bryant SE, Marcus DA, Rains JC, Penzien DB. Neuropsychology of migraine: present status and future directions. *Expert Rev Neurother* 2005; 5: 363–70.

[204] Lane R, Davies P. *Migraine.* New York, NY: Taylor & Francis, 2006: 124–5.

[205] Larner AJ. Unconscious driving phenomenon. *Adv Clin Neurosci Rehabil* 2011; 10(6): 26.

[206] Mulder EJ, Linssen WH, Passchier J, Orlebeke JF, de Geus EJ. Interictal and postictal cognitive changes in migraine. *Cephalalgia* 1999; 19: 557–65.

[207] Farmer K, Cady R, Bleiberg J, Reeves D. A pilot study to measure cognitive efficiency during migraine. *Headache* 2000; 40: 657–61.

[208] Jelicic M, van Boxtel MP, Houx PJ, Jolles J. Does migraine headache affect cognitive function in the elderly? Report from the Maastricht Aging Study (MAAS). *Headache* 2000; 40: 715–19.

[209] Mongini F, Keller R, Deregibus A, Barbalonga E, Mongini T. Frontal lobe dysfunction in patients with chronic migraine: a clinical-neuropsychological study. *Psychiatry Res* 2005; 133: 101–6.

[210] Le Pira F, Lanaia F, Zappala G, *et al.* Relationship between clinical variables and cognitive performances in migraineurs with and without aura. *Funct Neurol* 2004; 19: 101–5.

[211] Calandre EP, Bembibre J, Arnedo ML, Becerra D. Cognitive disturbances and regional cerebral blood flow abnormalities in migraine patients: their relationship with the clinical manifestation of the illness. *Cephalalgia* 2002; 22: 291–302.

[212] Kalaydjian A, Zandi PP, Swartz KL, Eaton WW, Lyketsos C. How migraines impact cognitive function. Findings from the Baltimore ECA. *Neurology* 2007; 68: 1417–24.

[213] Baars MA, van Boxtel MP, Jolles J. Migraine does not affect cognitive decline: results from the Maastricht aging study. *Headache* 2010; 50: 176–84.

[214] Rist PM, Dufouil C, Glymour MM, Tzourio C, Kurth T. Migraine and cognitive decline in the population-based EVA study. *Cephalalgia* 2011; 31: 1291–300.

[215] Rist PM, Kang JH, Buring JE, *et al.* Migraine and cognitive decline among women: prospective cohort study. *BMJ* 2012; 345: e5027.

[216] Freilinger T, Ackl N, Ebert A, *et al.* A novel mutation in CACNA1A associated with hemiplegic migraine, cerebellar dysfunction and late-onset cognitive decline. *J Neurol Sci* 2011; 300: 160–3.

[217] Karner E, Delazer M, Benke T, Bösch S. Cognitive functions, emotional behavior, and quality of life in familial hemiplegic migraine. *Cogn Behav Neurol* 2010; 23: 106–11.

[218] Guyotat MM, Courjon J. Les ictus amnesiques. *J Med Lyon* 1956; 37: 697–701.

[219] Fisher CM, Adams RD. Transient global amnesia. *Acta Neurol Scand* 1964; 40: 1–81.

[220] Quinette P, Guillery-Girard B, Dayan J, *et al.* What does transient global amnesia really mean? Review of the literature and thorough study of 142 cases. *Brain* 2006; 129: 1640–58.

[221] Bartsch T, Deuschl G. Transient global amnesia: functional anatomy and clinical implications. *Lancet Neurol* 2010; 9: 205–14.

[222] Lane R, Davies P. *Migraine*. New York, NY: Taylor & Francis, 2006; 125–30, 168.

[223] Olesen J, Jorgensen MB. Leao's spreading depression in the hippocampus explains transient global amnesia. A hypothesis. *Acta Neurol Scand* 1986; 73: 219–20.

[224] McCorry DJ, Crowley P. Transient global amnesia secondary to herpes simplex viral encephalitis. *QJM* 2005; 98: 154–5.

[225] Ung KYC, Larner AJ. Transient amnesia: epileptic or global? A differential diagnosis with significant implications for management. *Q J Med* 2012 [Epub ahead of print]

[226] Larner AJ. Transient global amnesia in the district general hospital. *Int J Clin Pract* 2007; 61: 255–8.

[227] Hodges JR, Ward CD. Observations during transient global amnesia. A behavioural and neuropsychological study of five cases. *Brain* 1989; 112: 595–620.

[228] Hodges JR. Transient semantic amnesia. *J Neurol Neurosurg Psychiatry* 1997; 63: 548–9.

[229] Guillery-Girard B, Desgranges B, Urban C, *et al.* The dynamic time course of memory recovery in transient global amnesia. *J Neurol Neurosurg Psychiatry* 2004; 75: 1532–40.

The epilepsies

4.1 Epilepsy and cognitive impairment

As far back as the seventeenth century, Thomas Willis (1621–1675), in some senses the father of neurology, recognized that chronic epilepsy could bring on "stupidity," a term roughly corresponding to our notion of dementia [1]. In the nineteenth century, authors such as Henry Maudsley (1835–1918) and William Gowers (1845–1915) regarded epileptics as prone to dementia or defective memory; indeed, Maudsley thought such decline inevitable [2]. These views may have been determined, at least in part, by clinical practice among patients with very severe seizure disorders, but regrettably brought with them stigmatizing notions of epilepsy as a marker of criminality, mental abnormality, and degeneration, also reflected in popular culture [3]. With the advent of effective antiepileptic drugs in the twentieth century, a more optimistic outlook for cognition in epilepsy generally prevailed. Now, however, cognitive impairment in epilepsy is once again a subject of increasing concern and investigation [4]. Rather than an "epileptic dementia," this problem is now better conceptualized as dementia or cognitive impairment in people with epilepsy [2], a syndrome with various possible causes.

Historically, epilepsy surgery has provided a critical insight into the relevance of certain brain structures to cognitive function. One of the most remarkable cases in the history of neuropsychology is that of Henry or HM (Henry Gustav Molaison, 1926–2008) who developed profound anterograde amnesia following surgical removal of the anterior temporal lobes bilaterally, including the hippocampus, for intractable seizures of temporal lobe origin [5,6]. Occasional cases of amnesia following unilateral surgery have also been reported, when there is subclinical damage in the unoperated, contralateral, temporal lobe, often as a result of birth asphyxia [7]. Cases such as these have demonstrated the critical relevance of the hippocampus in memory function.

The marked heterogeneity of epilepsy syndromes, with respect to factors such as site of seizure origin (generalized vs. partial, or localization-related), etiology (idiopathic vs. symptomatic), and pathology [8,9], means that definition of a specific profile of neuropsychological impairments is as untenable for epilepsy as it is for cerebrovascular disease (Chapter 3). Nonetheless, certain common patterns may be identified in particular epilepsy syndromes.

There are at least three possible reasons for an association between cognitive decline and epileptic seizures [10–15]:

- cognitive decline and epilepsy may be phenotypic expressions of a shared etiopathogenesis;
- epileptic seizures per se may lead to acquired cognitive impairment;
- antiepileptic drug therapy may cause cognitive decline.

These variables are not necessarily independent; specific brain diseases or brain injuries may be associated with a longer duration of seizure disorder and/or more frequent seizures, requiring polytherapy and/or higher doses of antiepileptic drugs. Because of this potential confounding, it is difficult to separate the various parameters. Indeed, most cognitive problems in patients with epilepsy are of multifactorial origin. Psychiatric comorbidity may also need to be taken into account; depression may contribute more to subjective memory complaints and poor quality of life in epilepsy than seizures per se. Brain plasticity and epilepsy surgery may also have cognitive consequences [13], but neither is considered further here.

Memory complaints in epilepsy patients are a subject of increasing concern in disease management, over and above simple reduction in seizure frequency and severity [4]. How appropriate standard neuropsychological tests are in the detection of cognitive impairments in epilepsy patients is open to question, particularly in the assessment of executive functions [16].

4.2 Cognitive decline and epilepsy: shared etiopathogenesis

Cognitive decline and epilepsy may both be phenotypic features of brain pathophysiology. A study of patients newly diagnosed with epilepsy and without known brain pathology found evidence that these individuals were cognitively compromised, particularly in the domains of memory and psychomotor speed. These deficits were unrelated to the number of seizures, type of epilepsy, or mood, and were present prior to treatment with antiepileptic drugs [17]. Furthermore, these cognitive domains, along with higher executive functioning, showed a decline in the first twelve months after epilepsy diagnosis in comparison to healthy volunteers, even if seizure remission was achieved [18]. These findings suggest that the phenotypic features of epilepsy and cognitive decline may possibly have a shared or overlapping etiopathogenesis. Five-year follow-up of a small cohort (n = 50) of newly diagnosed epilepsy patients found stability in the majority of cognitive measures but subtle declines in memory and psychomotor speed in around one-third of cases [19].

The symptomatic epilepsies include those due to brain tumor, stroke (infarct or hemorrhage), inflammation of autoimmune (demyelination) or infective (encephalitis, meningitis) etiology, and various dementia syndromes. The concurrence of seizures and cognitive impairment does not necessarily imply a causal link (i.e., seizures causing cognitive impairment) in these conditions. For example, seizures may sometimes be a feature of Huntington's disease (HD; Section 5.1.1), particularly early onset forms, but there is no suggestion that they are responsible for, or even contribute to, the cognitive deficits of HD. However, in other clinical situations, there may be a link, as for example in neurocysticercosis with mesial temporal sclerosis (Section 9.4.4) and tuberous sclerosis and the number of cortical tubers (Section 5.6.2). Epileptic seizures may be a symptomatic feature of various other pathologies associated with cognitive decline (e.g., encephalitides, mitochondrial disease, progressive myoclonic epilepsy syndromes, Hashimoto's encephalitis). The corollary of this observation is that treatment of the underlying disease, where possible, might ameliorate both seizures and cognitive decline.

Alzheimer's disease (AD) has long been recognized to be a risk factor for the development of late-onset epileptic seizures [20,21], of both partial and generalized onset [22]. Seizures become increasingly common with the progression of AD [23,24], although may sometimes occur in the earliest stages of the disease [25]. It was thought previously that seizures were epiphenomenal to the neurodegenerative changes of AD, but more recently animal model studies have prompted a view that subclinical seizures may be an integral part of the AD phenotype. Cognitive decline and seizures may reflect a shared pathogenesis in terms of neuronal disconnection [23,26], which in part may be genetically determined [27]. Likewise in Down syndrome, where AD-type pathology inevitably develops, there is a strong association between seizure onset or exacerbation and cognitive decline [28]. Whether treatment of seizures in AD might ameliorate cognitive decline remains unknown [29].

Early group studies suggested that epilepsy patients had reduced speed of mental processing, and reaction and response times [30], as well as impairments in remembering lists of words and geometric patterns [31]. Attention deficits may be more common in generalized than focal epilepsy [32,33], and memory difficulties more common in focal (temporal lobe) epilepsy.

4.2.1 Idiopathic generalized epilepsies

Idiopathic generalized epilepsies (IGE) are characterized by primary generalized seizures which, unlike localization-related epilepsies, occur in the absence of any macroscopic brain abnormalities [8,9]. Hence, IGEs may facilitate the study of the effect of seizures on cognitive function. Primary generalized seizures may take various forms, including generalized tonic-clonic seizures (GTCS), also known in the older literature as "grand mal," and absence seizures (AS) or "petit mal." One of the most common forms of IGE is juvenile myoclonic epilepsy (JME).

Controlled studies of cognitive function in homogeneous groups of adult IGE patients are relatively few. In one small study (n = 30; mean age 30+/– 12.6 years), IGE patients were reported to perform worse than controls on speed of information processing and in tests of memory encompassing word and face recognition and verbal and visual recall, with evidence from magnetic resonance (MR) spectroscopy that this correlated with neuronal dysfunction secondary to epileptic activity [34]. Children with IGE (AS and GTCS) showed poorer performance than healthy controls in attention, with verbal learning and memory and word fluency impairments in those children with AS [35]. Currently, there is no definitive answer as to whether verbal or nonverbal memory is more impaired in IGE.

Hommet *et al.* [36] suggested that disorders of social integration and personality in JME patients might suggest the presence of impaired executive functions, and that benign childhood epilepsy with centrotemporal spikes (BCECTS) might provide a useful model for the study of the relationship between epileptiform electroencephalographic (EEG) discharges in the perisylvian region and language functions. There are reports, in one study, of mild impairments of working memory, verbal fluency, abstract reasoning, planning, and mental flexibility in JME, suggesting frontal type dysfunction [37,38], but Roebling *et al.* [39] ascribed the slightly worse performance of JME patients in semantic and verbal fluency compared to controls to concurrent antiepileptic medication, which was not controlled for in some studies [38].

4.2.2 Localization-related (partial) epilepsies

Partial or focal seizures may be of temporal, frontal, or occipital lobe onset, with or without secondary generalization. These may be a consequence of defined pathological processes (e.g., tumor, stroke, inflammation), but many remain cryptogenic despite extensive investigation. Generally, cognitive deficits are those anticipated for the affected brain region. Thus, partial seizures with epileptic foci in the temporal lobes show lateralized material-specific deficits, left-sided lesions generally being associated with impaired verbal long-term memory, while right temporal lobe foci cause greater difficulty with visual long-term memory. Patients with well-controlled partial seizures, doing a regular job or attending a normal school, may be found on neuropsychological testing to have impairments in cognition [40]. Secondary generalized seizures may be associated with lower intelligence and a trend toward cognitive decline [41].

4.2.2.1 Temporal lobe epilepsy

Cognitive features have been most extensively investigated in temporal lobe epilepsy (TLE). Symptomatic TLE with the neuroradiological signature of hippocampal sclerosis or mesial temporal sclerosis (MTS), mesial temporal lobe epilepsy (MTLE), is thought to be the most common form of localization-related epilepsy [42]. Precipitating incidents such as febrile convulsions, brain trauma, ischemia, or intracranial infection are common, and most individuals have seizure onset in childhood or adolescence. Because of the involvement of structures important for memory processes in TLE, it has been logical to examine cognitive function in these patients.

Cognitive deficits, specifically memory disturbances, may be apparent even at disease onset in MTLE, suggesting that these are symptoms of the disease and not simply consequences of frequent seizures or the effects of antiepileptic drug therapy [43]. Left-sided (dominant hemisphere) MTLE is characterized by deficits in material-specific verbal memory [44], although this may disappear at older age [45]. Right-sided (nondominant hemisphere) MTLE is associated with

nonverbal/visual memory deficit, albeit less consistently [46], perhaps in part an artifact of the neuropsychological tests being insufficiently nonverbal in nature [47]. Other cognitive profiles are sometimes encountered in TLE; for example, relatively selective autobiographical amnesia [48]. Semantic memory deficits involving verbal and visual information may be found in left MTLE [49]. Examining cognitively based daily living skills (daily living tests from the Neuropsychological Assessment Battery), a test of "everyday cognition," TLE patients showed significant impairments in daily memory functioning [50].

In addition to these memory impairments, a phenomenon of accelerated forgetting of material despite normal learning and retention over 30 minutes has been described in patients with left temporal lobe epileptic foci, suggesting impaired memory consolidation processes [51].

Some quantitative MR imaging (MRI) studies have suggested that both the hippocampus and other related structures such as the fornix are atrophied in TLE patients [52]. Other studies could not relate cognitive impairments to hippocampal volume changes, but rather to reduced functional connectivity in prefrontal networks involving the anterior cingulate and middle and inferior frontal gyrus [53].

Some studies have indicated that higher seizure frequency and duration of MTLE are associated with more severe cognitive decline [54], but in a report on patients with MTLE undergoing temporal lobe resection, no correlation was found between disease-related parameters, such as cumulative number of seizures, and neuropsychological deficits, suggesting that factors other than repetitive seizures are responsible for cognitive dysfunction in these patients [55]. MTS is reported to be associated with poorer cognitive performance than other pathologies [45].

The question whether cognitive impairments in epilepsy may progress to dementia has been examined. It would seem that there is a negative interaction of cognitive impairment with mental ageing rather than progressively dementing decline [45,56].

MTLE may be complicated by the development of an interictal psychosis, which is reminiscent in some ways of schizophrenia (Section 12.2). Patients with the schizophrenia-like psychosis of epilepsy (SLPE) have been reported to show executive function deficits that lie intermediate between those of patients with schizophrenia and epilepsy/controls [57]. There may also be deficits in working memory and semantic memory in SLPE [58].

4.2.2.2 Frontal lobe epilepsy

The frontal lobe epilepsies (FLE), resulting from a primary epileptic focus anywhere within the frontal lobe, have various seizure patterns. Motor manifestations are more common than in seizures arising elsewhere; for example, simple focal motor seizures with or without Jacksonian march, and tonic posturing in seizures of supplementary motor area origin (fencer's posture, *en garde*, salutatory seizures). FLE may be idiopathic or symptomatic.

Early group studies found patients with unilateral frontal lobe seizure foci to be no different cognitively from controls [59,60]. However, more recent studies have provided evidence for frontal-type, executive, cognitive dysfunction in FLE, in terms of attention, working memory, planning, and psychomotor speed [61]. Problems with shifting cognitive sets, abstraction, and inhibition are also reported [62,63]. Elements of social cognition, such as humor appreciation and ability to detect emotional expression, but not tests of theory of mind, may also be impaired [64]. Examining cognitively based daily living skills, FLE patients showed significant impairments in daily memory functioning, like TLE patients, but no impairment in executive daily functioning; whether these tests are sufficiently sensitive to identify such deficits was questioned [50]. Unlike the situation in MTLE, encoding and retrieval memory functions may be normal in FLE, although memory processes related to attentional and executive function may be impaired.

A nocturnal variant of FLE may be either sporadic or inherited as an autosomal dominant disorder, the latter (autosomal dominant nocturnal frontal lobe epilepsy, ADNFLE) associated with mutations in at least two genes, CHRNA4 and CHRNB2 (OMIM#600513 #605375, respectively). ADNFLE associated with one point mutation (I312M) in CHRNB2, is reported to be associated with distinct memory deficits involving storage of verbal information [65,66].

4.2.3 Rasmussen's syndrome (chronic encephalitis and epilepsy)

A syndrome of chronic partial, often intractable, epileptic seizures attended by progressive focal sensorimotor neurological deficit and cognitive decline was described by Rasmussen *et al.* in 1958 [67]; a similar syndrome was described by Kozhevnikov in Russia in 1952. The pathogenesis of Rasmussen's syndrome, also known as chronic encephalitis and epilepsy, remains uncertain: possibilities include viral infection and autoimmune mechanisms [68,69]. Although typically a disorder with childhood onset [70], cases with adult onset have been described [71–74]. These appear to have a more protracted and milder clinical course with less in the way of residual functional deficits, lesser degrees of brain hemiatrophy, but with identical clinical, EEG, neuroimaging, and histopathology findings. Cases of NMDA-receptor encephalitis (Section 6.12.2) resembling Rasmussen's syndrome have been reported [75; W Pietkowicz, personal communication, 26/09/12].

Neuropsychological assessment of patients with Rasmussen's syndrome is subject to various biases, such as selected cohorts, ongoing seizures or even epilepsia partialis continua, and surgical interventions. Low IQ is typical in childhood-onset cases, usually with little change after surgery although exceptionally, improvement is noted. In adult-onset cases, McLachlan *et al.* [71] noted decline in IQ in two of their three patients, with greater left hemisphere dysfunction, consistent in one patient with exclusively left hemisphere involvement. Over an eight-year period, between the ages of 22 and 30 years, another adult-onset patient developed IQ decline, impaired auditory verbal memory, motor and sensory aphasia in association with left temporo-occipital cortical MRI change and EEG multifocal spike discharges in the left posterior quadrant [72]. Improvements in neuropsychological function, as well as in seizure frequency, have been recorded in adult-onset cases following cycles of treatment with human intravenous immunoglobulin [73].

4.3 Epileptic seizures causing acquired cognitive impairment

Epileptic seizures may lead unequivocally to cognitive impairment [76]. Deficits have been noted in psychomotor speed, attention, memory, and visuomotor tasks, which cannot be ascribed to the encephalopathy associated with status epilepticus, postictal state, or antiepileptic drug toxicity, and which are reversible with good seizure control. Longitudinal studies suggest a link between adverse cognitive change and number of seizures or presence of tonic-clonic status epilepticus [77].

Electroconvulsive therapy (ECT), a treatment for depression that aims to cause epileptic seizure through application of an electric current, is associated with subsequent impairments of episodic memory [78].

The impact of frequent interictal epileptiform discharges on cognitive function remains a subject of debate [76,79–81], specifically whether such discharges could be responsible for transitory cognitive impairment. It may be difficult to distinguish such EEG changes from subtle nonconvulsive seizures, but nonetheless, there is evidence that EEG discharges may be associated with brief effects on mental alertness and speed [81]. Whether drug treatment, with its attendant risk of adverse effects (Section 4.4), is indicated in these situations remains to be determined.

Amnesia for complex partial, primary and secondarily generalized seizures is the norm. Sometimes the effects of frequent complex partial seizures are sufficient to manifest as an amnesic or dementia syndrome, which may even be confused with AD [82–85]. The frequency of such "epileptic pseudodementia" is not known, but merits consideration in light of the fact that the incidence of complex partial seizures rises sharply after the age of 60 years. However, the classic example of epileptic seizures causing cognitive impairment is seen in the syndrome of transient epileptic amnesia (Section 4.3.1).

Progressive dementia does not seem to be a consequence of temporal lobe epilepsy [45].

4.3.1 Transient epileptic amnesia (TEA)

Attacks of transient amnesia of epileptic origin were first described by Hughlings Jackson (1835–1911) in the physician patient "Dr Z" in 1888 [86]. However, although occasional cases of epileptic amnesia were reported subsequently [87,88], it was not until the 1990s that the syndrome of transient epileptic amnesia (TEA) was characterized [89,90] and systematic studies undertaken [91–93].

Typically, TEA manifests with brief amnesic attacks, usually one hour or less in duration, often occurring on waking. Attacks have a high recurrence rate, and may be accompanied by other features suggestive of epilepsy, such as automatisms or olfactory hallucinations. Autobiographical amnesia may be prominent [94]. Many TEA patients also report interictal memory problems. An accelerated loss of new information (as in MTLE; Section 4.2.2.1; [51]) and impaired remote autobiographical memory has been demonstrated in TEA patients, but the etiology of these deficits remains uncertain, possibilities including ongoing seizure activity, seizure-induced medial temporal lobe damage, or subtle ischemic pathology [95]. Although usually idiopathic, cases of secondary or symptomatic TEA have been reported; for example, a case possibly associated with the onset of AD [96].

The EEG in TEA may be associated with clearcut seizure activity during amnesic episodes. Abnormalities may be found in interictal EEG recordings in about one-third of TEA patients, although sometimes sleep-deprived EEG may be required. Management may require not only antiepileptic drug therapy (TEA generally responds favorably to standard antiepileptic medications such as sodium valproate or carbamazepine), but also advice on appropriate lifestyle modifications, including reference to DVLA (Driver and Vehicle Licensing Agency) restrictions on driving [93].

Clinically, TEA resembles transient global amnesia (TGA; Section 3.6.2), but attacks are briefer and have a higher recurrence rate. The "absence of epileptic features" is one of the proposed diagnostic criteria for TGA [97], although EEG is seldom performed in TGA, other than fortuitously, and is normal [98].

4.3.2 Epileptic aphasia; ictal speech arrest

Aphasia is the principal symptom in the childhood epilepsy disorder of the Landau–Kleffner syndrome (acquired epileptic aphasia), possibly reflecting a verbal auditory agnosia [99].

Isolated epileptic aphasia is uncommon, perhaps obscured in some cases by ictal motor activity [100]. Nonconvulsive status epilepticus may manifest with aphasia ("status aphasicus"), usually with abrupt onset and rapid resolution with appropriate antiepileptic drug therapy, although persistent aphasia has also been reported [101,102]. Aphasic status most often reflects left-sided (frontotemporal or temporoparietal) pathology [103], as would be anticipated, although visual stimuli provoking an occipital lobe seizure spreading to the left inferior frontal lobe has been reported [104], as has a right-sided focus [101]. Parasagittal lesions confined to the left superior frontal gyrus (supplementary motor area) may be sufficient to cause the syndrome [105]. Other reported causes of epileptic aphasia include nonketotic hyperglycemia [106], AIDS-related toxoplasmosis [107], and multiple sclerosis

[108] (Section 6.1). Recurrent Wernicke-type aphasia of epileptic origin, misdiagnosed as transient ischemic attacks, has also been reported [109].

4.4 Antiepileptic drug therapy causing cognitive impairment

Although individuals developing epilepsy have evidence for cognitive compromise prior to treatment with antiepileptic drugs (AEDs) [17,43], reduction in seizure frequency as a consequence of AED treatment may improve cognitive function. However, AEDs feature in any list of medicines that are reported to cause cognitive decline or even dementia. It has even been claimed that patients were "reduced to practical dementia by bromides" [110]. The cognitive adverse effects of chronic AED therapy, to which elderly individuals are more susceptible, have long been a topic of research interest [111–114]. The vexed questions of the effects of AEDs, particularly sodium valproate, on the IQ of children exposed in utero during development remain highly topical but are not discussed here [115].

Sedation may be an important factor in adults receiving AEDs, as judged by increased reaction times [30] and specific deficits in attention and working memory observed in some but not all patients taking drugs such as phenobarbitone, phenytoin, and benzodiazepines, recognized to have sedative effects. Patients receiving monotherapy with phenytoin, sodium valproate, or carbamazepine, who were tested before and after changes in drug dosage, either up or down, showed deficits in cognitive performance in the high serum level group, especially those receiving phenytoin or sodium valproate, whereas the carbamazepine group showed no change or even a trend toward improvement in the high serum level group [116,117]. Volunteers receiving phenytoin, carbamazepine, sodium valproate, clonazepam, and clobazam have shown significant deficits, most marked with phenytoin and clonazepam. A large study in the U.S. that compared the efficacy and toxicity of monotherapy with four antiepileptic drugs (phenobarbitone, primidone, phenytoin, and carbamazepine) found that when controlling for age, education, and IQ, carbamazepine had fewer cognitive effects than the other drugs [118], confirming previous smaller studies. However, other studies have not found a difference between carbamazepine and phenytoin when drug levels have been taken into account [119]. Polypharmacy is certainly associated with more severe adverse consequences for cognitive function [120].

Newer AEDs generally have improved adverse effect profiles in comparison with previously used medications, but the increased scrutiny to which these medications have been subject has shown that they are not exempt from cognitive adverse effects [114,121]. Lamotrigine, probably the most extensively studied AED from the cognitive perspective, seems well tolerated [122], and the same is probably true of gabapentin [123] and oxcarbazepine [124]. However, impaired attention, psychomotor slowing, and memory deficits have been recorded with topiramate, which seems more prone to cognitive adverse effects than lamotrigine or gabapentin [18,125,126], although this may be related to rapid drug titration in some studies. Pragmatic comparative drug trials have shown that memory disturbance is a common symptom and one of the most common adverse effects to result in treatment failure; again this may be the case particularly with topiramate [127,128]. Currently there are few studies evaluating cognitive adverse effects of vigabatrin, levetiracetam, tiagabine, zonisamide, and lacosamide [114], with no evidence for significant cognitive problems with these drugs with the possible exception of zonisamide [129,130]. In the absence of randomized studies, patient self-reported symptoms may be used to gain insight into cognitive adverse effects [131].

4.5 Treatment of cognitive problems in epilepsy

Treatment of cognitive complaints needs to be individualized to each patient with epilepsy, but some general guidelines may be enunciated. Optimizing seizure control with AEDs that have a good adverse effect profile as far as cognitive function is concerned, and avoiding polypharmacy, is paramount. Treating confounding factors such as depression and sleep disorders is mandatory. However, it must be recognized that the underlying etiology of epileptic seizures is often a major contributing factor that may not be amenable to specific treatment [17,18].

Whether cognitive enhancers such as cholinesterase inhibitors, licensed for use in AD, have anything to offer in epilepsy-related cognitive impairment is uncertain [132], with only a few small studies having been reported. A pilot open-label study of donepezil over three months in 18 epilepsy patients found greater recall in the Buschke Selective Reminding Test, but no changes were noted in attention, visual sequencing, mental flexibility, or psychomotor speed. There was no significant increase in seizure frequency [133]. A randomized double-blind placebo-controlled trial of donepezil over three months in 23 patients was not associated with improvement in memory or other cognitive functions, nor with any increase in seizure frequency or severity [134]. A randomized trial of galantamine for 12 weeks in 28 patients again showed no significant differences in memory measures at retest [135]. The lack of effect seen in these trials may, in part, reflect underpowered trials, the brief dosing period, and the heterogeneous nature of epilepsy patients with subjective memory difficulty.

REFERENCES

[1] Zimmer C. *Soul Made Flesh. The Discovery of the Brain – and How it Changed the World.* London: Heinemann, 2004; 226.

[2] Brown SW, Vaughan M. Dementia in epileptic patients. In: Trimble MR, Reynolds EH (eds.). *Epilepsy, Behaviour and Cognitive Function.* Chichester: Wiley, 1988; 177–88.

[3] Larner AJ. Charles Dickens (1812–1870) and epilepsy. *Epilepsy Behav* 2012; 24: 422–5.

[4] Zeman A, Kapur N, Jones-Gotman M (eds.). *Epilepsy and Memory*. Oxford: Oxford University Press, 2012.

[5] Scoville W, Milner B. Loss of recent memory after bilateral hippocampal lesions. *J Neurol Neurosurg Psychiatry* 1957; 20: 11–21.

[6] Ogden JA. *Fractured Minds. A Case-Study Approach To Clinical Neuropsychology* (2nd edn.). Oxford: Oxford University Press, 2005; 46–63.

[7] Kapur N, Prevett M. Unexpected amnesia: are there lessons to be learned from cases of amnesia following unilateral temporal lobe surgery? *Brain* 2003; **126**: 2573–85.

[8] Panayiotopoulos CP. *A Clinical Guide to Epileptic Syndromes and their Treatment: Based on the ILAE Classifications and Practice Parameter Guidelines* (2nd edn.). London: Springer, 2007.

[9] Engel J, Pedley TA, Aicardi J (eds.). *Epilepsy. A Comprehensive Textbook* (2nd edn.). Philadelphia, PA: Lippincott Williams & Wilkins, 2008.

[10] Trimble MR, Reynolds EH (eds.). *Epilepsy, Behaviour and Cognitive Function*. Chichester: Wiley, 1988.

[11] Kwan P, Brodie MJ. Neuropsychological effects of epilepsy and antiepileptic drugs. *Lancet* 2001; 357: 216–22.

[12] Motamedi G, Meador K. Epilepsy and cognition. *Epilepsy Behav* 2003; 4: S25–38.

[13] Elger CE, Helmstaedter C, Kurthen M. Chronic epilepsy and cognition. *Lancet Neurol* 2004; 3: 663–72.

[14] Hermann B, Seidenberg M. Epilepsy and cognition. *Epilepsy Curr* 2007; 7: 1–6.

[15] Trimble M, Schmitz B (eds.). *The Neuropsychiatry of Epilepsy* (2nd edn.). Cambridge: Cambridge University Press, 2011; 135–85.

[16] Baker GA, Marson AG. Cognitive and behavioural assessments in clinical trials: what type of measure? *Epilepsy Res* 2001; 45: 163–7.

[17] Taylor J, Kolamunnage-Dona R, Marson AG, *et al.* Patients with epilepsy: cognitively compromised before the start of antiepileptic drug treatment? *Epilepsia* 2010; 51: 48–56.

[18] Baker GA, Taylor J, Aldenkamp AP, SANAD group. Newly diagnosed epilepsy: cognitive outcome after 12 months. *Epilepsia* 2011; 52: 1084–91.

[19] Taylor J, Baker GA. Newly diagnosed epilepsy: cognitive outcome at 5 years. *Epilepsy Behav* 2010; 18: 397–403.

[20] Hauser WA, Morris ML, Heston LL, Anderson VE. Seizures and myoclonus in patients with Alzheimer's disease. *Neurology* 1986; 36: 1226–30.

[21] Romanelli MF, Morris JC, Ashkin K, Coben LA. Advanced Alzheimer's disease is a risk factor for late onset seizures. *Arch Neurol* 1990; 47: 847–50.

[22] Hesdorffer DC, Hauser WA, Annegers JF, Kokmen E, Rocca WA. Dementia and adult-onset unprovoked seizures. *Neurology* 1996; 46: 727–30.

[23] Larner AJ. Epileptic seizures in AD patients. *Neuromolecular Med* 2010; 12: 71–7.

[24] Friedman D, Honig LS, Scarmeas N. Seizures and epilepsy in Alzheimer's disease. *CNS Neurosci Ther* 2012; 18: 285–94.

[25] Lozsadi DA, Larner AJ. Prevalence and causes of seizures at time of diagnosis of probable Alzheimer's disease. *Dement Geriatr Cogn Disord* 2006; 22: 121–4.

[26] Noebels J. A perfect storm: converging paths of epilepsy and Alzheimer's dementia in the hippocampal formation. *Epilepsia* 2011; 52: S39–46.

[27] Larner AJ. Presenilin 1 mutation Alzheimer's disease: a genetic epilepsy syndrome? *Epilepsy Behav* 2011; 21: 20–2.

[28] Lott IT, Doran E, Nguyen VQ, *et al.* Down syndrome and dementia: seizures and cognitive decline. *J Alzheimers Dis* 2012; 29: 177–85.

[29] Larner AJ, Marson AG. Epileptic seizures in Alzheimer's disease: another fine MESS? *J Alzheimers Dis* 2011; 25: 417–19.

[30] Bruhn P, Parsons OA. Reaction time variability in epileptic and brain-damaged patients. *Cortex* 1977; 13: 373–84.

[31] Loiseau P, Strube E, Broustet D, *et al.* Evaluation of memory function in a population of epileptic patients and matched controls. *Acta Neurol Scand Suppl* 1980; 80: 58–61.

[32] Mirsky AF, Primac DW, Marsan CA, Rosvold HE, Stevens JR. A comparison of the psychological test performance of patients with focal and non-focal epilepsy. *Exp Neurol* 1960; 2: 75–89.

[33] Kimura D. Cognitive deficit related to seizure patterns in centrencephalic epilepsy. *J Neurol Neurosurg Psychiatry* 1964; 27: 291–5.

[34] Dickson JM, Wilkinson ID, Howell SJL, Griffiths PD, Grünewald RA. Idiopathic generalised epilepsy: a pilot study of memory and neuronal dysfunction in the temporal lobes, assessed by magnetic resonance

spectroscopy. *J Neurol Neurosurg Psychiatry* 2006; 77: 834–40.

[35] Henkin Y, Sadeh M, Kivity S, *et al.* Cognitive function in idiopathic generalized epilepsy of childhood. *Dev Med Child Neurol* 2005; 47: 126–32.

[36] Hommet C, Sauerwein HC, De Toffol B, Lassonde M. Idiopathic epileptic syndromes and cognition. *Neurosci Biobehav Rev* 2006; 30: 85–96.

[37] Devinsky O, Gershengorn J, Brown E, *et al.* Frontal functions in juvenile myoclonic epilepsy. *Neuropsychiatry Neuropsychol Behav Neurol* 1997; 10: 243–6.

[38] Pascalicchio TF, de Araujo Filho GM, da Silva Noffs MH, *et al.* Neuropsychological profile of patients with juvenile myoclonic epilepsy: a controlled study of 50 patients. *Epilepsy Behav* 2007; 10: 263–7.

[39] Roebling R, Scheerer N, Uttner I, *et al.* Evaluation of cognition, structural, and functional MRI in juvenile myoclonic epilepsy. *Epilepsia* 2009; 50: 2456–65.

[40] Engelberts NHJ, Klein M, van der Ploeg HM, *et al.* Cognition and health-related quality of life in a well-defined subgroup of patients with partial epilepsy. *J Neurol* 2002; 249: 294–9.

[41] Vlooswijk MC, Jansen JF, Reijs RP, *et al.* Cognitive fMRI and neuropsychological assessment in patients with secondarily generalized seizures. *Clin Neurol Neurosurg* 2008; 110: 441–50.

[42] Wieser HG. Mesial temporal lobe epilepsy with hippocampal sclerosis. *Epilepsia* 2004; 45: 695–714.

[43] Aikia M, Salmenpera T, Partanen K, Kalviainen R. Verbal memory in newly diagnosed patients and patients with chronic left temporal lobe epilepsy. *Epilepsy Behav* 2001; 2: 20–7.

[44] Hermann BP, Seidenberg M, Schoenfeld J, Davies K. Neuropsychological characteristics of the syndrome of mesial temporal lobe epilepsy. *Arch Neurol* 1997; 54: 369–76.

[45] Helmstaedter C, Elger CE. Chronic temporal lobe epilepsy: a neurodevelopmental or progressively dementing disease? *Brain* 2009; 132: 2822–30.

[46] Gleissner U, Helmstaedter C, Elger CE. Right hippocampal contribution to visual memory: a presurgical and postsurgical study in patients with temporal lobe epilepsy. *J Neurol Neurosurg Psychiatry* 1998; 65: 665–9.

[47] Djordjevic J, Jones-Gotman M. Neuropsychological assessment of memory in patients with epilepsy. In: Zeman A, Kapur N, Jones-Gotman M (eds.). *Epilepsy and Memory.* Oxford: Oxford University Press, 2012; 177–88.

[48] Kapur N. Autobiographical amnesia and temporal lobe pathology. In: Parkin AJ (ed.). *Case Studies in the Neuropsychology of Memory.* Hove: Psychology Press, 1997; 37–62.

[49] Giovagnoli AR, Erbetta A, Villani F, Avanzini G. Semantic memory in partial epilepsy: verbal and non-verbal deficits and neuroanatomical relationships. *Neuropsychologia* 2005; 43: 1482–92.

[50] Cahn-Weiner DA, Wittenberg D, McDonald C. Everyday cognition in temporal and frontal lobe epilepsy. *Epileptic Disord* 2009; 11: 222–7.

[51] Blake R, Wroe S, Breen E, McCarthy R. Accelerated forgetting in patients with epilepsy: evidence for impairment in memory consolidation. *Brain* 2000; 123: 472–83.

[52] Kuzniecky R, Bilir E, Gilliam F, *et al.* Quantitative MRI in temporal lobe epilepsy: evidence for fornix atrophy. *Neurology* 1999; 53: 496–501.

[53] Vlooswijk MC, Jansen JF, Jeukens CR, *et al.* Memory processes and prefrontal network dysfunction in cryptogenic epilepsy. *Epilepsia* 2011; 52: 1467–75.

[54] Jokheit H, Ebner A. Long term effects of refractory temporal lobe epilepsy on cognitive abilities: a cross sectional study. *J Neurol Neurosurg Psychiatry* 1999; 67: 44–50.

[55] Kramer U, Kipervasser S, Neufeld MY, *et al.* Is there any correlation between severity of epilepsy and cognitive abilities in patients with temporal lobe epilepsy? *Eur J Neurol* 2006; 13: 130–4.

[56] Helmstaedter C, Elger CE. The phantom of progressive dementia in epilepsy. *Lancet* 1999; 354: 2133–4 [Erratum: *Lancet* 2000; **355**: 1020].

[57] Nathaniel-James DA, Brown RG, Maier M, *et al.* Cognitive abnormalities in schizophrenia and schizophrenia-like psychosis of epilepsy. *J Neuropsychiatry Clin Neurosci* 2004; 16: 472–9.

[58] Flugel D, O'Toole A, Thompson PJ, *et al.* A neuropsychological study of patients with temporal lobe epilepsy and chronic interictal psychosis. *Epilepsy Res* 2006; 71: 117–28.

[59] Làdavas E, Umiltà C, Provinciali L. Hemisphere-dependent cognitive performances in epileptic patients. *Epilepsia* 1979; 20: 493–502.

[60] Delaney RC, Rosen AJ, Mattson RH, Novelly RA. Memory function in focal epilepsy: a comparison of non-surgical, unilateral temporal lobe and frontal lobe samples. *Cortex* 1980; 16: 103–17.

[61] Patrikelis P, Angelakis E, Gatzonis S. Neurocognitive and behavioural functioning in frontal lobe epilepsy: a review. *Epilepsy Behav* 2009; 14: 19–26.

[62] McDonald CR, Delis DC, Norman MA, Tecoma ES, Iragui VJ. Discriminating patients with frontal-lobe epilepsy and temporal-lobe epilepsy: utility of a multilevel design fluency test. *Neuropsychology* 2005; 19: 806–13.

[63] McDonald CR, Delis DC, Norman MA, *et al.* Response inhibition and set shifting in patients with frontal lobe epilepsy or temporal lobe epilepsy. *Epilepsy Behav* 2005; 7: 438–46.

[64] Farrant A, Morris RG, Russell T, *et al.* Social cognition in frontal lobe epilepsy. *Epilepsy Behav* 2005; 7: 506–16.

[65] Bertrand D, Elmslie F, Hughes E, *et al.* The CHRNB2 mutation I312M is associated with epilepsy and distinct memory deficits. *Neurobiol Dis* 2005; 20: 799–804.

[66] Cho TW, Yi SD, Lim JG, Kim DK, Motamedi GK. Autosomal dominant nocturnal frontal lobe epilepsy and mild memory impairment associated with CHRNB2 mutation I312M in the neuronal nicotinic acetylcholine receptor. *Epilepsy Behav* 2008; 13: 361–5.

[67] Rasmussen T, Olszewski J, Lloyd-Smith D. Focal seizures due to chronic localized encephalitis. *Neurology* 1958; 8: 435–45.

[68] Larner AJ, Anderson M. Rasmussen's syndrome: pathogenetic theories and therapeutic strategies. *J Neurol* 1995; 242: 355–8.

[69] Bien CG, Granata T, Antozzi C, *et al.* Pathogenesis, diagnosis and treatment of Rasmussen encephalitis. A European consensus statement. *Brain* 2005; 128: 454–71.

[70] Andermann F (ed.). *Chronic Encephalitis and Epilepsy: Rasmussen's Syndrome.* Boston, MA: Butterworth-Heinemann, 1991.

[71] McLachlan RS, Girvin JP, Blume WT, Reichman H. Rasmussen's chronic encephalitis in adults. *Arch Neurol* 1993; 50: 269–74.

[72] Larner AJ, Smith SJM, Duncan JS, Howard RS. Late-onset Rasmussen's syndrome with first seizure during pregnancy. *Eur Neurol* 1995; 35: 172.

[73] Leach JP, Chadwick DW, Miles JB, Hart IK. Improvement in adult-onset Rasmussen's encephalitis with long-term immunomodulatory therapy. *Neurology* 1999; 52: 738–42.

[74] Nicholas RS, Scott AC, Hart IK. Two clinical presentations of adult onset Rasmussen's syndrome share common immunological and pathological features. *J Neurol Neurosurg Psychiatry* 2002; 72: 141.

[75] Greiner H, Leach JL, Lee KH, Krueger DA. Anti-NMDA receptor encephalitis presenting with imaging findings and clinical features mimicking Rasmussen syndrome. *Seizure* 2011; 20: 266–70.

[76] Aldenkamp AP. Effect of seizures and epileptiform discharges on cognitive function. *Epilepsia* 1997; 38: S52–5.

[77] Dodrill CB. Neuropsychological effects of seizures. *Epilepsy Behav* 2004; 5: S21–4.

[78] Söderlund H, Percy A, Levine B. Electroconvulsive therapy for depression and autobiographical memory. In: Zeman A, Kapur N, Jones-Gotman M (eds.). *Epilepsy and Memory.* Oxford: Oxford University Press, 2012; 244–58.

[79] Binnie CD. Cognitive impairment during epileptiform discharges: is it ever justifiable to treat the EEG? *Lancet Neurol* 2003; 2: 725–30.

[80] Aldenkamp AP, Arends J. Effects of epileptiform EEG discharges on cognitive function: is the concept of "transient cognitive impairment" still valid? *Epilepsy Behav* 2004; 5: S25–34.

[81] Aldenkamp AP. Effects of epileptiform EEG discharges on cognitive function. In: Zeman A, Kapur N, Jones-Gotman M (eds.). *Epilepsy and Memory.* Oxford: Oxford University Press, 2012; 160–74.

[82] Tatum WO, Ross J, Cole AJ. Epileptic pseudodementia. *Neurology* 1998; 50: 1472–5.

[83] Høgh P, Smith SJ, Scahill RI, *et al.* Epilepsy presenting as AD: neuroimaging, electroclinical features, and response to treatment. *Neurology* 2002; 58: 298–301.

[84] Sinforiani E, Manni R, Bernasconi L, Banchieri LM, Zucchella C. Memory disturbances and temporal lobe epilepsy simulating Alzheimer's disease: a case report. *Funct Neurol* 2003; 18: 39–41.

[85] Tombini M, Koch G, Placidi F, *et al.* Temporal lobe epileptic activity mimicking dementia: a case report. *Eur J Neurol* 2005; 12: 805–6.

[86] Jackson JH. On a particular variety of epilepsy (intellectual aura). One case with symptoms of organic brain disease. *Brain* 1888; 11: 179–207.

[87] Pritchard PB III, Holmstrom VL, Roitzsch JC, Giacinto J. Epileptic amnesic attacks: benefit from antiepileptic drugs. *Neurology* 1985; 35: 1188–9.

[88] Gallassi R, Morreale A, Di Sarro R, Lugaresi E. Epileptic amnesic syndrome. *Epilepsia* 1992; 33: S21–5.

[89] Kapur N. Transient epileptic amnesia: a clinical update and a reformulation. *J Neurol Neurosurg Psychiatry* 1993; 56: 1184–90.

[90] Zeman AZJ, Boniface SJ, Hodges JR. Transient epileptic amnesia: a description of the clinical and neuropsychological features in 10 cases and a review of the literature. *J Neurol Neurosurg Psychiatry* 1998; 64: 435–43.

[91] Butler CR, Graham KS, Hodges JR, *et al.* The syndrome of transient epileptic amnesia. *Ann Neurol* 2007; 61: 587–98.

[92] Butler CR, Zeman A. The causes and consequences of transient epileptic amnesia. *Behav Neurol* 2011; 24: 299–305.

[93] Zeman A, Butler C, Hodges J, Kapur N. The syndrome of transient epileptic amnesia. In: Zeman A, Kapur N, Jones-Gotman M (eds.). *Epilepsy and Memory*. Oxford: Oxford University Press, 2012: 139–59.

[94] Manes F, Hodges JR, Graham KS, *et al.* Focal autobiographical amnesia in association with transient epileptic amnesia. *Brain* 2001; 124: 499–509.

[95] Manes F, Graham KS, Zeman A, *et al.* Autobiographical amnesia and accelerated forgetting in transient epileptic amnesia. *J Neurol Neurosurg Psychiatry* 2005; 76: 1387–91.

[96] Krishnan K, Larner AJ. Concurrent onset of transient epileptic amnesia and Alzheimer's disease. *Eur J Neurol* 2009; 16(suppl 3): 468 (abstract p. 2386).

[97] Hodges JR, Warlow CP. Syndromes of transient amnesia: towards a classification. A study of 153 cases. *J Neurol Neurosurg Psychiatry* 1990; 53: 834–43.

[98] Ung KYC, Larner AJ. Transient amnesia: epileptic or global? A differential diagnosis with significant implications for management. *Q J Med* 2012 [Epub ahead of print]

[99] Paquier PF, Van Dongen HR, Loonen CB. The Landau–Kleffner syndrome or "acquired aphasia with convulsive disorder": long-term follow-up of six children and a review of the recent literature. *Arch Neurol* 1992; 49: 354–9.

[100] Rosenbaum DH, Siegel M, Barr WB, Rowan AJ. Epileptic aphasia. *Neurology* 1986; 36: 822–5.

[101] DeToledo JC, Minagar A, Lowe MR. Persisting aphasia as the sole manifestation of partial status epilepticus. *Clin Neurol Neurosurg* 2000; 102: 144–8.

[102] Chung PW, Seo DW, Kwon JC, Kim H, Na DL. Nonconvulsive status epilepticus presenting as a subacute progressive aphasia. *Seizure* 2002; 11: 449–54.

[103] Grimes DA, Guberman A. De novo aphasic status epilepticus. *Epilepsia* 1997; 38: 945–9.

[104] Kobayashi M, Takayama H, Mihara B, Sugishita M. Partial seizure with aphasic speech arrest caused by watching a popular animated TV program. *Epilepsia* 1999; 40: 652–4.

[105] Wieshmann UC, Niehaus L, Meierkord H. Ictal speech arrest and parasagittal lesions. *Eur Neurol* 1997; 38: 123–7.

[106] Carril JM, Guijarro C, Portocarrero JS, *et al.* Speech arrest as manifestation of seizures in non-ketotic hyperglycaemia. *Lancet* 1992; 340: 1227.

[107] Ozkaya G, Kurne A, Unal S, *et al.* Aphasic status epilepticus with periodic lateralized epileptiform discharges in a bilingual patient as a presenting sign of AIDS-toxoplasmosis complex. *Epilepsy Behav* 2006; 9: 193–6.

[108] Trinka E, Unterberger I, Spiegel M, *et al.* De novo aphasic status epilepticus as presenting symptom of multiple sclerosis. *J Neurol* 2002; 249: 782–3.

[109] Sahaya K, Dhand UK, Goyal MK, Soni CR, Sahota PK. Recurrent epileptic Wernicke aphasia. *J Neurol Sci* 2010; 291: 98–9.

[110] Stirling J. *Representing Epilepsy. Myth and Matter.* Liverpool: Liverpool University Press, 2010; 148.

[111] Devinsky O. Cognitive and behavioral effects of antiepileptic drugs. *Epilepsia* 1995; 36: 46–65.

[112] Vermeulen J, Aldenkamp AP. Cognitive side-effects of chronic antiepileptic drug treatment: a review of 25 years of research. *Epilepsy Res* 1995; 22: 65–95.

[113] Mula M, Trimble MR. Antiepileptic drug-induced cognitive adverse effects: potential mechanisms and contributing factors. *CNS Drugs* 2009; 23: 121–37.

[114] Taylor J, Baker GA. Anticonvulsants and memory. In: Zeman A, Kapur N, Jones-Gotman M (eds.). *Epilepsy and Memory*. Oxford: Oxford University Press, 2012; 397–410.

[115] Shallcross R, Bromley RL, Irwin B, *et al.* Child development following in utero exposure: levetiracetam vs sodium valproate. *Neurology* 2011; 76: 383–9.

[116] Thompson PJ, Trimble MR. Anticonvulsant drugs and cognitive functions. *Epilepsia* 1982; 23: 531–44.

[117] Thompson PJ, Trimble MR. Anticonvulsant serum levels: relationship to impairments of cognitive functioning. *J Neurol Neurosurg Psychiatry* 1983; 46: 227–33.

[118] Mattson RH, Cramer JA, Collins JF, *et al.* Comparison of carbamazepine, phenobarbital, phenytoin

and primidone in partial and secondarily generalized tonic-clonic seizures. *N Engl J Med* 1985; 313: 145–51.

[119] Dodrill CB, Troupin AS. Neuropsychological effects of carbamazepine and phenytoin: a reanalysis. *Neurology* 1991; 41: 141–3.

[120] Trimble MR. Anticonvulsant drugs and cognitive function: a review of the literature. *Epilepsia* 1987; 28: 37–45.

[121] Aldenkamp AP, De Krom M, Reijs R. Newer antiepileptic drugs and cognitive issues. *Epilepsia* 2003; 44: 21–9.

[122] Aldenkamp AP, Baker G. A systematic review of the effects of lamotrigine on cognitive function and quality of life. *Epilepsy Behav* 2001; 2: 85–91.

[123] Dodrill CB, Arnett JL, Hayes AG, *et al.* Cognitive abilities and adjustment with gabapentin: results of multi-site study. *Epilepsy Res* 1999; 35: 109–21.

[124] Donati F, Gobbi G, Campistol J, *et al.* Effects of oxcarbazepine on cognitive function in children and adolescents with partial seizures. *Neurology* 2006; 67: 679–82.

[125] Martin R, Kuzniecky R, Ho S, *et al.* Cognitive effects of topiramate, gabapentin, and lamotrigine in healthy young adults. *Neurology* 1999; 52: 321–7.

[126] Huppertz HJ, Quiske A, Schulze-Bonhage A. Cognitive impairments due to add-on therapy with topiramate [in German]. *Nervenarzt* 2001; 72: 275–80.

[127] Marson AG, Al-Kharusi AM, Alwaidh M, *et al.* The SANAD study of effectiveness of carbamazepine, gabapentin, lamotrigine, oxcarbazepine, or topiramate for the treatment of partial epilepsy: an unblinded randomised controlled trial. *Lancet* 2007; 369: 1000–15.

[128] Marson AG, Al-Kharusi AM, Alwaidh M, *et al.* The SANAD study of effectiveness of valproate, lamotrigine, or topiramate for generalised and unclassifiable epilepsy: an unblinded randomised controlled trial. *Lancet* 2007; 369: 1016–26.

[129] Park SP, Hwang YH, Lee HW, *et al.* Long-term cognitive and mood effects of zonisamide monotherapy in epilepsy patients. *Epilepsy Behav* 2008; 12: 102–8.

[130] White JR, Walczak TS, Marino SE, *et al.* Zonisamide discontinuation due to psychiatric and cognitive adverse events: a case-control study. *Neurology* 2010; 75: 513–18.

[131] Wieshmann UC, Tan GM, Baker G. Self-reported symptoms in patients on antiepileptic drugs in monotherapy. *Acta Neurol Scand* 2011; 124: 355–8.

[132] Larner AJ. Cholinesterase inhibitors–beyond Alzheimer's disease. *Expert Rev Neurother* 2010; 10: 1699–705.

[133] Fisher RS, Bortz JJ, Blum DE, Duncan B, Burke H. A pilot study of donepezil for memory problems in epilepsy. *Epilepsy Behav* 2001; 2: 330–4.

[134] Hamberger MJ, Palmese CA, Scarmeas N, *et al.* A randomized double-blind placebo-controlled trial of donepezil to improve memory in epilepsy. *Epilepsia* 2007; 48: 1283–91.

[135] Griffith HR, Martin R, Andrews S, *et al.* The safety and tolerability of galantamine in patients with epilepsy and memory difficulties. *Epilepsy Behav* 2008; 13: 376–80.

Neurogenetic disorders

Although great advances have been made in elucidating the genetic basis of neurological disorders in recent years, with profound implications not only for diagnosis but also for beginning to understand disease pathogenesis, a clinical rather than a pathogenetic classification of disorders is used here, in part because the pathogenetic pathway or pathways from mutant gene to disease phenotype remain uncertain in many instances.

5.1 Hereditary dementias

Dementia syndromes with a confirmed genetic basis, with or without additional neurological features, and which have not been discussed elsewhere, are included under this rubric. Other hereditary dementias include familial (autosomal dominant) Alzheimer's disease (AD) (Section 2.1.1) and frontotemporal dementias (e.g., FTDP-17; Section 2.2.5.1), and hereditary forms of prion disease (Section 2.5.3), CADASIL (Section 3.5.1), and some of the hereditary cerebral amyloid angiopathies (Section 3.5.3).

5.1.1 Huntington's disease (HD)

In the 1872 description of the disorder that now bears his name, George Huntington not only delineated the movement disorder, most usually chorea (cortical myoclonus and parkinsonism may also occur), the neuropsychiatric features, and the mode of inheritance, but also alluded to the gradually

progressive impairment of the mind [1]. Cognition is one of the four characteristics, along with motor function, behavior, and functional abilities, assessed by the Unified Huntington's Disease Rating Scale (UHDRS), which has now become the universal scale for measuring HD function [2].

HD results from a trinucleotide (CAG, polyglutamine, polyQ) repeat expansion in the IT15 gene on chromosome 4 (OMIM#143100), which encodes the huntingtin protein [3]. A significant inverse relationship exists between the CAG repeat length and age at clinical onset. Clinical phenotype also varies with age of onset; juvenile disease (Westphal variant; onset before the age of 20 years) has a prominent parkinsonian syndrome and sometimes epileptic seizures whereas very late-onset disease may be associated with chorea and little intellectual impairment. Neuropathologically, there is a loss of medium spiny neurons and gliosis in the caudate nucleus and putamen, resulting in shrinkage of the caudate that may be observed on structural brain imaging, as well as degenerative change in the cortex and hippocampus. Intranuclear inclusions immunopositive for huntingtin and ubiquitin are found [4]. The availability of a diagnostic neurogenetic test has made possible not only definitive diagnosis of symptomatic cases but also the detection of presymptomatic cases in at-risk family members. Such predictive testing should only be undertaken with appropriate genetic counseling under the auspices of accredited clinical genetics services, guidelines for which exist [5].

HD phenocopies, without trinucleotide repeats in the huntingtin gene, are described [6]. These

Table 5.1. Typical neuropsychological deficits in Huntington's disease

Attention	↓ Divided, sustained attention; impaired working memory
Memory	"Subcortical pattern": impaired encoding and retrieval, recognition better than recall; impaired skill learning. Semantic memory relatively spared
Language	Naming errors. Impaired oral and reading comprehension. Letter fluency worse than category fluency
Perception	Visuoperceptual problems: defects in judging distance, spatial relationships
Praxis	Ideomotor apraxia
Executive function	Dysexecutive syndrome (impaired Stroop, Wisconsin Card Sorting Test); may contribute to many of the observed neuropsychological deficits

Huntington's disease-like (HDL) syndromes include insertions in the prion protein PRNP gene (Section 2.5.3), and expansions in the genes encoding JPH3 junctophilin or the TATA box-binding protein gene (TBP), the latter allelic with spinocerebellar ataxia (SCA) type 17 (Section 5.2.1.9). SCA8 may also cause a HD phenocopy syndrome occasionally (Section 5.2.1.6). Other conditions that enter the differential diagnosis of HD include dentatorubropallidoluysian atrophy (Section 5.1.2), neuroferritinopathy (Section 5.4.5), pantothenate-kinase-associated neurodegeneration (Section 5.4.3), and neuroacanthocytosis (Section 5.4.4) [6].

As yet, no curative treatment is available for HD and symptomatic treatments are limited in their effect. The natural history is one of relentless progression. Cell-based treatments (neural transplantation) remain experimental [7].

Neuropsychological profile (Table 5.1)

The cognitive disorder of HD has been investigated extensively [8]. Following the characterization of "subcortical dementia" in progressive supranuclear palsy (Sections 1.3.3.1 and 2.4.3) [9], the core deficits in HD were also labeled as subcortical [10], and subsequent investigations have confirmed a pattern of cognitive deficits distinct from that in AD. Using the Mini-Mental State Examination (MMSE), HD patients perform worse than AD patients on the attention item (serial sevens) but better on the orientation in time and memory items [11]. Likewise, HD patients administered the Mattis

Dementia Rating Scale show more impairment on the initiation/perseveration subtest and less impairment on the memory subtest than AD patients [12]. Reviewing a large number of studies of HD patients, Zakzanis [13] reported deficits in memory acquisition and delayed recall, cognitive flexibility, abstraction, attention, and concentration. It may be that a dysexecutive syndrome accounts for the poor performance in many areas, reflective of pathological involvement of the basal ganglia and frontostriatal connections. The natural history of cognitive function is one of decline, but the rate is variable as are the different domains affected. In one longitudinal study, significant decline was detected over a one-year period in low-level psychomotor tasks, object recall, and verbal fluency whereas executive function (Wisconsin Card Sorting Test; WCST) remained stable [14]. However, in a group of mild to moderate HD patients studied over a three-year period, progressive impairments were noted in attention, executive function, immediate memory, and timed tests of psychomotor skill while semantic memory and delayed recall memory were relatively preserved [15]. Cognitive decline may also occur early in the course of juvenile HD [16].

Attention

Attentional control mechanisms are compromised in symptomatic HD [11], as attested to by poor performance on Wechsler Adult Intelligence Scale (WAIS) subtests such as Digit Span and Digit Symbol, which probe attention and working memory.

Shifting of attention to new information may be particularly impaired, whereas attention to previously learned information is maintained with perseveration on previously correct responses [17]. This may be manifested in the clinical observation that HD patients perform worse when required to divide attention between tasks or stimuli. Selective and progressive attentional and executive dysfunctions are features of early HD [15], and assessment of attentional tasks has been used to monitor disease progression [18].

Neglect, an attentional deficit resulting in a failure to orient or respond to stimuli in one side of space, has rarely been reported in HD [19].

Memory

Learning and memory difficulties are a common complaint of HD patients and their relatives. There is a problem with information encoding and retrieval, as verbal recognition memory is preserved relative to recall [20]. This may relate to inefficient encoding strategies, itself reflective of executive dysfunction. Retention of information over a delay period is relatively intact, hence there is no abnormal forgetting [21], and on remote memory tests there is no temporal gradient. Compared to AD individuals, HD patients matched for overall level of dementia had less impairment of delayed verbal and figural episodic memory but were worse on letter fluency, suggesting a double dissociation of semantic and episodic memory impairment [22]. Semantic memory and delayed recall memory are relatively unaffected in early HD [15] but visuospatial memory may be impaired [17].

Implicit memory as tested by skill learning is impaired in HD, indicating a role for the basal ganglia in such learning processes, particularly "open-loop" skills, a finding which possibly may be related to working memory deficits.

Language

Naming errors in HD seem to be largely visually based, reflecting disrupted perceptual analysis, while phonemic processes remain relatively intact [23]. This contrasts with the semantic breakdown observed in AD, and is corroborated by verbal fluency tests showing greater impairment in letter fluency rather than semantic fluency in HD, even early in the disease [22,24], presumably related to frontostriatal dysfunction. Late deficits in confrontation naming are more likely due to visuoperceptual deficits and retrieval slowing rather than a disintegration of semantic knowledge. In a systematic study of language function in HD, compared to controls impairments in oral comprehension, repetition, oral agility, and reading comprehension as well as poorer verbal fluency were noted [25].

The motor disorder of HD may affect phonation, speech output becoming increasingly limited as the disease progresses. Apathy and psychomotor slowing may also contribute to this loss of speech. Additionally, there may be impaired comprehension of affective and propositional speech prosody [26].

Perception

Visuospatial disorder may be evident on object assembly and block design tasks and tests of pattern and spatial recognition memory, but again these deficits may reflect problems with other processes such as planning [27]. A defect in the perception of personal (egocentric) space has been documented consistently, with difficulty judging distances and the spatial relationship to other objects [28], the clinical correlate of which is a tendency to bump into things; it may contribute to falls. Impaired contrast sensitivity for moving sinusoidal gratings has also been noted [29].

Praxis

Although the assessment of praxis may be difficult in the context of the motor disorder of HD, nonetheless occasional studies have been undertaken. Shelton and Knopman [30] found ideomotor apraxia to be common in a small cohort of patients with long-standing disease (mean duration >10 yr), particularly for imitation of nonsymbolic movements, whereas recognition of gestures was preserved. These changes were thought to be primarily subcortical in origin. However, Hamilton *et al.* [31] found apraxia to be more common in patients with greater neurological involvement and longer disease duration, suggesting that apraxia resulted from damage to corticostriate pathways rather than restricted basal ganglia involvement as in early disease, which fits better with the notion of apraxia as a feature of cortical dementias. Hödl *et al.* [32] confirmed the high frequency of ideomotor limb apraxia in HD, which they found to be independent of cognitive decline and the severity of most neurological symptoms.

Executive function

Progressive impairment in executive function is found in early HD [17,19] and is associated with bilateral striatal (caudate) and extrastriatal (insular) atrophy [33]. Typical of patients with executive deficits, verbal fluency tests show poor category fluency but worse letter fluency, the reverse of the pattern seen in AD [24], plus impairments on the Stroop Test and the WCST [18]. This dysexecutive syndrome may account for many of the cognitive impairments documented in HD, due to striatal and corticostriatal involvement. Assessment of executive functions may be used to monitor progression of disease [18].

Presymptomatic gene mutation carriers

With the characterization of the CAG trinucleotide repeat expansion on chromosome 4 as deterministic for HD [3], testing of presymptomatic, perhaps better termed premanifest carriers of the HD gene mutation has become possible. Such studies have indicated that cognitive impairment may be present at least 15 years prior to motor diagnosis [8], yet in clinical practice, HD almost invariably presents as a consequence of movement disorder rather than because of cognitive decline [34].

While premanifest HD patients show little cognitive deterioration compared to controls [35,36], those nearing clinical onset may show deficits in sustained attention and mental processing speed. There is an association between CAG repeat length and poorer performance on learning and memory tests, suggesting that cognitive deficits may be an early, subclinical manifestation of disease [37]. In one study, these premanifest deficits were suggested to be highly specific for attentional set shifting and semantic verbal fluency, reflecting impaired striatofrontal mechanisms [38]. In another study, carriers performed worse on digit symbol, picture arrangement, and arithmetic tests, and also showed mild impairment on reaction time tasks [39]. A prospective study of genetically defined disease carriers found impairments in attentional and visuoperceptual and executive functions compared to controls [18]. Clearly, these observations of cognitive impairments in premanifest carriers have implications for preventive therapeutic strategies and monitoring of the efficacy of therapeutic measures.

5.1.2 Dentatorubropallidoluysian atrophy (DRPLA)

This autosomal dominant trinucleotide repeat disorder due to a CAG (polyglutamine) expansion in the gene encoding atrophin-1 on chromosome 12p13.31 (OMIM#125370) often has a clinical presentation identical to HD, with movement disorders including chorea, dystonia, myoclonus, and parkinsonism, as well as cerebellar ataxia, psychosis, and epilepsy; the latter may be more common than in HD. Likewise, cognitive dysfunction similar to that in HD may be seen, including slowed thinking, difficulty retrieving information, and in sequencing tasks, progressing to a more severe dementia; in other words, a subcortical pattern of deficits [40,41]. Chiefly described in reports from Japan, DRPLA has also been seen in European and North American families, in which clinical features are noted to be heterogeneous even within individual families.

5.1.3 Familial British dementia (FBD) and familial Danish dementia (FDD)

Familial British dementia (FBD), previously known as Worster–Drought syndrome, is an autosomal dominant progressive dementia syndrome, with associated cerebellar ataxia and spastic paraparesis with pathological evidence of deposition of cerebrovascular amyloid distinct from that observed in AD [42,43]. Familial Danish dementia (FDD), originally known as heredopathia ophthalmo-oto-encephalica, is an autosomal dominant disorder characterized by cataracts and ocular hemorrhages occurring around the age of 30 years, impaired hearing and hearing loss in the 40s–50s, cerebellar ataxia in the 40s, and paranoid psychosis and dementia in the 50s [44]. Both FBD and FDD result from mutations in the ITM2B gene (previously known as the BRI gene) on chromosome 13q14.2 (OMIM#176500 and #117300, respectively), in which substitution in a stop codon increases the length of the open reading frame, resulting in the production of amyloidogenic C-terminal peptides [45,46]. These conditions are sometimes classified with the cerebral amyloid angiopathies (Section 3.5.3).

Memory impairment early in the course of FBD is marked, ultimately progressing to global dementia. Personality change, either irritability or depression, may also be an early manifestation [43]. In a study of patients at risk, cognitive problems were identified in some patients thought to be affected clinically (with limb/gait ataxia, mild spastic paraparesis). Impairments in delayed recognition and, particularly, recall memory were found, with additional impairments in delayed visual recall in some patients. General intelligence, naming, frontal lobe functions, and perception were preserved. These changes were associated with deep white matter hyperintensities and lacunar infarcts on MRI of the brain [47].

5.1.4 Familial encephalopathy with neuroserpin inclusion bodies (FENIB)

This rare autosomal dominant disorder is one of the serpinopathies linked to a point mutation in the gene on chromosome 3 encoding neuroserpin (OMIM#604218), a serine proteinase inhibitor, the mutant protein undergoing polymerization. FENIB is characterized pathologically by cytoplasmic neuroserpin inclusions (Collins bodies) within the deep cortical layers, substantia nigra, and subcortical nuclei. Clinical phenotype is determined by genotype; neuroserpin mutations causing greater conformational change (G392E) result in early onset progressive myoclonus epilepsy, whereas lesser degrees of conformational change (S49P) cause dementia in the fifth decade of life [48,49].

Neuropsychological assessment of patients with the S49P mutation in the neuroserpin gene showed frontal or frontosubcortical impairment in mildly to moderately affected individuals, with impaired attention, concentration, and response regulation functions, while recall memory was not as affected as other cognitive domains. A more global pattern of impairment was seen in more severely affected individuals. This pattern was corroborated by single-photon emission computed tomography (SPECT) imaging studies, which showed exclusively frontal anomalies in the less affected patients, with more global but patchy hypoperfusion in the more severely affected individuals [50].

5.1.5 Polycystic lipomembranous osteodysplasia with sclerosing leukoencephalopathy (PLOSL); Nasu–Hakola disease; presenile dementia with bone cysts

This autosomal recessive disorder, described in both Japan and Finland, is characterized by large-scale destruction of cancellous bone, resulting in bone cysts in the third decade of life that cause pain, swelling, and sometimes fracture of the wrists and ankles; and presenile dementia in the fourth decade, sometimes with epileptic seizures. MRI of the brain reveals frontal myelin loss and massive gliosis ("sclerosing leukoencephalopathy") as well as basal ganglia calcification. The condition is genetically heterogeneous, with mutations being identified in the TYROBP (also known as DAP12) gene on chromosome 19q13.12 (deletions, point mutations, and single base deletions) in some families, and in the TREM2 gene on chromosome 6p21.1 in others (OMIM#221770). Both genes encode subunits of a multisubunit receptor complex, resulting in an identical phenotype [51].

The cognitive impairment in PLOSL may be of the frontal lobe type, sometimes without preceding osseous symptoms [52]. Healthy subjects heterozygous for a TREM2 mutation have been reported with a deficit of visuospatial memory, with basal ganglia hypoperfusion on functional neuroimaging (SPECT), not seen in homozygotes for the wild-type allele [53].

5.2 Hereditary ataxias

Classically, the cerebellum has been viewed as a component of the motor system, with damage resulting in motor signs of localizing value (ataxia, dysdiadochokinesia, nystagmus), first clearly defined by Gordon Holmes (1876–1965) [54]. A role for the cerebellum in cognition has been acknowledged increasingly in recent times (Section 1.3.3.2), particularly since the description of a "cerebellar cognitive affective syndrome" in association with posterior lobe and vermis lesions, characterized by executive dysfunction (in set-shifting, planning, verbal fluency, abstract reasoning, working memory) and difficulties with spatial cognition, memory, and language, as well as personality change [55]. In this section, hereditary ataxias are considered according to their pattern of inheritance, although a pathogenetic classification of the hereditary ataxias may be more appropriate eventually [56]. So-called idiopathic late-onset cerebellar ataxias, possibly with added cognitive problems, may be caused by multiple system atrophy (MSA-C; Section 2.4.5), fragile-X tremor/ataxia syndrome (FXTAS; Section

5.4.1), or gluten sensitivity with or without celiac disease (Section 8.2.1.3).

5.2.1 Autosomal dominant cerebellar ataxias (ADCA); spinocerebellar ataxias (SCA)

The phenotypic classification of autosomal dominant cerebellar ataxias (ADCA) proposed by Anita Harding (1952–1995) acknowledged the concurrence of dementia in some patients with these conditions, specifically in type I, whereas type II was characterized by pigmentary maculopathy and type III by a pure ataxia [57]. This nosology has been superseded by a genotypic classification of the SCAs based on the discovery of gene loci and specific genetic mutations responsible for some of these syndromes. At the time of writing, over 30 loci had been defined. SCAs are characterized by ataxia of gait and limb, ataxic dysarthria, spasticity, and decreased vibration perception, with additional parkinsonism, tremor, neuropathy, ophthalmoparesis, and epileptic seizures, with cognitive impairment in some cases. Marked cerebellar atrophy, sometimes with cerebral cortical atrophy, is seen on structural brain imaging. Variability of phenotype despite identical genetic mutation may occur. Several SCAs may fall within the old clinical classification of ADCA type I (i.e., with cognitive impairment), including SCAs 1–4, 12, and 17. Clues to the particular SCA may be obtained from clinical examination; the presence of early and/or prominent dementia suggests that SCA2 or SCA17 may be the cause. Guidelines for the molecular genetic testing of SCAs have appeared [58].

The differential diagnosis of hereditary ataxias also includes the episodic ataxias, channelopathies, the prion disease Gerstmann–Straussler–Scheinker disease (GSS; Section 2.5.3), and vanishing white matter disease (Section 5.5.2.6). Although episodic ataxia type 2 (EA2) is allelic with one form of familial hemiplegic migraine (Section 3.6.1) and with SCA6 (Section 5.2.1.4), both of which have been associated with cognitive impairments, at the time of writing no report of cognitive dysfunction in EA2 had been identified.

5.2.1.1 SCA1

SCA1 is associated with a CAG/polyQ mutation in the ataxin-1 gene at 6p22.3 (OMIM#164400). Generally, intellect remains intact until the late stages of disease when behavioral changes and a frontal lobe-like syndrome may occur. One study found impairments of verbal memory and executive dysfunction with relative preservation of visuospatial memory and attention, a pattern labeled as typical of frontosubcortical dementia [59]. As for other SCAs, cognitive impairments were not related to age of onset, disease duration, or trinucleotide repeat length.

5.2.1.2 SCA2

SCA2 is associated with a CAG/polyQ mutation in the ataxin-2 gene at 12q24.12 (OMIM#183090); expansions in this gene are also associated with the development of motor neuron disease. Although ataxia is the chief sign, SCA2 may also produce a levodopa-responsive parkinsonism, and cognitive changes are sometimes prominent. In one series, 25% of patients were demented, and cognitive defects were also apparent in nondemented individuals [60]. Impairments have been noted in frontal executive function, as measured by the Stroop Test, verbal fluency, and WCST. Attention and verbal and visual memory are sometimes affected [61,62]. Various studies have reached different conclusions as regards correlations between cognitive deficits and age at disease onset, clinical severity, and motor disability [60–65].

5.2.1.3 SCA3, Machado–Joseph disease (MJD)

This is probably the most common dominantly inherited ataxia worldwide, resulting from a CAG/polyQ mutation in the ataxin-3 gene at 14q32.12 (OMIM#109150). In addition to ataxia, there is levodopa-responsive parkinsonism, and variable peripheral involvement, ophthalmoparesis, and lingual and facial fasciculations. Cognitive

impairments have also been described, sometimes amounting to a mild dementia [66]. Deficits in visual attentional function with slowed processing of visual information were reported using a computerized test battery, along with inability to shift attention to previously irrelevant stimuli; learning and visual memory were normal. A fronto-subcortical pattern of impairments was claimed, apparently independent of motor dysfunction [67]. Abnormal behavior, uncooperativeness, crying, slow thought processes, hallucinations, and delusions were reported in four Japanese patients, developing disease after the age of 40 years and progressing to dementia [68]. Deficits in memory, executive functions, naming, and attention, with preserved calculation and visuospatial processing have also been reported in SCA3 [69]. Depressive symptoms have been said to characterize SCA3 [70].

5.2.1.4 SCA6

SCA6 results from a CAG/polyQ mutation in the alpha1A voltage-dependent calcium channel (CACNA1A) gene at chromosome 19p13.2 (OMIM#183086), and is allelic with some cases of familial hemiplegic migraine (Section 3.6.1) and episodic ataxia type 2. This common SCA is generally a "pure" cerebellar ataxia, hence originally classified as ADCA type III [57], and thus provides an intriguing opportunity to examine possible contributions of the cerebellum to cognitive functioning.

A case of SCA6 with slowly progressive mental disorders labeled as schizophrenia and dementia has been reported [71]. A more systematic study found deficits in memory, executive functions, naming, and attention but with preserved calculation and visuospatial processing [69]. In a Japanese study, verbal fluency and immediate visual memory were markedly impaired, independent of ataxic motor dysfunction [72]. The largest study reported to date (n = 27) found no intellectual or memory decline in SCA6 but executive dysfunction, involving cognitive flexibility, inhibition of response, and verbal reasoning and abstraction. These data were felt to support a role for the cerebellum in cognitive processes [73]. Imaging studies in this cohort have suggested the specific cerebellar subregions that may play a role in verbal working memory [74]. The memory symptoms seen in other SCA groups are said to be relatively spared in SCA6 [70].

5.2.1.5 SCA7

SCA7 results from a CAG/polyQ mutation in the ataxin-7 gene at chromosome 3p14.1 (OMIM#164500). The clinical phenotype is marked by progressive visual loss due to retinal dystrophy, hence the condition was originally classified as ADCA type II [57]. Dementia has been mentioned as a symptom in some cases [75].

5.2.1.6 SCA8

SCA8 results from a CTA/CTG expansion in the ataxin-8 gene at chromosome 13q21 (OMIM#608768). Two of seven patients with SCA8 in a case series reported from Portugal were said to have mild to moderate memory impairment [76]. A study of ten patients in Finland noted deficits in executive functions, with memory and visuoperceptual functions preserved [77]. A dysexecutive syndrome was also noted in SCA8 patients from Scotland [78]. A Greek patient with HD phenocopy syndrome was found to have a SCA8 expansion; memory decline and impairment of frontal assessment tests were associated with choreiform movements and psychiatric symptoms [79].

5.2.1.7 SCA12

SCA12 results from a CAG expansion in the PPP2R2B gene at chromosome 5q32 (OMIM#604326). Dementia has been reported in some patients in the later stages of SCA12. Disorientation, memory loss, inability to calculate, and perseveration were the reported clinical features [80].

5.2.1.8 SCA15

In an Italian family with SCA15, a disorder resulting from mutations or deletions of the ITPR1 gene on chromosome 3p26 (OMIM#606658), all affected members presented with cognitive impairment as well as gait ataxia, dysarthria, and impaired balance, with or without involuntary movements [81].

5.2.1.9 SCA 17

Cognitive decline and dementia, as well as extrapyramidal features are common in SCA17 [82], resulting from a CAG/polyQ mutation in the TATA binding protein gene (TBP or TFIID) at chromosome 6q27 (OMIM#607136). Behavioral disorder and dementia may dominate the early stages of disease. This is one of the Huntington's disease-like (HDL) syndromes (Section 5.1.1) [6]. In a study of 15 Italian patients, 9 of 11 symptomatic individuals had cognitive impairment, but no further neuropsychological characterization was presented [83]. A frontal picture with distractibility, poor judgment, and impaired verbal fluency has been reported [84].

5.2.1.10 SCA19

Frontal executive dysfunction has been recorded in a Dutch family with SCA19, linked to chromosome 1p21-q21, with some members developing global cognitive impairment [85].

5.2.1.11 SCA21

Mild cognitive impairment has been reported in a French family with SCA21, linked to chromosome 7p21.3-p15.1 [86].

5.2.2 Autosomal recessive hereditary ataxias

5.2.2.1 Friedreich's ataxia (FA)

The most common autosomal recessive cause of ataxia, Friedreich's ataxia (FA) is a disorder characterized by ataxia, dysarthria, axonal polyneuropathy, and pyramidal weakness of the legs (absent ankle jerks and upgoing plantar reflexes), optic atrophy, scoliosis, and cardiac conduction abnormalities, usually with onset before the age of 20 years. Intronic trinucleotide (GAA) repeat expansions in the frataxin gene on chromosome 9q13 (OMIM#229300) are the cause of FA, resulting in disordered mitochondrial function. Some FA patients are compound heterozygotes with GAA expansion on one allele and a point mutation on the other. The clinical phenotype has broadened as a result of the discovery of the causative genetic mutations [87].

Any assessment of neuropsychological function in FA must take account of possible confounders such as dysarthria and fatigue, and any educational shortcomings as a consequence of physical disability. Nonetheless, studies suggest that FA is attended by cognitive impairments, such as lengthened mental reaction times and color–word interference in the Stroop task. One study found no impairment in tests sensitive to neocortical (particularly prefrontal cortex) function, including verbal fluency, WCST, Tower of Hanoi, and picture arrangement [88], whereas another found deficits in letter fluency, as well as impaired acquisition and consolidation of verbal information, and alterations in visuoperceptual and visuoconstructive abilities [89]. All studies agree that cerebellar degeneration and interruption of cerebellar afferent and efferent connections is probably responsible for these findings.

5.2.2.2 Ataxia telangiectasia (AT)

This childhood onset autosomal recessive syndrome is characterized by progressive ataxia, oculomotor apraxia requiring head thrusts to achieve ocular fixation, dysarthria, telangiectasia, and a tendency to develop recurrent infections (especially sinopulmonary) and malignancies. The molecular defect is in the ATM gene on chromosome 11 (OMIM#208900), which encodes a protein required for DNA repair.

Cognitive status is said to be normal in most cases, some patients completing university level education, and significant neuropsychological impairments have been said to be uncommon. However, Colvin and Lennox [90] reported frontal lobe dysfunction in a series of 18 AT patients as assessed with WCST, Tower of London Test, verbal fluency, and similarities. Impairments of visual memory assessed with the Warrington Recognition Memory Test, and failure on some elements of the Visual Object and Space Perception Battery (VOSP), were attributed to impaired oculomotor function. Mild to moderate cognitive impairment was detected in eight children with AT, with deficits in attention, nonverbal memory, and verbal fluency [91].

5.2.2.3 Autosomal recessive spastic ataxia of Charlevoix–Saguenay (ARSACS)

This autosomal recessive disorder of childhood, initially reported from northeastern Quebec in Canada, is characterized by childhood onset of a slowly progressive pyramidal syndrome, dysarthria, ataxia, abnormal eye movements (nystagmus), retinal striation (i.e., hypermyelinated retinal fibers), sphincter involvement, mitral incompetence, and motor neuropathy. It has been classified variously as either a "complicated" hereditary spastic paraplegia (Section 5.3) or as an early onset autosomal recessive cerebellar ataxia with retained reflexes. Pedigrees from Quebec and Tunisia showed linkage to chromosome 13q11–12, whence positional cloning techniques permitted characterization of the sacsin gene (OMIM#270550). Many sacsin gene mutations have now been reported from pedigrees throughout the world, expanding the spectrum of sacsinopathies [92]. Cognitive function is usually not affected but two siblings reported from Japan had a unique phenotype of dementia, ophthalmoplegia, and absence of prominent retinal myelinated fibers [93]. The cerebellar cognitive affective syndrome [55] has been reported in two siblings with ARSACS, one of whom presented with behavioral disinhibition [94].

5.2.2.4 Ataxia with vitamin E deficiency (AVED)

This autosomal recessive disorder manifests as spinocerebellar ataxia and polyneuropathy without evidence of cognitive impairment, suggesting that vitamin E may not be crucial to cognitive function.

5.3 Hereditary spastic paraplegia (HSP)

The hereditary spastic paraplegias (HSP) are a heterogeneous group of inherited motor system disorders, typically presenting with lower limb spasticity and, to a lesser extent, weakness. Clinically, HSP may be divided into pure (uncomplicated; mostly autosomal dominant) and complicated (mostly autosomal recessive) types, the latter manifesting other neurological features in addition to spasticity, such as epileptic seizures, amyotrophy, extrapyramidal signs, peripheral neuropathy, and cognitive impairment sometimes amounting to dementia. Subtle cognitive deficits have also been detected in so-called "pure" HSP types. Cognitive impairment has been noted in both autosomal recessive [95] and autosomal dominant [96] HSP.

At the time of writing, approaching 50 genetic loci linked to HSP had been described, with dominant, recessive, and X-linked patterns of inheritance, and deterministic mutations have been described in more than a dozen genes, encoding the proteins L1-CAM, proteolipid protein (PLP), atlastin, spastin, CYP7B1, NIPA1, paraplegin, strumpellin, spatacsin, spastizin, spartin, maspardin, hsp60, and KIF5A. Guidelines for the molecular genetic testing of HSPs have appeared [97].

Spastic paraparesis may be a feature of other monogenic Mendelian disorders, which may also be associated with cognitive impairment, such as some examples of autosomal dominant AD (Section 2.1.1) associated with certain of the presenilin-1 mutations [98], some of the hereditary cerebral amyloid angiopathies (Section 3.5.3), and autosomal recessive spastic ataxia of Charlevoix–Saguenay (ARSACS; Section 5.2.2.3). Spastic paraparesis has also been reported in Krabbe disease (Section 5.5.2.5).

5.3.1 SPG4

The most common form of autosomal dominant HSP is that linked to the SPG4 locus encoding the spastin gene on chromosome 2p22 (OMIM#182601). Although classified as a pure form of HSP, cognitive deficits have been noted in patients, sometimes amounting to a global dementia with a profile similar to that in subcortical dementias. Mild cognitive problems may be the first clinical manifestation in spastin gene carriers. Studies in Irish families reported cognitive decline affecting orientation, memory, and language, which was age-dependent and progressive over time [99–101], whereas in a French study, cognitive decline was found to be correlated with disease progression and not with age [102]. This study found only mild, asymptomatic, cognitive loss, particularly affecting executive functions, that was more frequently observed in patients with missense rather than truncating spastin mutations.

5.3.2 SPG21, Mast syndrome

Mast syndrome, also known as SPG21, is an autosomal recessive, complicated form of HSP with a clinical phenotype of paraplegia, dysarthria, athetosis, and dementia, with onset in the second decade of life. It was originally described in the Old Order Amish community [103], but possible non-Amish cases have been reported with a phenotype of bradyphrenia and comprehension difficulties in the patients' 40s, progressing to rare and inappropriate single syllable answers in their 50s [104]. SPG21 is slowly progressive, with cerebellar and extrapyramidal features emerging in advanced disease. It maps to chromosome 15q22.31 and frameshift mutations have been identified in a gene named maspardin [105].

5.4 Hereditary movement disorders

The focus here is largely on movement disorders that show a monogenic Mendelian pattern of inheritance with identified genetic mutations. Restless legs syndrome, which may have genetic determinants, is discussed with sleep-related disorders (Section 11.5.1); Tourette syndrome, which is frequently accompanied by obsessive-compulsive disorders, is discussed with psychiatric disorders (Section 12.4.1).

5.4.1 Fragile-X syndrome (FRAX), fragile-X tremor/ataxia syndrome (FXTAS)

Fragile-X-associated disorders include the fragile-X syndrome (FRAX) and the fragile-X tremor/ataxia syndrome (FXTAS) [106,107].

FRAX is the most common genetically determined cause of intellectual disability in males [108], resulting from a trinucleotide (CGG) repeat expansion in the 5′ promoter region of the fragile site mental retardation 1 (FMR1) gene, located on the X chromosome (OMIM#300624) [109]. Various mechanisms may mediate the effects of this mutation, including effects on the cytoplasmic protein FMRP, which has RNA-binding properties, and on synaptic plasticity [107]. Healthy male patients with FRAX have been reported to show poorer attention and short-term memory function than a comparison group of Down's syndrome patients [110]. Women with FRAX are worse than controls on tests of executive function [111].

Lesser numbers of CGG repeats in the FMR1 gene, 50–200, are termed premutations and are associated with the fragile-X tremor/ataxia syndrome (FXTAS; OMIM#300623) [106,107]. Clinically, FXTAS is characterized by progressive cerebellar ataxia and tremor (which may be postural, action, or resting), with or without parkinsonism, peripheral neuropathy, and autonomic features, symptoms which do not occur in FRAX and which have caused frequent misdiagnosis of FXTAS, for example, as other tremor or ataxia syndromes [112]. MRI of the brain typically shows high signal intensity lesions on T_2-weighted images in the cerebellar peduncles and in white matter inferior and lateral to the deep cerebellar nuclei, with additional cerebellar and cortical atrophy [113,114].

Cognitive impairment and dementia may also be a feature of FXTAS, which has been misdiagnosed as a dementia syndrome of the Alzheimer or vascular type [112], although one study found no cognitive deficits in premutation carriers under the age of 50 years old [115]. In those who develop cognitive problems, deficits in the domains of short-term memory and executive function were specified initially and included in suggested diagnostic criteria [114]. A study of over 100 patients found that men with FXTAS scored worse than normal controls in measures of intelligence, working memory, remote recall, declarative learning and memory, information processing speed, and executive function, but with relative sparing of language and verbal comprehension, while asymptomatic carriers of the premutation were worse than controls in declarative learning and memory, and executive function [116]. The profile was dissimilar to that seen in mild AD [117].

FXTAS has also been described in women. Some were reported to perform poorly on certain tests of visual selective attention [118], but initially it was thought that dementia did not occur [119]. More recent studies have identified women who develop dementia [120,121], some with typical AD pathology suggesting a possible synergistic effect [121].

5.4.2 Wilson's disease (hepatolenticular degeneration)

Wilson's disease is an autosomal recessive disorder of copper metabolism resulting from mutations in the ATP7B gene on chromosome 13q14.3–q21.1 (OMIM#277900), which encodes a copper-binding membrane-bound ATPase, resulting in elevated blood and urine copper and reduced blood ceruloplasmin levels. The condition usually presents in young adults with hepatic and/or neurological disease due to accumulation of copper in affected tissues. In the brain, although copper deposition occurs throughout, it is the basal ganglia that are particularly vulnerable, resulting in movement disorders (parkinsonism, dystonia, grimacing, excessive salivation); likewise the cerebellum (ataxia, wing-beating tremor, dysarthria). Copper deposition in the eye in Descemet's membrane may be observed as Kayser–Fleischer rings, a reliable sign of brain copper deposition. Neuropsychiatric features are also common, such as personality change, depression, and occasionally psychosis. Motor and neuropsychiatric features might possibly confound neuropsychological testing in Wilson's disease.

In his seminal paper on the disorder that now bears his name, Kinnier Wilson [122] noted a distinct pattern of neurobehavioral disturbances without agnosia, apraxia, or severe memory loss in association with disease of the basal ganglia. The cognitive impairments in patients with neurological and/or hepatic symptoms may be mild [123], or involvement may be widespread, including impaired memory, visuospatial processing, attention, and frontal-executive functions [124–126]. Rate of information processing may be spared, although response latencies are prolonged, probably as a consequence of the motor disorder [127]. Neuropsychological deficits may be present early in the course of the disease [128], but patients with exclusive hepatic involvement do not differ from controls, and adequate early treatment may prevent cognitive decline [129]. If untreated, dementia develops with disease progression, hence the need to screen all younger patients with movement disorders for abnormalities of copper metabolism. Once established, the dementia is generally held to be irreversible, although anecdotal reports of cognitive (as well as motor) improvement after chelation therapy [130] and liver transplantation ([131], case 2) have appeared.

5.4.3 Neurodegeneration with brain iron accumulation (NBIA); pantothenate-kinase-associated neurodegeneration (PKAN)

Mutations in the gene encoding pantothenate kinase (PANK2) on chromosome 20p13 (OMIM#234200) have been identified in the disorder variously known as neurodegeneration with brain iron accumulation (NBIA) or pantothenate-kinase-associated neurodegeneration (PKAN) [132]. Typically, this is a disorder of either familial or sporadic origin with childhood onset with a fairly homogeneous phenotype of dystonia, dysarthria, rigidity, choreoathetosis, and pigmentary retinopathy. "Atypical" cases are usually of later onset (second to third decade of life), with speech difficulty, with or without extrapyramidal and pyramidal signs, and in some cases cognitive decline that is said to be reminiscent of FTD with personality change, impulsivity, violent outbursts, and emotional lability. Neuropathological findings are of pallidal iron deposition, axonal spheroids, and gliosis. T_2-weighted MRI scans of the brain may show decreased signal intensity in the pallidal nuclei with central hyperintensity, the "eye-of-the-tiger" sign, which is highly suggestive of the diagnosis although not specific. PANK2 mutations have been found in both classic cases and in around one-third of atypical late-onset cases [133,134].

Historically, PKAN has been associated with cognitive decline, but a recent study of childhood cases has questioned whether, in fact, such findings are confounded by dystonia [135]. A neuropsychological profile of bradyphrenia, reduced verbal fluency, judgment difficulties, and attentional impairment, but with relative preservation of memory (i.e., of frontosubcortical type, as might be expected) has been reported. Phenotype may be variable, even in siblings sharing the same mutation [136].

5.4.4 Neuroacanthocytosis

There are various neuroacanthocytosis syndromes [137], of which chorea–acanthocytosis is a multisystem neurodegenerative disorder inherited as an autosomal recessive condition linked to chromosome 9q21 and associated with mutations in the VPS13A gene encoding the protein chorein (OMIM#200150). The clinical phenotype includes movement disorders (orofaciolingual dystonia, chorea, parkinsonism), axonal polyneuropathy, epileptic seizures, and neuropsychiatric abnormalities, as well as cognitive impairments. Salient investigation findings are acanthocytes on fresh blood films (more than one film may need to be examined) and raised creatine phosphokinase, but there is no abnormality of lipid metabolism [138].

Personality change such as impulsive and distractible behavior or apathy and loss of insight may be observed, and is sometimes sufficient to prompt legal intervention [139]. Consistent with this suggestion of frontal lobe dysfunction, tests of executive function may be impaired enough to amount to a subcortical dementia [140]. Hence, in both its clinical and neuropsychological features, neuroacanthocytosis may resemble HD (Section 5.1.1).

5.4.5 Neuroferritinopathy

Mutations in the gene encoding ferritin light polypeptide or ferritin light chain (FTL) located on chromosome 19q13.33 (OMIM#606159) have been associated with a variety of autosomal dominant movement disorders, including dystonia, chorea, and akinetic-rigid syndrome. The extrapyramidal features may resemble HD or parkinsonism. There is a low serum ferritin with brain aggregates of ferritin and iron [141,142].

Cognitive decline is associated with neuroferritinopathy in some instances. In one case, frontal lobe function was particularly affected (perseveration, poor cognitive estimates, impaired nonverbal abstract reasoning, and some word retrieval difficulties), although the patient had been treated with high-dose anticholinergic agents for the movement disorder before cognitive decline occurred [143]. In a French family, two of the seven members had a frontal syndrome and another was demented [144], and in another family, the index case had a frontal syndrome and dementia [142]. The index case in a Portuguese family had nonprogressive mental retardation with an IQ of 60 [145]. Overall, cognitive impairment seems to be absent or subtle in the early stages, unlike the situation in HD, with subcortical-frontal dysfunction developing in the later stages [146].

5.4.6 Aceruloplasminemia

Aceruloplasminemia is an autosomal recessive condition resulting from the absence of ceruloplasmin ferroxidase activity due to mutations in the ceruloplasmin gene on chromosome 3q24-q25 (OMIM#604290), with subsequent effects on iron metabolism. There is low serum iron, raised ferritin, absent ceruloplasmin, and increased liver iron on biopsy. Although serum copper is low, this is in proportion to reduced ceruloplasmin, as normal urine and liver copper indicate that there is no copper overload (cf., Wilson's disease, Section 5.4.2). Diabetes mellitus is a common feature. Unlike the situation with hemochromatosis, another iron-related disorder (Section 5.5.5), neurological presentations are common in aceruloplasminemia, usually with a movement disorder (dystonia, chorea, ataxia), with imaging evidence of iron deposition in the brain, particularly the basal ganglia. A role for ceruloplasmin in brain iron metabolism is likely, therefore [147].

Dementia has been reported in association with aceruloplasminemia [147–149]. The limited information available on the pattern of cognitive impairments indicates defects in immediate and delayed recall of verbal material, inability to learn new verbal material, but with preservation of long-term memory, at least initially. The findings were said to be "similar to subcortical dementia" [147,149].

5.4.7 Kufor–Rakeb syndrome (PARK9)

Unlike the clinically similar pallidopyramidal syndrome [150], dementia may be a feature of Kufor–Rakeb syndrome, a very rare autosomal recessive nigrostriatal-pallidopyramidal degeneration syndrome [151] linked to chromosome 1p36 (designated PARK9), and resulting from mutations in a neuronal P-type ATPase gene, ATP13A2, the product of which may be located in lysosomes (OMIM#606693). Detailed description of the dementia has not been identified, but considering the topography of disease, a frontosubcortical pattern might be anticipated. Juvenile-onset dementia has been described [152].

5.4.8 Fahr's disease (bilateral striatopallidodentate calcinosis)

This rubric encompasses a heterogeneous group of conditions, both familial and sporadic, characterized variably by calcification of the basal ganglia, dentate nucleus, and deeper cortical layers, which may be detected radiologically or sonographically. The calcinosis may be asymptomatic or associated with any combination of movement disorder (parkinsonism, dystonia, tremor, ataxia), epileptic seizures, and cognitive decline or dementia, with or without endocrine parathyroid disorder of calcium metabolism.

The familial idiopathic syndrome may often be associated with intellectual decline, with impairment of recent memory and memory retention, as well as parkinsonism and cerebellar ataxia [153]. Cases of Fahr's disease presenting with subacute dementia and without a movement disorder have been reported [154,155], characterized in one case by executive deficits, anterograde amnesia, attentional impairment, and neuropsychiatric features, with the functional imaging correlate of reduced glucose metabolism in the basal ganglia and frontal lobes [154]. One wonders if there might be overlap here with polycystic lipomembranous osteodysplasia with sclerosing leukoencephalopathy (Nasu–Hakola disease), a condition characterized by presenile dementia with basal ganglia calcification (Section 5.1.5).

5.4.9 Urbach–Wiethe disease (lipoid proteinosis)

This rare autosomal recessive condition is characterized by bilateral calcification of the anterior medial temporal lobe, especially the amygdala, but with sparing of the hippocampus, thus permitting an analysis of the contribution of the amygdala to cognitive function. It results from mutation in the extracellular matrix protein 1 (ECM1) gene on chromosome 1q21 (OMIM#247100). Clinical studies suggest impaired learning and recall of odor–figure associations but no amnesia as such [156], and also impairments in emotional judgment and memory [157].

5.4.10 Myoclonus–dystonia syndrome (MDS), DYT11

Myoclonus–dystonia syndrome (MDS) is an autosomal dominant disorder most often resulting from mutations in the epsilon-sarcoglycan gene on chromosome 7q21.3 (DYT11; OMIM#159900). In addition to myoclonus and dystonia, alcohol responsiveness and psychiatric symptoms are characteristic. Cognitive impairment has been reported [158].

5.4.11 Essential tremor (ET)

Classic hereditary essential tremor (ET), in which similarly affected family members are found in at least three generations, is typified by early onset, complete penetrance by the age of 65 years, invariable onset of tremor in the hands, and absence of rigidity, rest tremor, persistent unilateral tremor, and isolated head, tongue, voice, jaw, or leg tremor [159]. The role of genetic factors has been confirmed by the demonstration of the linkage of ET to various chromosomal loci (e.g., 3q13, 2p24.1, 6p23). However, many cases clinically labeled as ET lack either a family history (nonfamilial or sporadic ET), suggesting that environmental factors may contribute to the etiology, or vary from the classical clinical phenotype. Such cases are sometimes labeled as "possible ET," although other diagnoses need to be borne in mind, such as enhanced physiological tremor, early Parkinson's disease (PD), or dystonic tremor [160,161]. Pathological examinations in ET cases are few, but have suggested cerebellar involvement.

ET was previously considered a monosymptomatic tremor disorder, but administration of neuropsychological tests has revealed subclinical impairments in tests sensitive to frontal lobe function. One early study noted impaired verbal fluency, naming, mental set-shifting, verbal memory, and working memory. Deficits did not correlate with tremor severity. Prefrontal cortical involvement, perhaps encompassing frontocerebellar circuits, was surmised [162]. Impairments in attentional and conceptual thinking tasks were noted in a further study, akin to those seen in idiopathic PD, prompting the suggestion that this frontal lobe dysfunction may reflect dysregulation of frontosubcortical dopamine pathways [163]. There is reasonable evidence of an epidemiological association between ET and neurodegenerative disorders, specifically PD and AD [164], and the occasional concurrence of familial ET and restless legs syndrome [165] may support the idea of dopaminergic dysfunction. Attentional problems were also identified in another study [166].

Lacritz *et al.* [167] found mild cognitive impairment in about half of a small cohort of ET patients being evaluated for tremor surgery (hence, a highly selected group), with deficits identified in cognitive flexibility, figural fluency, and selective attention. A population-based study from Spain has found that older-onset ET (>65 yr) is associated with mild cognitive impairment and with an increased risk of incident dementia, supporting the hypothesis that cognitive impairments are part of the core ET phenotype [168,169].

5.4.12 Dystonia

The dystonias constitute a heterogeneous group of hyperkinetic movement disorders characterized by involuntary sustained muscle contractions that produce abnormal postures and repetitive movements. These may be primary (idiopathic) or secondary (symptomatic), genetic or sporadic, focal or generalized [170].

Although principally manifested as a movement disorder, there may be subtle cognitive impairments associated with dystonias. Attentional-executive deficits were identified in a heterogeneous group of 14 primary dystonia patients, although speed of information processing, language, spatial, memory, and general intellectual skills were well preserved [171]. However, another study found no difference from controls in any measure of executive function other than category word fluency in 10 patients with idiopathic dystonia [172]. In patients with focal dystonias, Ochudlo *et al.* [173] reported impairments on the Frontal Assessment Battery in cervical dystonia, Meige's syndrome, and blepharospasm.

5.5 Hereditary metabolic disorders

This section encompasses those disorders once styled, after Archibald Garrod, as "inborn errors of metabolism." Another condition that might be included within this rubric is cobalamin C disease (Section 8.2.1.2).

5.5.1 Mitochondrial disorders

Mitochondrial disorders are a heterogeneous group with respect to both phenotype and genotype. Both peripheral and central nervous systems may be affected, the former including myopathy and peripheral neuropathy, the CNS features including epilepsy, migraine, stroke-like episodes, ophthalmoplegia, ataxia, and spasticity, as well as cognitive impairment. There may also be involvement of other body systems, with clinical features including cardiomyopathy, diabetes mellitus, pigmentary retinal degeneration, and sensorineural hearing loss. Various more or less characteristic phenotypes or syndromes associated with mitochondrial dysfunction may be identified, including Kearns–Sayre syndrome (KSS), chronic progressive external ophthalmoplegia (CPEO), the syndrome of mitochondrial encephalomyopathy, lactic acidosis and stroke-like episodes (MELAS), and the syndrome of myoclonic epilepsy and ragged red fibers (MERRF), but so-called "non-syndromic" forms also occur. At the level of genotype, mitochondrial disorders may result from mutations (deletions, point mutations) within the small mitochondrial genome or within nuclear genes (autosomal, X-linked) that encode mitochondrial respiratory chain proteins. Guidelines for the molecular genetic testing of mitochondrial disorders have appeared [174].

The possibility that neuropsychological deficits might be common in mitochondrial disorders was suggested by Kartsounis *et al.* [175], who noted in a series of 36 patients with myopathies and encephalomyopathies that 14 patients were thought to be cognitively impaired on clinical grounds, but 21 were found to have general intellectual decline on testing, and a further five of the remaining 15 had focal cognitive deficits in the domains of language, memory, or perception (frontal lobe tests were not administered in this series). Turconi *et al.* [176] found no global cognitive decline in 16 patients with mitochondrial encephalomyopathies but selective impairments of visuospatial skills and short-term memory, unrelated to clinical phenotype and genetic mutations. Kornblum *et al.* [177] studied 18 patients with CPEO and KSS. None had general intellectual deterioration but disturbances were identified in visual construction, vigilance and concentration, abstraction/flexibility, and verbal/visual memory, suggesting the presence of frontal and parieto-occipital deficits. Evolution of cognitive deficits in MELAS in the absence of stroke-like episodes has been reported [178], perhaps reflecting the alterations in cerebral oxygen and glucose metabolism in this condition [179].

Cognitive decline or dementia ("mitochondrial dementia") is said to have been reported in various mitochondrial syndromes, including MELAS, MERRF, CPEO, KSS, Leber's hereditary optic neuropathy (LHON), mitochondrial neurogastrointestinal encephalopathy (MNGIE), NARP syndrome, Leigh syndrome, and Alpers–Huttenlocher disease [180,181]. Occasionally, dementia has been reported as a prominent feature in nonsyndromic mitochondrial disorders [182].

5.5.2 Leukodystrophies

Leukodystrophies are genetic metabolic disorders that generally present in early childhood, often at the time of brain myelination. Occasionally, however, these disorders may present in adulthood [183], and dementia may be one feature of the clinical phenotype. These conditions may be autosomal recessive (e.g., metachromatic leukodystrophy) or sex-linked (e.g., X-linked adrenoleukodystrophy) in their inheritance pattern. This is a heterogeneous group, including both lysosomal and peroxisomal disorders. Cerebrotendinous xanthomatosis (Section 5.5.4) is classified sometimes with the leukodystrophies. White matter change as a consequence of treatment with radiotherapy may be described occasionally as a leukodystrophy (Section 7.1.8).

5.5.2.1 Metachromatic leukodystrophy (MLD)

In metachromatic leukodystrophy (MLD), reduced enzymatic activity of arylsulfatase A (ARSA) results in accumulation of sulfatides (sulfogalactosylceramides) in Schwann cells and oligodendroglia with peripheral and central demyelination, causing peripheral neuropathy and leukodystrophy, respectively. Depending on the degree of residual enzyme activity, disease may range from severe with late-infantile onset to mild with adult onset. Classically, MLD is due to deficiency of the lysosomal hydrolase arylsulfatase A (also known as cerebroside sulfate sulfatase) associated with mutations in the arylsulfatase A gene on chromosome 22q13.31 (OMIM#250100). The normal catalytic function of arylsulfatase A requires a sphingolipid activator protein, saposin B, deficiency of which may be associated with mutations in the prosaposin gene on chromosome 10q21 (OMIM#249900).

Cases of MLD with adult-onset dementia have been reported. These may vary in the pattern of cognitive impairment; cases with amnesia, visuospatial dysfunction, and attentional difficulties, with medial temporal and frontal cortical hypometabolism on functional imaging, are reported [184], as are cases with typical frontal features of behavioral change, apathy, psychosis akin to schizophrenia, and with frontal hypoperfusion on functional imaging [185,186], sometimes simulating FTD [187]. Concurrent peripheral neuropathy may be a clue to the diagnosis of MLD although cases with adult-onset dementia without neuropathy have been reported [187,188]. It has been suggested that Alzheimer's first patient, in fact, had MLD [189,190].

5.5.2.2 X-linked adrenoleukodystrophy (X-ALD)

X-linked adrenoleukodystrophy (X-ALD) is a peroxisomal disorder associated with mutations in the ATP-binding cassette (ABCD1) gene, which encodes a peroxisomal membrane protein (OMIM#300100). The clinical phenotype varies, dependent on the age of presentation; children most often have rapidly progressive cerebral disease, whereas adults most often present with adrenomyeloneuropathy (AMN), these two phenotypes accounting for more than 75% of all cases. Adult cerebral disease is the least frequently observed phenotype [191].

X-ALD cases presenting with adult-onset dementia have only occasionally been reported. Features suggestive of frontal lobe dysfunction have been prominent in many of these cases [192–197], some with confirmed ABCD1 gene mutations [196,197]. X-ALD patients presenting with marked personality change and labeled as having manic-depressive psychosis [198] or mania with disinhibition, impulsivity, hypersexuality, and perseveration [199] possibly may represent the same phenotype. Presentation with Balint's syndrome and dementia has also been described [200]. The pathogenesis of these features is presumably the functional disconnection (Section 1.3.4) of cortical regions by an advancing wave of inflammatory demyelination, either anterior or posterior, which is the typical pathological substrate of X-ALD. A correlation between frontal type dementia and an anterior pattern of white matter change on MRI has been noted in one case [196].

With developments in diagnostic techniques, particularly neuroimaging and neurogenetic testing, X-ALD now may be diagnosed in asymptomatic at-risk individuals. Study of neurologically and radiologically asymptomatic boys has shown overall normal cognitive function, with the emergence of subtle visual perceptual and visuomotor deficits with age in a few [201]. In a family with the R152C ABCD1 mutation, the proband of which had presented with a frontal dementia [196], two asymptomatic individuals who had been treatment compliant since childhood showed neither neuroradiological nor neuropsychological evidence of subclinical disease [202]. Early therapeutic intervention might be predicted to preserve cognitive function in such cases. Options include Lorenzo's oil [203] and hematopoietic cell transplantation [204].

5.5.2.3 Alexander's disease and Rosenthal fiber encephalopathy (RFE)

Alexander's disease is typically a disorder of childhood characterized by megalencephaly and relentless neurological deterioration, with a leukodystrophy and the neuropathological finding of Rosenthal fibers, eosinophilic cytoplasmic inclusions within astrocyte processes adjacent to areas of demyelination. These are immunopositive for glial fibrillary acidic protein (GFAP), ubiquitin, and heat shock proteins such as hsp27 and αβcrystallin. Mutations in the gene encoding GFAP on chromosome 17 have been associated with the condition (OMIM#203450) [205], including occasional adult-onset cases [206].

Rosenthal fiber encephalopathy (RFE) is the name used for a condition in which the pathological finding of Rosenthal fibers occurs without clinical features of demyelinating lesions typical of Alexander's disease. Rosenthal fibers are typically found in subependymal, subpial, and perivascular regions, often confined to the brainstem, and often in the context of systemic illness [207].

Adult-onset cases of Alexander's disease and RFE have been described [206,208,209], some with dementia; for example, in a patient with learning disability who developed further cognitive decline, ataxia, and dysarthria [210]. A review of adult-onset cases [208] suggested that dementia was more common in RFE (4/11) than in Alexander's disease (2/15). A nationwide questionnaire-based survey of Alexander's disease in Japan found that 4/16 cases (25%) with the adult form had dementia, and reported that "three cases with clinical findings similar to FTD were mentioned in the free comments section of the questionnaire" [209].

5.5.2.4 Pelizaeus–Merzbacher disease (PMD)

Pelizaeus-Merzbacher disease (PMD) is an X-linked recessive disorder of myelin due to deficiency of proteolipid protein (PLP), which usually presents in the first months of life with a combination of a movement disorder (head tremor, laryngeal stridor, choreoathetosis, spastic paraparesis) and intellectual decline. Various forms have been described, including a late-onset form known as Löwenberg–Hill syndrome [211]. Point mutations, duplications and deletions of the PLP gene on chromosome Xq 22.2 have been identified (OMIM#312080), as have cases with the clinical phenotype of PMD but normal PLP gene, suggesting that other regulatory genes may also be involved in disease pathogenesis [212].

Adult cases of PMD with dementia and movement disorder are unusual. Cases with or without PLP gene mutation have been described, as has a case of dementia and gait disorder with MRI evidence of leukodystrophy in the mother of a man with PMD, presumably a manifesting carrier [213–215]. In a Cajun kindred, heterozygous females developed progressive gait disturbances and cognitive deterioration starting in the fourth decade of life [216].

5.5.2.5 Krabbe disease (globoid cell leukodystrophy)

This autosomal recessive leukodystrophy results from deficiency of the lysosomal enzyme galactocerebroside β-galactosidase (GALC) due to mutations in the encoding gene located on chromosome 14q24.3-q32.1 (OMIM#245200). In addition to infantile and late-infantile/juvenile forms, which account for most cases, an adult form is described manifesting with spastic paraparesis. Dementia, optic atrophy, and peripheral neuropathy also

develop, although a protracted course with apparently preserved intellect has been reported [217].

5.5.2.6 Vanishing white matter disease (VWMD)

Vanishing white matter disease (VWMD) encompasses a group of disorders with leukoencephalopathy or leukodystrophy resulting from mutations in the eIF2B gene (OMIM#603896), usually dominated clinically by cerebellar ataxia [218]. Presenile dementia has been reported as an unusual presentation [219–221].

5.5.2.7 18q deletion (18q-) syndrome

Deletion of the long arm of chromosome 18, also known as de Grouchy syndrome (OMIM#601808), produces a variable phenotype encompassing learning disability, short stature, variable dysmorphism, and neurological symptoms and signs [222]. Brain MRI shows white matter abnormalities with incomplete myelination and poor differentiation of gray and white matter, features ascribed to loss of the myelin basic protein (MBP) gene which lies on chromosome 18q. For this reason, the condition has been classified with the leukodystrophies, although rare deletions in which the MBP gene is retained have normal appearing white matter. Occasional cases presenting in adult life have been reported, but these are due to a seizure disorder rather than cognitive decline [223]. Lower cognitive ability predicts larger 18q deletion size [224].

5.5.2.8 Hereditary diffuse leukoencephalopathy with axonal spheroids (HDLS)

Hereditary diffuse leukoencephalopathy with spheroids (HDLS) is a rare autosomal-dominant CNS white matter disease, which may present with cognitive, behavioral, epileptic, and motor features (both pyramidal and extrapyramidal). The differential diagnosis includes FTD, multiple sclerosis (patchy or diffuse white matter changes are seen on MRI of the brain), atypical Parkinson's disease, AD, and CADASIL. Diagnosis has relied on examination of brain tissue, showing loss of myelin sheaths, axonal destruction, axonal spheroids, gliosis, and autofluorescent lipid-laden macrophages. Recently, mutations in the colony stimulating factor 1 receptor (CSF1R) on chromosome 5q have been demonstrated in HDLS [225].

5.5.3 Lysosomal storage disorders

Around 40 lysosomal storage disorders affecting the brain are described [226]. Learning disability/mental retardation is a feature in many of these disorders, but some may present in adulthood with cognitive impairment as a feature. Some of these are mentioned elsewhere; for example, metachromatic leukodystrophy (Section 5.5.2.1), Krabbe disease (Section 5.5.2.5).

5.5.3.1 Acid maltase deficiency (glycogenosis type IIb, Pompe's disease)

This autosomal recessive lysosomal disorder of glycogen storage results from deficiency of the lysosomal enzyme acid α-glucosidase, or acid maltase, due to mutation of the gene located on chromosome 17 that encodes this protein (OMIM#232300). The clinical phenotype is variable, with age of onset ranging from infancy to adulthood, and clinical features may include myopathy, cardiomyopathy, and organomegaly. Adult-onset disease (Engel's disease) may present with respiratory failure due to diaphragmatic involvement [227]. Enzyme replacement therapy is now available [228].

One case of adult-onset acid maltase deficiency (AMD) associated with low IQ and impairments of frontal lobe function has been reported; other family members with AMD did not have dementia. As the authors point out, this may be a fortuitous association, but equally, acid maltase is expressed in brain as well as in muscle and brain levels may be low [229]. A review of 225 published cases of "non-classic" Pompe's disease noted abnormal mental development in only three, and no other reports of dementia [230].

5.5.3.2 Fabry's disease (Anderson–Fabry disease; angiokeratoma corporis diffusum; hereditary dystonic lipidosis)

This autosomal recessive lysosomal storage disorder is due to mutations in the gene encoding α-galactosidase A (OMIM#301500), with resultant enzyme deficiency leading to accumulation of glycosphingolipids, such as ceramide trihexoside in the vascular endothelium and smooth muscle cells of visceral tissues including brain, and in body fluids. The resultant multisystem disease has a broad phenotype, with neurological (peripheral and central nervous system), dermatological, renal, ocular, gastroenterological, cardiac, and respiratory features with variable age at diagnosis [231].

A slowly progressive vascular dementia (Chapter 3) has been described in Fabry's disease with multiple cognitive deficits including memory impairment, anomia, perseveration, and visuospatial difficulties, with additional behavioral changes. This was a result of multiple subcortical strokes and diffuse ischemic white matter disease due to pathological involvement of small penetrating arteries, hypertension (secondary to renal disease), and cardiogenic emboli [232]. An autopsy case of a demented Fabry patient confirmed ischemic changes [233]. Although this is an extremely rare presentation of Fabry's disease, a case-registry series reported dementia in 18% of patients, in all cases associated with recurrent strokes or transient ischemic attacks [234]. Prevention may be feasible with enzyme replacement therapy [231].

5.5.3.3 GM2 gangliosidosis, Tay–Sachs disease

GM2 gangliosidosis or Tay–Sachs disease, resulting from autosomal recessive hexosaminidase A deficiency (OMIM#272800), is usually a relentlessly progressive disease of infancy with paralysis, blindness, and mental retardation. The condition may sometimes have adult onset. Cognitive dysfunction has been reported in about half of adult patients, with impaired executive and memory function, although studies disagree as to whether dementia occurs at all [235] or is common [236].

5.5.3.4 Gaucher's disease, type III

A rare subacute neuronopathic form (type III) of this autosomal recessive disease, due to deficiency of β-glucocerebrosidase (GBA; OMIM#231000), which presents in juveniles and adults [237], is recognized as causing an akinetic-rigid syndrome, supranuclear gaze palsy, myoclonus, epileptic seizures, and cognitive decline. There is elevated serum acid phosphatase and bone marrow infiltration with lipid-laden fibroblasts known as Gaucher's cells.

Multiple studies have identified an association between GBA mutations and synucleinopathies (parkinsonism and other Lewy body disorders; Section 2.4), including dementia with Lewy bodies [238].

5.5.3.5 Neuronal ceroid lipofuscinosis (NCL); Kufs disease

The neuronal ceroid lipofuscinoses (NCL) constitute a large group of neurodegenerative disorders with onset between infancy and adulthood, characterized by accumulation of autofluorescent inclusion bodies in neurons and other tissues. Various genetic loci and mutations have been defined in NCLs, with both autosomal recessive and dominant patterns of inheritance [239].

Kufs disease is the name which has often been applied to adult-onset NCL variants, which may be sporadic or inherited, and manifest with a progressive myoclonus epilepsy (Type A), or with cognitive decline and dementia with movement disorders (Type B). Families with disease onset in the fourth decade of life, heralded by epileptic seizures and with subsequent dementia, have been reported [240]. In addition to the various pathological inclusions (fingerprint, curvilinear, rectilinear, granular, osmiophilic), neuritic plaques and possibly neurofibrillary tangles may be seen in Kufs disease,

prompting the suggestion of an overlapping pathogenesis with AD [241]. Mutations in the CLN6 gene on chromosome 15 seem to be a common cause of type A Kufs disease (OMIM#204300) [242].

5.5.3.6 Niemann–Pick disease type C

This autosomal recessive neurovisceral disorder is a lipidosis, resulting from a defect in intracellular trafficking of cholesterol and glycosphingolipids leading to their accumulation in late endosomes/lysosomes in the brain and other tissues. It results from mutations in the genes NPC1 (around 95% of cases) on chromosome 18q11.2 (type C1; OMIM#257220) and NPC2 (around 5% of cases) on chromosome 14q24.3 (type C2; OMIM#607625). The clinical phenotype is similar in both forms, including dystonia, supranuclear gaze palsy, ataxia, dysarthria, epileptic seizures, and progressive cognitive decline, with onset from the first to the fifth decade of life [243,244]. Mutations in the gene encoding the cholesterol-binding protein HE1 (NPC2) have been reported to cause dementia in the 30s with focal frontal involvement. Tau-positive neurofibrillary tangles as well as lysosomal inclusions were seen at postmortem [245]. Although rare, the diagnosis should be considered as disease-specific therapy with miglustat is now available [246], to which end a "Suspicion Index" to facilitate early diagnosis has been developed [247].

5.5.3.7 Sanfilippo syndrome (mucopolysaccharidosis III)

This autosomal recessive disorder associated with excessive urinary excretion of heparan sulfate comes in four biochemical and genetic variants, all due to deficiencies of different enzymes, usually causing childhood-onset dementia and neurobehavioral problems. The clinical phenotype is variable, and type B cases (OMIM#252920) with dementia onset in the third decade of life or later have been reported [248,249].

5.5.4 Cerebrotendinous xanthomatosis (CTX)

Cerebrotendinous xanthomatosis (CTX) is an auto-somal recessive lipid-storage disorder resulting from mutations in the mitochondrial enzyme 27-sterol hydroxylase located on chromosome 2p (OMIM#213700), causing impaired bile acid synthesis. Brain imaging shows global atrophy and demyelination, such that some authorities classify CTX with the leukodystrophies. Spasticity, ataxia, and peripheral neuropathy, as well as dementia are included among the neurological features, with onset in the third decade of life.

A survey of 32 CTX patients found low IQ in 66%, and in 81% of 181 patients reported in the literature [250,251]. No detailed neuropsychological profile has been identified, although a subcortical pattern might be expected. Occasional patients with a FTD phenotype have been reported [252,253]. Resolution of cognitive deficits in 10/17 patients treated with CDA (chenodeoxycholic acid) was claimed by Berginer *et al.* [254], but not all patients show a cognitive response to CDA [253].

5.5.5 Hemochromatosis

Genetic, primary, or hereditary hemochromatosis is an autosomal recessive disorder characterized by iron overload with pathological deposition in the liver and pancreas, with resulting impairment of liver function and diabetes mellitus, respectively. Iron does not normally cross the blood–brain barrier, and elevated brain iron content is rarely, if ever, a feature of hemochromatosis, the clinical correlate being that neurological symptoms are also rare, despite systemic iron overload equivalent to that seen in aceruloplasminemia (Section 5.4.6), with which hemochromatosis may be misdiagnosed [255]. Cognitive features may be seen in hereditary movement disorders associated with abnormal iron metabolism (e.g., neuroferritinopathy, aceruloplasminemia; Sections 5.4.5 and 5.4.6), and iron content is reported to be increased in the striatum in

HD and in the posterior putamen in parkinsonian-type MSA.

Cases of hemochromatosis presenting with dementia and ataxia have been documented in the context of advanced liver disease, progressing to death within two years of the onset of neurological features [256]. Two cases with mild systemic features and concurrent dementia of frontotemporal type (one semantic dementia, one frontal variant) have been reported, with the suggestion that this may reflect linkage of genetic diseases, rather than a toxic consequence of abnormal iron metabolism, although in the absence of brain pathology the question remained unresolved [257]. One patient had sensorineural hearing loss, which may be significant (see Superficial siderosis of the nervous system, Section 3.3.3).

The association of these cases may be no more than chance concurrence. It has been argued that movement disorders occurring in the context of hereditary hemochromatosis should prompt a search for another cause [258], and the same is probably true of cognitive impairment, although this might be anticipated as a consequence of complications of the disease, such as hepatic failure and/or diabetes mellitus.

5.5.6 Polyglucosan body disease (PGBD)

Glycogen storage disease type IV (GSDIV), also known as amylopectinosis or Andersen's disease, is an autosomal recessive disorder associated with a deficiency of the glycogen branching enzyme (GBE) encoded on chromosome 3p14. The clinical phenotype of GSDIV is extremely heterogeneous, ranging from progressive liver cirrhosis and death in childhood, through cardiomyopathic and benign myopathic variants, to an adult-onset neurodegenerative disorder, polyglucosan body disease (PGBD; OMIM#263570). This latter condition is a rare disorder, often characterized by a combination of upper and lower motor neuron signs, the latter due to an axonal sensorimotor peripheral neuropathy, along with urinary incontinence and other motor disorders. Nerve biopsy may be diagnostic, showing the typical polyglucosan bodies, which may also be seen in dermal sweat glands or brain tissue [259].

Cognitive impairment and dementia have been reported in PGBD, apparently of frontal type, sometimes associated with white matter changes on MRI, and sometimes nonprogressive [260–263]. Familial cases have been reported [264]. Mild cognitive impairment has been documented in an individual heterozygous for a point mutation in the GBE gene, and with other clinical features suggesting manifesting heterozygote status [265]. An "AD-type" has also been presented [266], emphasizing the clinical phenotypic heterogeneity of PGBD.

5.5.7 Lafora body disease

This autosomal recessive progressive myoclonic epilepsy syndrome typically presents in the 10–18-year-old age group with epileptic seizures, myoclonus, and neurological deterioration with cognitive impairment and eventually dementia, with typical Lafora body inclusions in the brain, liver, skin, and muscle. Deterministic mutations have been demonstrated in two genes, EPM2A and EPM2B, encoding the proteins laforin and malin, respectively (OMIM#254780), which colocalize to the endoplasmic reticulum.

Delayed onset of Lafora body disease up to about the age of 25 years has been reported infrequently [267] and presenile dementia has been described in the older literature [268].

5.5.8 Myoclonic epilepsy of Unverricht and Lundborg (Baltic myoclonus)

This autosomal recessive condition due to mutations in the cystatin B gene on chromosome 21q22.3 (OMIM#254800) enters the differential diagnosis of progressive myoclonic epilepsy along with Lafora body disease, neuronal ceroid lipofuscinosis, and mitochondrial disorders, among others. In addition to the polymyoclonus and cerebellar ataxia, there is said to be minimal or no cognitive decline [269], but

the phenotype may include a mild and slowly progressive dementia occasionally [270].

5.5.9 Porphyria

Although a recognized cause of various neurological and neuropsychiatric syndromes, including delirium in response to precipitating factors such as infection or drugs [271,272], it is not clear that any one of the porphyrias causes or leads to dementia, although there may be complaints of poor memory. The popular association of porphyria with the madness of King George III (1738–1820) seems to have no compelling evidence to support it [272].

5.6 Hereditary neurocutaneous syndromes (phakomatoses)

Inherited disorders in this category are characterized by involvement of ectodermal structures (nervous system, skin, eyes) with slow evolution during childhood and adolescence with a tendency to the formation of benign tumors or hamartomas. The terminology may also be taken to include conditions with cutaneous angiomatosis and CNS abnormalities, such as ataxia telangiectasia (Section 5.2.2.2) and Fabry disease (Section 5.5.3.2).

5.6.1 Neurofibromatosis

Neurofibromatosis type 1 (NF1) is one of the most common monogenic Mendelian disorders seen in general neurology outpatient practice, but reasons for consultation may often be incidental to the diagnosis of NF1 [34], although there are many possible neurological problems that may be encountered in both NF1 and NF2 [273,274].

In a series of 103 NF1 patients aged between six and 75 years, IQ was lower than in control patients, although the impairment was generally mild. NF1 patients had poorer reading and impaired short-term memory, and on computerized tests had slower reaction times, higher error rates, and impaired attention. However, no particular profile emerged [275]. Intellectual problems in NF1 are not thought to be progressive. Severe impairments are unusual and should mandate a search for another cause, either related to NF1 such as cerebral tumor or hydrocephalus, or unrelated.

Deficits of spatial memory and navigation associated with bilateral hippocampal atrophy have been reported in bilateral vestibulopathy associated with NF 2 (Section 6.16).

5.6.2 Tuberous sclerosis

Tuberous sclerosis was identified initially as a syndrome of mental retardation, epilepsy, and facial angiofibroma, with the neuropathological finding of tubers. It is now recognized to be an autosomal dominant condition that is clinically and genetically heterogeneous, with chromosomal linkage to two loci, at 9q34.13 (TSC1) encoding hamartin and at 16p13.3 (TSC2) encoding tuberin (OMIM#191100).

Neuropsychological studies have confirmed variability in cognitive function, with a possible emphasis on executive tasks related to prefrontal pathology [276]. Many patients have normal cognition. Refractory seizures and presence of the TSC2 mutation have been associated with adverse cognitive outcome [277]. In children, a negative correlation has been found between the number of tubers and IQ [278]. Mutation location may also be significant; TSC1 mutations in the tuberin interaction domain were associated with lower intellectual outcomes as were TSC2 protein-truncating and hamartin interaction domain mutations, whereas TSC2 missense mutations and small in-frame deletions were associated with higher IQ [279].

5.7 Sex chromosome aneuploidies

Although these disorders might be classified as learning disability syndromes, nonetheless patients with these conditions may be seen in adult cognitive disorders clinics occasionally, hence their inclusion here.

5.7.1 Turner syndrome

Turner syndrome is characterized by complete (XO) or partial monosomy for the X-chromosome in a phenotypic female. As well as characteristic morphological abnormalities, these women have cognitive deficits that persist into adult life. The cognitive profile is typically one of relatively weak visuospatial, executive, and social cognitive domains but with intact intellectual function and verbal abilities [280]. Despite estrogen replacement therapy, adult patients have been found to have difficulty on spatial and perceptual skills, visual memory, visuomotor integration, attention, and executive function, but have normal verbal IQ [281].

5.7.2 Klinefelter syndrome (47,XXY) and 47,XYY syndrome

Klinefelter syndrome is characterized by an extra X chromosome (47,XXY) in a phenotypic male. As well as typical morphological abnormalities, there is a characteristic cognitive profile with increased risk of language disorders and reading disabilities, with a reduction in overall IQ, possibly with executive function deficits as well [282].

Boys with the 47,XYY genotype have more severe and pervasive language impairment than Klinefelter boys, although they also show below average performance on tests of verbal memory, attention, and executive function [283].

REFERENCES

[1] Huntington G. On chorea. *Med Surg Rep* 1872; 26: 317–21.

[2] Huntington's Study Group. Unified Huntington's Disease Rating Scale: reliability and consistency. *Mov Disord* 1996; 11: 136–42.

[3] Huntington's Disease Collaborative Research Group. A novel gene containing a trinucleotide repeat that is expanded and unstable on Huntington's disease chromosomes. *Cell* 1993; 72: 971–83.

[4] Vonsattel JPG, Lianski M. Huntington's disease. In: Esiri MM, Lee VM-Y, Trojanowski JQ (eds.). *The*

Neuropathology of Dementia (2nd edn.). Cambridge: Cambridge University Press, 2004: 376–401.

[5] Harbo HF, Finsterer J, Baets J, *et al.* EFNS guidelines on the molecular diagnosis of neurogenetic disorders: general issues, Huntington's disease, Parkinson's disease and dystonias. *Eur J Neurol* 2009; 16: 777–85 [Erratum *Eur J Neurol* 2010; 17: 339].

[6] Schneider SA, Walker RH, Bhatia KP. The Huntington's disease-like syndromes: what to consider in patients with a negative Huntington's disease gene test. *Nat Clin Pract Neurol* 2007; 3: 517–25.

[7] Dunnett SB, Rosser AE. Cell-based treatments for Huntington's disease. *Int Rev Neurobiol* 2011; 98: 483–508.

[8] Paulsen JS. Cognitive impairment in Huntington disease: diagnosis and treatment. *Curr Neurol Neurosci Rep* 2011; 11: 474–83.

[9] Albert ML, Feldman RG, Willis AL. The "subcortical dementia" of progressive supranuclear palsy. *J Neurol Neurosurg Psychiatry* 1974; 37: 121–30.

[10] McHugh PR, Folstein MF. Psychiatric symptoms of Huntington's chorea: a clinical and phenomenological study. In: Benson DF, Blumer D (eds.). *Psychiatric Aspects of Neurological Disease.* New York, NY: Raven Press, 1975; 267–85.

[11] Brandt J, Folstein SE, Folstein MF. Differential cognitive impairment in Alzheimer's disease and Huntington's disease. *Ann Neurol* 1988; 23: 555–61.

[12] Rosser AE, Hodges JR. The Dementia Rating Scale in Alzheimer's disease, Huntington's disease and progressive supranuclear palsy. *J Neurol* 1994; 241: 531–6.

[13] Zakzanis KK. The subcortical dementia of Huntington's disease. *J Clin Exp Neuropsychol* 1998; 20: 565–78.

[14] Snowden J, Craufurd D, Griffiths H, Thompson J, Neary D. Longitudinal evaluation of cognitive disorder in Huntington's disease. *J Int Neuropsychol Soc* 2001; 7: 33–44.

[15] Ho AK, Sahakian BJ, Brown RG, *et al.* Profile of cognitive progression in early Huntington's disease. *Neurology* 2003; 61: 1702–6.

[16] Ribai P, Nguyen K, Hahn-Barma V, *et al.* Psychiatric and cognitive difficulties as indicators of juvenile Huntington disease onset in 29 patients. *Arch Neurol* 2007; 64: 813–19.

[17] Lawrence AD, Sahakian BJ, Hodges JR, *et al.* Executive and mnemonic functions in early Huntington's disease. *Brain* 1996; 119: 1633–45.

[18] Lemiere J, Decruyenaere M, Evers-Kiebooms G, Vandenbussche E, Dom R. Cognitive changes in patients with Huntington's disease (HD) and asymptomatic carriers of the HD mutation. A longitudinal follow-up study. *J Neurol* 2004; 251: 935–42.

[19] Ho AK, Manly T, Nestor PJ, *et al.* A case of unilateral neglect in Huntington's disease. *Neurocase* 2003; 9: 261–73.

[20] Butters N, Wolfe J, Granholm E, Martone M. An assessment of verbal recall, recognition, and fluency abilities in patients with Huntington's disease. *Cortex* 1986; 22: 11–32.

[21] Massman PJ, Delis DC, Butters N, Levin BE, Salmon DP. Are all subcortical dementias alike? Verbal learning and memory in Parkinson's and Huntington's disease patients. *J Clin Exp Neuropsychol* 1990; 12: 729–44.

[22] Hodges JR, Salmon DP, Butters N. Differential impairment of semantic and episodic memory in Alzheimer's and Huntington's diseases: a controlled prospective study. *J Neurol Neurosurg Psychiatry* 1990; 53: 1089–95.

[23] Hodges JR, Salmon DP, Butters N. The nature of the naming deficit in Alzheimer's and Huntington's disease. *Brain* 1991; 114: 1547–58.

[24] Rosser AE, Hodges JR. Initial letter and semantic category fluency in Alzheimer's disease, Huntington's disease and progressive supranuclear palsy. *J Neurol Neurosurg Psychiatry* 1994; 57: 1389–94.

[25] Azambuja MJ, Radanovic M, Haddad MS, *et al.* Language impairment in Huntington's disease. *Arq Neuropsiquiatr* 2012; 70: 410–15.

[26] Speedie LJ, Brake N, Folstein SE, Bowers D, Heilman KM. Comprehension of prosody in Huntington's disease. *J Neurol Neurosurg Psychiatry* 1990; 53: 607–10.

[27] Lawrence AD, Watkins LH, Sahakian BJ, *et al.* Visual object and visuospatial cognition in Huntington's disease: implications for information processing in corticostriatal circuits. *Brain* 2000; 123: 1349–64.

[28] Brouwers P, Cox C, Martin A, Chase T, Fedio P. Differential perceptual-spatial impairment in Huntington's and Alzheimer's dementia. *Arch Neurol* 1984; 41: 1073–6.

[29] O'Donnell BF, Blekher TM, Weaver M, *et al.* Visual perception in prediagnostic and early stage Huntington's disease. *J Int Neuropsychol Soc* 2008; 14: 446–53.

[30] Shelton PA, Knopman DS. Ideomotor apraxia in Huntington's disease. *Arch Neurol* 1991; 48: 35–41.

[31] Hamilton JM, Haaland KY, Adair JC, Brandt J. Ideomotor limb apraxia in Huntington's disease: implications for corticostriate involvement. *Neuropsychologia* 2003; 41: 614–21.

[32] Hödl AK, Hödl E, Otti DV, *et al.* Ideomotor limb apraxia in Huntington's disease: a case-control study. *J Neurol* 2008; 255: 331–9.

[33] Peinemann A, Schuller S, Pohl C, *et al.* Executive dysfunction in early stages of Huntington's disease is associated with striatal and insular atrophy: a neuropsychological and voxel-based morphometric study. *J Neurol Sci* 2005; 239: 11–19.

[34] Larner AJ. Monogenic Mendelian disorders in general neurological practice. *Int J Clin Pract* 2008; 62: 744–6.

[35] Campodonico JR, Codori AM, Brandt J. Neuropsychological stability over two years in asymptomatic carriers of the Huntington's disease mutation. *J Neurol Neurosurg Psychiatry* 1996; 61: 621–4.

[36] Stout JC, Jones R, Labuschagne I, *et al.* Evaluation of longitudinal 12 and 24 month cognitive outcomes in premanifest and early Huntington's disease. *J Neurol Neurosurg Psychiatry* 2012; 83: 687–94.

[37] Hahn-Barma V, Deweer B, Dürr A, *et al.* Are cognitive changes the first symptoms of Huntington's disease? A study of gene carriers. *J Neurol Neurosurg Psychiatry* 1998; 64: 172–7.

[38] Lawrence AD, Hodges JR, Rosser AE, *et al.* Evidence for specific cognitive deficits in preclinical Huntington's disease. *Brain* 1998; 121: 1329–41.

[39] Kirkwood SC, Siemers E, Hodes ME, *et al.* Subtle changes among presymptomatic carriers of the Huntington's disease gene. *J Neurol Neurosurg Psychiatry* 2000; 69: 773–9.

[40] Naito H, Oyanagi S. Familial myoclonus epilepsy and choreoathetosis: hereditary dentatorubral-pallidoluysian atrophy. *Neurology* 1982; 32: 798–807.

[41] Farmer TW, Wingfield MS, Lynch SA, *et al.* Ataxia, chorea, seizures, and dementia: pathologic features of a newly defined familial disorder. *Arch Neurol* 1989; 46: 774–9.

[42] Worster-Drought C, Hill TR, McMenemey WH. Familial presenile dementia with spastic paralysis. *J Neurol Psychopathol* 1933; 14: 27–34.

[43] Plant GT, Ghiso J, Holton JL, Frangione B, Revesz T. Familial and sporadic cerebral amyloid angiopathies associated with dementia and the BRI dementias. In: Esiri MM, Lee VM-Y, Trojanowski JQ (eds.). *The Neuropathology of Dementia* (2nd edn.). Cambridge: Cambridge University Press, 2004; 330–52.

[44] Holton JL, Lashley T, Ghiso J, *et al.* Familial Danish dementia: a novel form of cerebral amyloidosis associated with deposition of both amyloid-Dan and amyloid-β. *J Neuropathol Exp Neurol* 2002; 61: 254–67.

[45] Vidal R, Frangione B, Rostagno A, *et al.* A stop-codon mutation in the *BRI* gene associated with familial British dementia. *Nature* 1999; 399: 776–81.

[46] Vidal R, Revesz T, Rostagno A, *et al.* A decamer duplication in the 3-prime region of the BRI gene originates an amyloid peptide that is associated with dementia in a Danish kindred. *Proc Natl Acad Sci USA* 2000; 97: 4920–5.

[47] Mead S, James-Galton M, Revesz T, *et al.* Familial British dementia with amyloid angiopathy: early clinical, neuropsychological and imaging findings. *Brain* 2000; 123: 975–91.

[48] Davis RL, Shrimpton AE, Holohan PD, *et al.* Familial dementia caused by polymerization of mutant neuroserpin. *Nature* 1999; 401: 376–9.

[49] Davis RL, Shrimpton AE, Carrell RW, *et al.* Association between conformational mutations in neuroserpin and onset and severity of dementia. *Lancet* 2002; 359: 2242–7 [Erratum: *Lancet* 2002; 360: 1102].

[50] Bradshaw CB, Davis RL, Shrimpton AE, *et al.* Cognitive deficits associated with a recently reported familial neurodegenerative disease: familial encephalopathy with neuroserpin inclusion bodies. *Arch Neurol* 2001; 58: 1429–34.

[51] Klünemann HH, Ridha BH, Magy L, *et al.* The genetic causes of basal ganglia calcification, dementia, and bone cysts: DAP12 and TREM2. *Neurology* 2005; 64: 1502–7.

[52] Paloneva J, Autti T, Raininko R, *et al.* CNS manifestations of Nasu–Hakola disease: a frontal dementia with bone cysts. *Neurology* 2001; 56: 1552–8.

[53] Montalbetti L, Ratti MT, Greco B, *et al.* Neuropsychological tests and functional nuclear neuroimaging provide evidence of subclinical impairment in Nasu–Hakola disease heterozygotes. *Funct Neurol* 2005; 20: 71–5.

[54] Holmes G. The Croonian lectures on the clinical symptoms of cerebellar disease and their interpretation. *Lancet* 1922; i: 1177–82, 1231–7; ii: 59–65, 111–5.

[55] Schmahmann JD, Sherman JC. The cerebellar cognitive affective syndrome. *Brain* 1998; 121: 561–79.

[56] De Michele G, Coppola G, Cocozza S, Filla A. A pathogenetic classification of hereditary ataxias: is the time ripe? *J Neurol* 2004; 251: 913–22.

[57] Harding AE. *The Hereditary Ataxias and Related Disorders*. Edinburgh: Churchill Livingstone, 1984.

[58] Sequeiros J, Martindale J, Seneca S, *et al.* EMQN best practice guidelines for molecular genetic testing of SCAs. *Eur J Hum Genet* 2010; 18: 1173–6 [Erratum *Eur J Hum Genet* 2010; 18: 1176–7].

[59] Bürk K, Bosch S, Globas C, *et al.* Executive dysfunction in spinocerebellar ataxia type 1. *Eur Neurol* 2001; 46: 43–8.

[60] Bürk K, Globas C, Bösch S, *et al.* Cognitive deficits in spinocerebellar ataxia 2. *Brain* 1999; 122: 769–77.

[61] Le Pira F, Zappala G, Saponara R, *et al.* Cognitive findings in spinocerebellar ataxia type 2: relationship to genetic and clinical variables. *J Neurol Sci* 2002; 201: 53–7.

[62] Valis M, Masopust J, Bazant J, *et al.* Cognitive changes in spinocerebellar ataxia type 2. *Neuro Endocrinol Lett* 2011; 32: 354–9.

[63] Storey E, Forrest SM, Shaw JH, *et al.* Spinocerebellar ataxia type 2. Clinical features of a pedigree displaying prominent frontal-executive dysfunction. *Arch Neurol* 1999; 56: 43–50.

[64] Boesch SM, Globas C, Bürk K, Poewe W, Dichgans J. Cognitive deficits in spinocerebellar ataxia type 2 (SCA2): a comparative study in two founder populations. *Mov Disord* 2000; 15: 235 (abstract P1092).

[65] Le Pira F, Giuffrida S, Maci T, *et al.* Dissociation between motor and cognitive impairments in SCA2: evidence from a follow-up study. *J Neurol* 2007; 254: 1455–6.

[66] Giunti P, Sweeney MG, Harding AE. Detection of the Machado–Joseph disease/spinocerebellar ataxia three trinucleotide repeat expansion in families with autosomal dominant motor disorders, including the Drew family of Walworth. *Brain* 1995; 118: 1077–85.

[67] Maruff P, Tyler P, Burt T, *et al.* Cognitive deficits in Machado–Joseph disease. *Ann Neurol* 1996; 40: 421–7.

[68] Ishikawa A, Yamada M, Makino K, *et al.* Dementia and delirium in 4 patients with Machado–Joseph disease. *Arch Neurol* 2002; 59: 1804–8.

[69] Garrard P, Martin NH, Giunti P, Cipolotti L. Cognitive and social cognitive functioning in spinocerebellar ataxia: a preliminary characterization. *J Neurol* 2008; 255: 398–405.

[70] McMurtray AM, Clark DG, Flood MK, Perlman S, Mendez MF. Depressive and memory symptoms as presenting features of spinocerebellar ataxia. *J Neuropsychiatry Clin Neurosci* 2006; 18: 420–2.

[71] Tashiro H, Suzuki SO, Hitotsumatsu T, Iwaki T. An autopsy case of spinocerebellar ataxia type 6 with mental symptoms of schizophrenia and dementia. *Clin Neuropathol* 1999; 18: 198–204.

[72] Suenaga M, Kawai Y, Watanabe H, *et al.* Cognitive impairment in spinocerebellar ataxia type 6. *J Neurol Neurosurg Psychiatry* 2008; 79: 496–9.

[73] Cooper FE, Grube M, Elsegood KJ, *et al.* The contribution of the cerebellum to cognition in spinocerebellar ataxia type 6. *Behav Neurol* 2010; 23: 3–15.

[74] Cooper FE, Grube M, Von Kriegstein K, *et al.* Distinct critical cerebellar subregions for components of verbal working memory. *Neuropsychologia* 2012; 50: 189–97.

[75] Walker M, Farrell D. Spinocerebellar ataxia type 7 (SCA7). *Pract Neurol* 2006; 6: 44–7.

[76] Silveira I, Alonso I, Guimaraes L, *et al.* High germinal instability of the (CTG)n at the SCA8 locus of both expanded and normal alleles. *Am J Hum Genet* 2000; 66: 830–40.

[77] Lilja A, Hamalainen P, Kaitaranta E, Rinne R. Cognitive impairment in spinocerebellar ataxia type 8. *J Neurol Sci* 2005; 237: 31–8.

[78] Torrens L, Burns E, Stone J, *et al.* Spinocerebellar ataxia type 8 in Scotland: frequency, neurological, neuropsychological and neuropsychiatric findings. *Acta Neurol Scand* 2008; 117: 41–8.

[79] Koutsis G, Karadima G, Pandraud A, *et al.* Genetic screening of Greek patients with Huntington's disease phenocopies identifies an SCA8 expansion. *J Neurol* 2012; 259: 1874–8.

[80] O'Hearn E, Holmes SE, Calvert PC, Ross CA, Margolis RL. SCA-12: tremor with cerebellar and cortical atrophy is associated with a CAG repeat expansion. *Neurology* 2001; 56: 299–303.

[81] Castrioto A, Prontera P, Di Gregorio E, *et al.* A novel spinocerebellar ataxia type 15 family with involuntary movements and cognitive decline. *Eur J Neurol* 2011; 18: 1263–5.

[82] Rolfs A, Koeppen AH, Bauer I, *et al.* Clinical features and neuropathology of autosomal dominant spinocerebellar ataxia (SCA17). *Ann Neurol* 2003; 54: 367–75.

[83] Mariotti C, Alpini D, Fancellu R, *et al.* Spinocerebellar ataxia type 17 (SCA17): oculomotor phenotype and clinical characterization of 15 Italian patients. *J Neurol* 2007; 254: 1538–46.

[84] Bruni AC, Takahashi-Fujigasaki J, Maltecca F, *et al.* Behavioral disorder, dementia, ataxia, and rigidity in a large family with TATA Box-binding protein mutation. *Arch Neurol* 2004; 61: 1314–20.

[85] Schelhaas JH, van de Warrenburg BP, Hageman G, *et al.* Cognitive impairment in SCA-19. *Acta Neurol Belg* 2003; 103: 199–205.

[86] Delplanque J, Devos D, Vuillaume I, *et al.* Slowly progressive spinocerebellar ataxia with extrapyramidal signs and mild cognitive impairment (SCA21). *Cerebellum* 2008; 7: 179–83.

[87] Pandolfo M. Friedreich ataxia. *Arch Neurol* 2008; 65: 1296–1303.

[88] White M, Lalonde R, Botez-Marquard T. Neuropsychologic and neuropsychiatric characteristics of patients with Friedreich's ataxia. *Acta Neurol Scand* 2000; 102: 222–6.

[89] Wollmann T, Barroso J, Monton F, Nieto A. Neuropsychological test performance of patients with Friedreich's ataxia. *J Clin Exp Neuropsychol* 2002; 24: 677–86.

[90] Colvin IB, Lennox GG. Cognitive function in ataxia telangiectasia. *J Neurol Neurosurg Psychiatry* 1997; 62: 210.

[91] Vinck A, Verhagen MM, Gerven M, *et al.* Cognitive and speech–language performance in children with ataxia telangiectasia. *Dev Neurorehabil* 2011; 14: 315–22.

[92] Gomez CM. ARSACS goes global. *Neurology* 2004; 62: 10–11.

[93] Hara K, Onodera O, Endo M, *et al.* Sacsin-related autosomal recessive ataxia without prominent retinal myelinated fibers in Japan. *Mov Disord* 2005; 20: 380–2.

[94] Verhoeven WM, Egger JI, Ahmed AI, *et al.* Cerebellar cognitive affective syndrome and autosomal recessive spastic ataxia of Charlevoix–Saguenay: a report of two male sibs. *Psychopathology* 2012; 45: 193–9.

[95] Ferrer I, Olivé M, Rivera R, *et al.* Hereditary spastic paraparesis with dementia, amyotrophy and peripheral neuropathy. A neuropathological study. *Neuropathol Appl Neurobiol* 1995; 21: 255–61.

[96] Webb S, Hutchinson M. Cognitive impairment in families with pure autosomal dominant hereditary spastic paraparesis. *Brain* 1998; 121: 923–9.

[97] Gasser T, Finsterer J, Baets J, *et al.* EFNS guidelines on the molecular diagnosis of ataxias and spastic paraplegias. *Eur J Neurol* 2010; 17: 179–88.

[98] Larner AJ, Doran M. Clinical phenotypic heterogeneity of Alzheimer's disease associated with mutations of the presenilin-1 gene. *J Neurol* 2006; 253: 139–58.

[99] Byrne P, McMonagle P, Webb S, *et al.* Age-related cognitive decline in hereditary spastic paraparesis linked to chromosome 2p. *Neurology* 2000; 54: 1510–17.

[100] McMonagle P, Byrne P, Hutchinson M. Further evidence of dementia in SPG4-linked autosomal dominant hereditary spastic paraplegia. *Neurology* 2004; 62: 407–10.

[101] Murphy S, Gorman G, Beetz C, *et al.* Dementia in SPG4 hereditary spastic paraplegia: clinical, genetic, and neuropathologic evidence. *Neurology* 2009; 73: 378–84.

[102] Tallaksen CME, Guichart-Gomez E, Verpillat P, *et al.* Subtle cognitive impairment but no dementia in patients with spastin mutations. *Arch Neurol* 2003; 60: 1113–18.

[103] Cross HE, McKusick VA. The Mast syndrome: a recessively inherited form of pre-senile dementia with motor disturbances. *Arch Neurol* 1967; 16: 1–13.

[104] D'Hooge M. Probable cases of Mast syndrome in a non-Amish family. *J Neurol Neurosurg Psychiatry* 1992; 55: 1210.

[105] Simpson MA, Cross H, Proukakis C, *et al.* Maspardin is mutated in Mast syndrome, a complicated form of hereditary spastic paraplegia associated with dementia. *Am J Hum Genet* 2003; 73: 1147–56.

[106] Jacquemont S, Hagerman RJ, Hagerman PJ, Leehey MA. Fragile-X syndrome and fragile-X-associated tremor/ataxia syndrome: two faces of FMR1. *Lancet Neurology* 2007; 6: 45–55.

[107] Gallagher A, Hallahan B. Fragile X-associated disorders: a clinical overview. *J Neurol* 2012; 259: 401–13.

[108] Davies KE (ed.). *The Fragile X Syndrome*. Oxford: Oxford University Press, 1989.

[109] Verkerk AJ, Pieretti M, Sutcliffe JS, *et al.* Identification of a gene (FMR1) containing a CGG repeat coincident with a breakpoint cluster region exhibiting length variation in fragile X syndrome. *Cell* 1991; 65: 905–14.

[110] Schapiro MB, Murphy DG, Hagerman RJ, *et al.* Adult fragile X syndrome: neuropsychology, brain anatomy,

and metabolism. *Am J Med Genet* 1995; 60: 480–93.

[111] Bennetto L, Pennington BF, Porter D, Taylor AK, Hagerman RJ. Profile of cognitive functioning in women with the fragile X mutation. *Neuropsychology* 2001; 15: 290–9.

[112] Hall DA, Berry KE, Jacquemont S, *et al.* Initial diagnoses given to persons with the fragile X associated tremor/ataxia syndrome (FXTAS). *Neurology* 2005; 65: 299–301.

[113] Brunberg JA, Jacquemont S, Hagerman RJ, *et al.* Fragile X premutation carriers: characteristic MR imaging findings of adult male patients with progressive cerebellar and cognitive dysfunction. *AJNR Am J Neuroradiol* 2002; 23: 1757–66.

[114] Jacquemont S, Hagerman RJ, Leehey M, *et al.* Fragile X premutation tremor/ataxia syndrome: molecular, clinical and neuroimaging correlates. *Am J Hum Genet* 2003; 72: 869–78.

[115] Hunter JE, Allen EG, Abramowitz A, *et al.* No evidence for a difference in neuropsychological profile among carriers and non-carriers of the FMR1 premutation in adults under the age of 50. *Am J Hum Genet* 2008; 83: 692–702.

[116] Grigsby J, Brega AG, Engle K, *et al.* Cognitive profile of fragile X premutation carriers with and without fragile X-associated tremor/ataxia syndrome. *Neuropsychology* 2008; 22: 48–60.

[117] Seritan AL, Nguyen DV, Farias ST, *et al.* Dementia in fragile X-associated tremor/ataxia syndrome (FXTAS): comparison with Alzheimer's disease. *Am J Med Genet B Neuropsychiatr Genet* 2008; 147B: 1138–44.

[118] Steyaert J, Legius E, Borghgraef M, Fryns JP. A distinct neurocognitive phenotype in female fragile-X premutation carriers assessed with visual attention tasks. *Am J Med Genet A* 2003; 116: 44–51.

[119] Hagerman RJ, Leavitt BR, Farzin F, *et al.* Fragile X-associated tremor/ataxia syndrome (FXTAS) in females with the FMR1 premutation. *Am J Hum Genet* 2004; 74: 1051–6.

[120] Karmon Y, Gadoth N. Fragile X-associated tremor/ataxia syndrome (FXTAS) with dementia in a female harbouring FMR1 premutation. *J Neurol Neurosurg Psychiatry* 2008; 79: 738–9.

[121] Tassone F, Greco CM, Hunsaker MR, *et al.* Neuropathological, clinical and molecular pathology in female fragile X premutation carriers with and without FXTAS. *Genes Brain Behav* 2012; 11: 577–85.

[122] Wilson SAK. Progressive lenticular degeneration: a familial nervous disease associated with cirrhosis of the liver. *Brain* 1912; 34: 295–509.

[123] Rathbun JK. Neuropsychological aspects of Wilson's disease. *Int J Neurosci* 1996; 85: 221–9.

[124] Medalia A, Isaacs Glaberman K, Scheinberg IH. Neuropsychological impairment in Wilson's disease. *Arch Neurol* 1988; 45: 502–4.

[125] Seniów J, Bak T, Gajda J, Poniatowska R, Czlonkowska A. Cognitive functioning in neurologically symptomatic and asymptomatic forms of Wilson's disease. *Mov Disord* 2002; 17: 1077–83.

[126] Hegde S, Sinha S, Rao SL, Taly AB, Vasudev MK. Cognitive profile and structural findings in Wilson's disease: a neuropsychological and MRI-based study. *Neurol India* 2010; 58: 708–13.

[127] Littman E, Medalia A, Senior G, Scheinberg IH. Rate of information processing in patients with Wilson's disease. *J Neuropsychiatry Clin Neurosci* 1995; 7: 68–71.

[128] Goldstein NP, Ewert JC, Randall RV, Gross JB. Psychiatric aspects of Wilson's disease (hepatolenticular degeneration): results of psychometric tests during long-term therapy. *Am J Psychiatry* 1968; 124: 1555–61.

[129] Lang C, Müller D, Claus D, Druschky KF. Neuropsychological findings in treated Wilson's disease. *Acta Neurol Scand* 1990; 81: 75–81.

[130] Rosselli M, Lorenzana P, Rosselli A, Vergara I. Wilson's disease, a reversible dementia: case report. *J Clin Exp Neuropsychol* 1987; 9: 399–406.

[131] Polson RJ, Rolles K, Calne RY, Williams R, Marsden D. Reversal of severe neurological manifestations of Wilson's disease following orthotopic liver transplantation. *Q J Med* 1987; 64: 685–91.

[132] Zhou B, Westaway SK, Levinson B, *et al.* A novel pantothenate kinase gene is defective in Hallervorden–Spatz syndrome. *Nat Genet* 2001; 28: 345–9.

[133] Hayflick SJ, Westaway SK, Levinson B, *et al.* Genetic, clinical, and radiographic delineation of Hallervorden–Spatz syndrome. *N Engl J Med* 2003; 348: 33–40.

[134] Gregory A, Polster BJ, Hayflick SJ. Clinical and genetic delineation of neurodegeneration with brain iron accumulation. *J Med Genet* 2009; 46: 73–80.

[135] Mahoney S, Selway R, Lin JP. Cognitive functioning in children with pantothenate-kinase-associated neurodegeneration undergoing deep brain stimulation. *Dev Med Child Neurol* 2011; 53: 275–9.

[136] Marelli C, Piacentini S, Garavaglia B, Girotti F, Albanese A. Clinical and neuropsychological correlates in two brothers with pantothenate kinase-associated neurodegeneration. *Mov Disord* 2005; 20: 208–12.

[137] Danek A (ed.). *Neuroacanthocytosis Syndromes.* Dordrecht: Springer, 2004.

[138] Hardie RJ, Pullon HW, Harding AE, *et al.* Neuroacanthocytosis. A clinical, haematological and pathological study of 19 cases. *Brain* 1991; 114: 13–49.

[139] Doran M, Harvie AK, Larner AJ. Antisocial behaviour disorders: the need to consider underlying neuropsychiatric disease. *Int J Clin Pract* 2006; 60: 861–2.

[140] Kartsounis LD, Hardie RJ. The pattern of cognitive impairments in neuroacanthocytosis. *Arch Neurol* 1996; 53: 77–80.

[141] Curtis AR, Fey C, Morris CM, *et al.* Mutation in the gene encoding ferritin light polypeptide causes dominant adult-onset basal ganglia disease. *Nat Genet* 2001; 28: 350–4.

[142] Vidal R, Ghetti B, Takao M, *et al.* Intracellular ferritin accumulation in neural and extraneural tissue characterizes a neurodegenerative disease associated with a mutation in the ferritin light polypeptide gene. *J Neuropath Exp Neurol* 2004; 63: 363–80.

[143] Wills AJ, Sawle GV, Guilbert PR, Curtis ARJ. Palatal tremor and cognitive decline in neuroferritinopathy. *J Neurol Neurosurg Psychiatry* 2002; 73: 91–2.

[144] Chinnery P, Curtis A, Fey C, *et al.* Neuroferritinopathy in a French family with late onset dominant dystonia. *J Med Genet* 2003; 40: e69.

[145] Maciel P, Cruz VT, Constante M, *et al.* Neuroferritinopathy: missense mutation in FTL causing early-onset bilateral pallidal involvement. *Neurology* 2005; 65: 603–5.

[146] Chinnery PF, Crompton DE, Birchall D, *et al.* Clinical features and natural history of neuroferritinopathy caused by the FTL1 460InsA mutation. *Brain* 2007; 130: 110–19.

[147] Harris ZL, Migas MC, Hughes AE, Logan JI, Gitlin JD. Familial dementia due to a frameshift mutation in the caeruloplasmin gene. *Q J Med* 1996; 89: 355–9.

[148] Morita H, Inoue A, Yanagisawa N. A case of caeruloplasmin deficiency which showed dementia, ataxia and iron deposition in the brain [in Japanese]. *Rinsho Shinkeigaku* 1992; 32: 483–7.

[149] Logan JI, Harveyson KB, Wisdom GB, Hughes AE, Archbold GPR. Hereditary caeruloplasmin deficiency, dementia and diabetes mellitus. *Q J Med* 1994; 87: 663–70.

[150] Davidson C. Pallido-pyramidal disease. *J Neuropathol Exp Neurol* 1954; 13: 50–9.

[151] Al-Din NAS, Wriekat A, Mubaidin A, Dasouki M, Hiari M. Pallido-pyramidal degeneration, supranuclear upgaze paresis and dementia: Kufor–Rakeb syndrome. *Acta Neurol Scand* 1994; 89: 347–52.

[152] Crosiers D, Ceulemans B, Meeus B, *et al.* Juvenile dystonia–parkinsonism and dementia caused by a novel ATP13A2 frameshift mutation. *Parkinsonism Relat Disord* 2011; 17: 135–8.

[153] Kobari M, Nogawa S, Sugimoto Y, Fukuuchi Y. Familial idiopathic brain calcification with autosomal dominant inheritance. *Neurology* 1997; 48: 645–9.

[154] Benke T, Karner S, Seppi K, *et al.* Subacute dementia and imaging correlates in a case of Fahr's disease. *J Neurol Neurosurg Psychiatry* 2004; 75: 1163–5.

[155] Modrego PJ, Mojonero J, Serrano M, Fayed N. Fahr's syndrome presenting with pure and progressive presenile dementia. *Neurol Sci* 2005; 26: 367–9.

[156] Markowitsch HJ, Calabrese P, Würker M, *et al.* The amygdala's contribution to memory–a study on two patients with Urbach-Wiethe disease. *Neuroreport* 1994; 5: 1349–52.

[157] Siebert M, Markowitsch HJ, Bartel P. Amygdala, affect and cognition: evidence from 10 patients with Urbach–Wiethe disease. *Brain* 2003; 126: 2627–37.

[158] Dale RC, Nasti JJ, Peters GB. Familial 7q21.3 microdeletion involving epsilon-sarcoglycan causing myoclonus dystonia, cognitive impairment, and psychosis. *Mov Disord* 2011; 26: 1774–5.

[159] Bain PG, Findley LJ, Thompson PD, *et al.* A study of hereditary essential tremor. *Brain* 1994; 117: 805–24

[160] Plumb M, Bain P. *Essential Tremor: The Facts.* Oxford: Oxford University Press, 2007.

[161] Louis ED. Essential tremor. *Handb Clin Neurol* 2011; 100: 433–48.

[162] Lombardi WJ, Woolston DJ, Roberts JW, Gross RE. Cognitive deficits in patients with essential tremor. *Neurology* 2001; 57: 785–90.

[163] Gasparini M, Bonifati V, Fabrizio E, *et al.* Frontal lobe dysfunction in essential tremor. A preliminary study. *J Neurol* 2001; 248: 399–402.

[164] LaRoia H, Louis ED. Association between essential tremor and other neurodegenerative diseases: what

is the epidemiological evidence? *Neuroepidemiology* 2011; 37: 1–10.

[165] Larner AJ, Allen CMC. Hereditary essential tremor and restless legs syndrome. *Postgrad Med J* 1997; 73: 254.

[166] Duane DD, Vermilion KJ. Cognitive deficits in patients with essential tremor. *Neurology* 2002; 58: 1706.

[167] Lacritz LH, Dewey R Jr, Giller C, Cullum CM. Cognitive functioning in individuals with benign essential tremor. *J Int Neuropsychol Soc* 2002; 8: 125–9.

[168] Benito-Leon J, Louis ED, Mitchell AJ, Bermejo-Pareja F. Elderly-onset essential tremor and mild cognitive impairment: a population-based study (NEDICES). *J Alzheimers Dis* 2011; 23: 727–35.

[169] Bermejo-Pareja F, Louis ED, Benito-Leon J. Risk of incident dementia in essential tremor: a population-based study. *Mov Disord* 2007; 22: 1573–80.

[170] Phukan J, Albanese A, Gasser T, Warner T. Primary dystonia and dystonia-plus syndromes: clinical characteristics, diagnosis, and pathogenesis. *Lancet Neurol* 2011; 10: 1074–85.

[171] Scott RB, Gregory R, Wilson J, *et al*. Executive cognitive deficits in primary dystonia. *Mov Disord* 2003; 18: 539–50.

[172] Jahanshahi M, Rowe J, Fuller R. Cognitive executive function in dystonia. *Mov Disord* 2003; 18: 1470–81.

[173] Ochudlo S, Wisniewska K, Opala G. Executive dysfunction in focal dystonia. *Neurodegen Dis* 2009; 6 (Suppl 1): 1756.

[174] Finsterer J, Harbo HF, Baets J, *et al*. EFNS guidelines on the molecular diagnosis of mitochondrial disorders. *Eur J Neurol* 2009; 16: 1255–64.

[175] Kartsounis LD, Truong DD, Morgan Hughes JA, Harding AE. The neuropsychological features of mitochondrial myopathies and encephalomyopathies. *Arch Neurol* 1992; 49: 158–60.

[176] Turconi AC, Benti R, Castelli E, *et al*. Focal cognitive impairment in mitochondrial encephalomyopathies: a neuropsychological and neuroimaging study. *J Neurol Sci* 1999; 170: 57–63.

[177] Kornblum C, Bosbach S, Wagner M, *et al*. Neuropsychological testing of patients with PEO and Kearns–Sayre syndrome reveals distinct frontal and parieto-occipital deficits. *J Neurol* 2000; 247: III/73 (abstract P266).

[178] Sartor H, Loose R, Tucha O, Klein HE, Lange KW. MELAS: a neuropsychological and radiological follow-up study. Mitochondrial encephalomyopathy, lactic acidosis and stroke. *Acta Neurol Scand* 2002; 106: 309–13.

[179] Lindroos MM, Borra RJ, Parkkola R, *et al*. Cerebral oxygen and glucose metabolism in patients with mitochondrial m3243A>G mutation. *Brain* 2009; 132: 3274–84.

[180] Finsterer J. Mitochondrial disorders, cognitive impairment and dementia. *J Neurol Sci* 2009; 283: 143–8.

[181] Salsano E, Giovagnoli AR, Morandi L, *et al*. Mitochondrial dementia: a sporadic case of progressive cognitive and behavioural decline with hearing loss due to the rare m.3291T>C MELAS mutation. *J Neurol Sci* 2011; 300: 165–8.

[182] Young TM, Blakely EL, Swalwell H, *et al*. Mitochondrial transfer RNA(Phe) mutation associated with a progressive neurodegenerative disorder characterized by psychiatric disturbance, dementia, and akinesia-rigidity. *Arch Neurol* 2010; 67: 1399–402.

[183] Baumann N, Turpin J-C. Adult-onset leukodystrophies. *J Neurol* 2000; 247: 751–9.

[184] Johannsen P, Ehlers L, Hansen HJ. Dementia with impaired temporal glucose metabolism in late-onset metachromatic leukodystrophy. *Dement Geriatr Cogn Disord* 2001; 12: 85–8.

[185] Fukutani Y, Noriki Y, Sasaki K, *et al*. Adult-type metachromatic leukodystrophy with a compound heterozygote mutation showing character change and dementia. *Psychiatry Clin Neurosci* 1999; 53: 425–8.

[186] Salmon E, van der Linden M, Maerfens-Noordhout A, *et al*. Early thalamic and cortical hypometabolism in adult-onset dementia due to metachromatic leukodystrophy. *Acta Neurol Belg* 1999; 99: 185–8.

[187] Kozian R, Sieber N, Thiergart S. Frontotemporal dementia in metachromatic leukodystrophy [in German]. *Fortschr Neurol Psychiatr* 2007; 75: 549–51.

[188] Marcão AM, Wiest R, Schindler K, *et al*. Adult onset metachromatic leukodystrophy without electroclinical peripheral nervous system involvement: a new mutation in the ARSA gene. *Arch Neurol* 2005; 62: 309–13.

[189] Amaducci L, Sorbi S, Piacentini S, Bick KL. The first Alzheimer disease case: a metachromatic leukodystrophy? *Dev Neurosci* 1991; 13: 186–7.

[190] Amaducci L. Alzheimer's original patient. *Science* 1996; 274: 328.

[191] Moser HW, Raymond GV, Dubey P. Adrenoleukodystrophy: new approaches to a neurodegenerative disease. *JAMA* 2005; 294: 3131–4.

[192] Powers JM, Schaumburg HH, Gaffney CL. Kluver-Bucy syndrome caused by adreno-leukodystrophy. *Neurology* 1980; 30: 1231–2.

[193] Esiri MM, Hyman NM, Horton WL, Lindenbaum RH. Adrenoleukodystrophy: clinical, pathological and biochemical findings in two brothers with the onset of cerebral disease in adult life. *Neuropath Appl Neurobiol* 1984; 10: 429–45.

[194] Sereni C, Ruel M, Iba-Zizen T, *et al.* Adult adrenoleukodystrophy: a sporadic case? *J Neurol Sci* 1987; 80: 121–8.

[195] Panegyres PK, Goldswain P, Kakulas BA. Adult-onset adrenoleukodystrophy manifesting as dementia. *Am J Med* 1989; 87: 481–3.

[196] Larner AJ. Adult-onset dementia with prominent frontal lobe dysfunction in X-linked adrenoleukodystrophy with R152C mutation in ABCD1 gene. *J Neurol* 2003; 250: 1253–4.

[197] Sutovsky S, Petrovic R, Chandoga J, Turcani P. Adult onset cerebral form of X-linked adrenoleukodystrophy with dementia of frontal lobe type with new L160P mutation in ABCD1 gene. *J Neurol Sci* 2007; 263: 149–53.

[198] Angus B, de Silva R, Davidson R, Bone I. A family with adult-onset cerebral adrenoleucodystrophy. *J Neurol* 1994; 241: 497–9.

[199] Garside S, Rosebush PI, Levinson AJ, Mazurek MF. Late-onset adrenoleukodystrophy associated with long-standing psychiatric symptoms. *J Clin Psychiatry* 1999; 60: 460–8.

[200] Uyama E, Iwagoe H, Maeda J, *et al.* Presenile onset cerebral adrenoleukodystrophy presenting as Balint's syndrome and dementia. *Neurology* 1993; 43: 1249–51.

[201] Cox CS, Dubey P, Raymond GV, *et al.* Cognitive evaluation of neurologically asymptomatic boys with X-linked adrenoleukodystrophy. *Arch Neurol* 2005; 63: 69–73.

[202] Larner AJ. Asymptomatic X-linked adrenoleukodystrophy with the R152C mutation: neuropsychological and neuroimaging findings. *Eur J Neurol* 2008; 15 (Suppl 3): 293 (abstract p. 2323).

[203] Moser HW, Raymond GV, Lu SE, *et al.* Follow-up of 89 asymptomatic patients with adrenoleukodystrophy treated with Lorenzo's oil. *Arch Neurol* 2005; 62: 1073–80.

[204] Mahmood A, Raymond GV, Dubey P, Peters C, Moser HW. Survival analysis of haematopoietic cell transplantation for childhood cerebral X-linked adrenoleukodystrophy: a comparison study. *Lancet Neurol* 2007; 6: 687–92.

[205] Brenner M, Johnson AB, Boespflug-Tanguy O, *et al.* Mutations in GFAP, encoding glial fibrillary acidic protein, are associated with Alexander disease. *Nat Genet* 2001; 27: 117–20.

[206] Namekawa M, Takiyama Y, Aoki Y, *et al.* Identification of GFAP gene mutation in hereditary adult-onset Alexander's disease. *Ann Neurol* 2002; 52: 779–85.

[207] Wilson SP, Al-Sarraj S, Bridges LR. Rosenthal fiber encephalopathy presenting with demyelination and Rosenthal fibers in a solvent abuser: adult Alexander's disease? *Clin Neuropathol* 1996; 15: 13–16.

[208] Jacob J, Robertson NJ, Hilton DA. The clinicopathological spectrum of Rosenthal fibre encephalopathy and Alexander's disease: a case report and review of the literature. *J Neurol Neurosurg Psychiatry* 2003; 74: 807–10.

[209] Yoshida T, Sasaki M, Yoshida M, *et al.* Nationwide survey of Alexander disease in Japan and proposed new guidelines for diagnosis. *J Neurol* 2011; 258: 1998–2008.

[210] Walls TJ, Jones RA, Cartlidge NEF, Saunders M. Alexander's disease with Rosenthal fibre formation in an adult. *J Neurol Neurosurg Psychiatry* 1984; 47: 399–403.

[211] Bruyn GW, Weenink HR, Bots GT, Teepen JL, van Wolferen WJ. Pelizaeus–Merzbacher disease. The Löwenberg–Hill type. *Acta Neuropathol* 1985; 67: 177–89.

[212] Garbern J, Cambi F, Shy M, Kamholz J. The molecular pathogenesis of Pelizaeus–Merzbacher disease. *Arch Neurol* 1999; 56: 1210–14.

[213] Saito Y, Ando T, Doyu M, Takahashi A, Hashizume Y. An adult case of classical Pelizaeus–Merzbacher disease–magnetic resonance images and neuropathological findings [in Japanese]. *Rinsho Shinkeigaku* 1993; 33: 187–93.

[214] Nance MA, Boyadjiev S, Pratt VM, *et al.* Adult-onset neurodegenerative disorder due to proteolipid protein gene mutation in the mother of a man with Pelizaeus–Merzbacher disease. *Neurology* 1996; 47: 1333–5.

[215] Sasaki A, Miyanaga K, Ototsuji M, *et al.* Two autopsy cases with Pelizaeus–Merzbacher disease phenotype

of adult onset, without mutation of proteolipid protein gene. *Acta Neuropathol* 2000; 99: 7–13.

[216] Marble M, Voeller KS, May MM, *et al.* Pelizaeus–Merzbacher syndrome: neurocognitive function in a family with carrier manifestations. *Am J Med Genet* 2007; 143A: 1442–7.

[217] Jardim LB, Giugliani R, Pires RF, *et al.* Protracted course of Krabbe disease in an adult patient bearing a novel mutation. *Arch Neurol* 1999; 56: 1014–17.

[218] van der Knapp MS, Pronk JC, Scheper GC. Vanishing white matter disease. *Lancet Neurol* 2006; 5: 413–23.

[219] Prass K, Bruck W, Schroder NW, *et al.* Adult-onset leukoencephalopathy with vanishing white matter presenting with dementia. *Ann Neurol* 2001; 50: 665–8.

[220] Ohtake H, Shimohata T, Terajima K, *et al.* Adult-onset leukoencephalopathy with vanishing white matter with a missense mutation in EIF2B5. *Neurology* 2004; 62: 1601–3.

[221] Gascon-Bayarri J, Campdelacreu J, Sanchez-Castaneda C, *et al.* Leukoencephalopathy with vanishing white matter presenting with presenile dementia. *J Neurol Neurosurg Psychiatry* 2009; 80: 810–11.

[222] De Grouchy J, Royer P, Salmon C, Lamy M. Deletion partielle des bras longs du chromosome 18. *Pathol Biol* 1964; 12: 579–82.

[223] Adab N, Larner AJ. Adult-onset seizure disorder in 18q deletion syndrome. *J Neurol* 2006; 253: 527–8.

[224] Semrud Clikeman M, Thompson NM, Schaub BL, *et al.* Cognitive ability predicts degree of genetic abnormality in participants with 18q deletions. *J Int Neuropsychol Soc* 2005; 11: 584–90.

[225] Rademakers R, Baker M, Nicholson AM, *et al.* Mutations in the colony stimulating factor 1 receptor (CSF1R) gene cause hereditary diffuse leukoencephalopathy with spheroids. *Nat Genet* 2011; 44: 200–5.

[226] Platt FM, Walkley SU (eds.). *Lysosomal Disorders of the Brain. Recent Advances in Molecular and Cellular Pathogenesis and Treatment*. Oxford: Oxford University Press, 2004.

[227] Trend PStJ, Wiles CM, Spencer GT, *et al.* Acid maltase deficiency in adults. *Brain* 1985; 108: 845–60.

[228] Sells RA, Larner AJ. From symptoms to causes: progress in the treatment of neurological disease. *Br J Hosp Med* 2011; 72: 350–1.

[229] Prevett M, Enevoldson TP, Duncan JS. Adult onset acid maltase deficiency associated with epilepsy and dementia: a case report. *J Neurol Neurosurg Psychiatry* 1992; 55: 509.

[230] Winkel LPF, Hagemans MLC, van Doorn PA, *et al.* The natural course of non-classic Pompe's disease: a review of 225 published cases. *J Neurol* 2005; 252: 875–84.

[231] Mehta A, Beck M, Eyskens F, *et al.* Fabry disease: a review of current management strategies. *Q J Med* 2010; 103: 641–59.

[232] Mendez MF, Stanley TM, Medel NM, Li Z, Tedesco DT. The vascular dementia of Fabry's disease. *Dement Geriatr Cogn Disord* 1997; 8: 252–7.

[233] Okeda R, Nisihara M. An autopsy case of Fabry disease with neuropathological investigation of the pathogenesis of associated dementia. *Neuropathology* 2008; 28: 532–40.

[234] MacDermott KD, Holmes A, Miners AH. Anderson–Fabry disease: clinical manifestations and impact of disease in a cohort of 98 hemizygous males. *J Med Genet* 2001; 38: 750–60.

[235] Zaroff CM, Neudorfer O, Morrison C, *et al.* Neuropsychological assessment of patients with late onset GM2 gangliosidosis. *Neurology* 2004; 62: 2283–6.

[236] Frey LC, Ringel SP, Filley CM. The natural history of cognitive dysfunction in late-onset GM2 gangliosidosis. *Arch Neurol* 2005; 62: 989–94.

[237] Guimarães J, Amaral O, Sá Miranda MC. Adult-onset neuronopathic form of Gaucher's disease: a case report. *Parkinsonism Relat Disord* 2003; 9: 261–4.

[238] Clark LN, Kartsaklis LA, Wolf Gilbert R, *et al.* Association of glucocerebrosidase mutations with dementia with Lewy bodies. *Arch Neurol* 2009; 66: 578–83.

[239] Williams RE, Mole SE. New nomenclature and classification scheme for the neuronal ceroid lipofuscinoses. *Neurology* 2012; 79: 183–91.

[240] Josephson SA, Schmidt RE, Millsap P, McManus DQ, Morris JC. Autosomal dominant Kufs' disease: a cause of early onset dementia. *J Neurol Sci* 2001; 188: 51–60.

[241] Larner AJ. Alzheimer's disease, Kufs disease, tellurium, and selenium. *Med Hypotheses* 1996; 47: 73–5.

[242] Arsov T, Smith KR, Damiano J, *et al.* Kufs disease, the major adult form of neuronal ceroid lipofuscinosis, caused by mutations in CLN6. *Am J Hum Genet* 2011; 88: 566–73.

[243] Uc EY, Wenger DA, Jankovic J. Niemann–Pick disease type C: two cases and an update. *Mov Disord* 2000; 15: 1199–203.

[244] Battisti C, Tarugi P, Dotti MT, *et al.* Adult onset Niemann–Pick type C disease: a clinical, neuroimaging and molecular genetic study. *Mov Disord* 2003; 18: 1405–9.

[245] Klünemann HH, Elleder M, Kaminski WE, *et al.* Frontal lobe atrophy due to a mutation in the cholesterol binding protein HE1/NPC2. *Ann Neurol* 2002; 52: 743–9.

[246] Patterson MC, Hendriksz CJ, Walterfang M, *et al.* Recommendations for the diagnosis and management of Niemann–Pick disease type C: an update. *Mol Genet Metab* 2012; 106: 330–44.

[247] Wijburg FA, Sedel F, Pineda M, *et al.* Development of a suspicion index to aid diagnosis of Niemann–Pick disease type C. *Neurology* 2012; 78: 1560–7.

[248] van Schrojenstein-de Valk HMJ, van de Kamp JJP. Follow-up on seven adult patients with mild Sanfilippo B disease. *Am J Med Genet* 1987; 28: 125–30.

[249] Verhoeven WM, Csepan R, Marcelis CL, *et al.* Sanfilippo B in an elderly female psychiatric patient: a rare but relevant diagnosis in presenile dementia. *Acta Psychiatr Scand* 2010; 122; 162–5.

[250] Verrips A, Hoefsloot LH, Steenbergen GCH, *et al.* Clinical and molecular genetic characteristics of patients with cerebrotendinous xanthomatosis. *Brain* 2000; 123: 908–19.

[251] Verrips A, van Engelen BGM, Wevers RA, *et al.* Presence of diarrhea and absence of tendon xanthomas in patients with cerebrotendinous xanthomatosis. *Arch Neurol* 2000; 57: 520–4.

[252] Sugama S, Kimura A, Chen W, *et al.* Frontal lobe dementia with abnormal cholesterol metabolism and heterozygous mutation in sterol 27-hydroxylase gene (CYP27). *J Inherit Metab Dis* 2001; 24: 379–92.

[253] Guyant-Marechal L, Verrips A, Girard C, *et al.* Unusual cerebrotendinous xanthomatosis with fronto-temporal dementia phenotype. *Am J Med Genet A* 2005; 139A: 114–17.

[254] Berginer VM, Salen G, Shefer S. Long-term treatment of cerebrotendinous xanthomatosis with chenodeoxycholic acid. *N Engl J Med* 1984; 311: 1649–52.

[255] Fasano A, Bentivoglio AR, Colosimo C. Movement disorder due to aceruloplasminemia and incorrect diagnosis of hereditary hemochromatosis. *J Neurol* 2007; 254: 113–14.

[256] Jones HR, Hedley-Whyte ET. Idiopathic hemochromatosis (IHC): dementia and ataxia as presenting signs. *Neurology* 1983; 33: 1479–83.

[257] Harvey RJ, Summerfield JA, Fox NC, Warrington EK, Rossor MN. Dementia associated with haemochromatosis: a report of two cases. *Eur J Neurol* 1997; 4: 318–22.

[258] Russo N, Edwards M, Andrews T, O'Brien M, Bhatia KP. Hereditary haemochromatosis is unlikely to cause movement disorders. A critical review. *J Neurol* 2004; 251: 849–52.

[259] Moses SW, Parvari R. The variable presentations of glycogen storage disease type IV: a review of clinical, enzymatic and molecular studies. *Curr Mol Med* 2002; 2: 177–88.

[260] Boulan Predseil P, Vital A, Brochet B, *et al.* Dementia of frontal lobe type due to adult polyglucosan body disease. *J Neurol* 1995; 242: 512–16.

[261] Robertson NP, Wharton S, Anderson J, Scolding NJ. Adult polyglucosan body disease associated with extrapyramidal syndrome. *J Neurol Neurosurg Psychiatry* 1998; 65: 788–90.

[262] Berkhoff M, Weis J, Schroth G, Sturzenegger M. Extensive white-matter changes in case of adult polyglucosan body disease. *Neuroradiology* 2001; 43: 234–6.

[263] Savage G, Ray F, Halmagyi M, Blazely A, Harper C. Stable neuropsychological deficits in adult polyglucosan body disease. *J Clin Neurosci* 2007; 14: 473–7.

[264] Bigio EH, Weiner MF, Bonte FJ, White CL. Familial dementia due to adult polyglucosan body disease. *Clin Neuropathol* 1997; 16: 227–34.

[265] Ubogu EE, Hong STK, Akman HO, *et al.* Adult polyglucosan body disease: a case report of a manifesting heterozygote. *Muscle Nerve* 2005; 32: 675–81.

[266] Segers K, Kadhaim H, Colson C, Duttmann R, Glibert G. Adult polyglucosan body disease masquerading as "ALS with dementia of the Alzheimer type": an exceptional phenotype in a rare pathology. *Alzheimer Dis Assoc Disord* 2012; 26: 96–9.

[267] Baykan B, Striano P, Gianotti S, *et al.* Late-onset and slow-progressing Lafora disease in four siblings with EPM2B mutation. *Epilepsia* 2005; 46: 1695–7.

[268] Stam FC, Wigboldus JM, Bots GT. Presenile dementia–a form of Lafora disease. *J Am Geriatr Soc* 1980; 28: 237–40.

[269] Ramachandran N, Girard JM, Turnbull J, Minassian BA. The autosomal recessively inherited progressive myoclonus epilepsies and their genes. *Epilepsia* 2009; 50: S29–36.

[270] Mazarib A, Xiong L, Neufeld MY, *et al.* Unverricht–Lundborg disease in a five-generation Arab family: instability of dodecamer repeats. *Neurology* 2001; 57: 1050–4.

[271] Crimlisk HL. The little imitator–porphyria: a neuropsychiatric disorder. *J Neurol Neurosurg Psychiatry* 1997; 62: 319–28.

[272] Peters TJ, Sarkany R. Porphyria for the general physician. *Clin Med* 2005; 5: 275–81.

[273] Huson SM, Hughes RAC (eds.). *The Neurofibromatoses: A Pathogenetic and Clinical Overview.* London: Chapman & Hall, 1994.

[274] Korf BR, Rubenstein AE. *Neurofibromatosis: A Handbook for Patients, Families, and Health Care Professionals* (2nd edn.). New York, NY: Thieme, 2005.

[275] Ferner RE, Hughes RAC, Weinman J. Intellectual impairment in neurofibromatosis 1. *J Neurol Sci* 1996; 138: 125–33.

[276] Harrison JE, Bolton PF. Cognitive dysfunction in tuberous sclerosis and other neuronal migration disorders. In: Harrison JE, Owen AM (eds.). *Cognitive Deficits in Brain Disorders.* London: Martin Dunitz, 2002; 325–39.

[277] Winterkorn EB, Pulsifer MB, Thiele EA. Cognitive prognosis of patients with tuberous sclerosis complex. *Neurology* 2007; 68: 62–4.

[278] Kassiri J, Snyder TJ, Bhargava R, Wheatley BM, Sinclair DB. Cortical tubers, cognition, and epilepsy in tuberous sclerosis. *Pediatr Neurol* 2011; 44: 328–32.

[279] van Eeghen AM, Black ME, Pulsifer MB, Kwiatkowski DJ, Thiele EA. Genotype and cognitive phenotype of patients with tuberous sclerosis complex. *Eur J Hum Genet* 2012; 20: 510–15.

[280] Hong D, Scaletta Kent J, Kesler S. Cognitive profile of Turner syndrome. *Dev Disabil Res Rev* 2009; 15: 270–8.

[281] Ross JL, Stefanatos GA, Kushenr H, *et al.* Persistent cognitive deficits in adult women with Turner syndrome. *Neurology* 2002; 58: 218–25.

[282] Boada R, Janusz J, Hutaff-Lee C, Tartaglia N. The cognitive phenotype in Klinefelter syndrome: a review of the literature including genetic and hormonal factors. *Dev Disabil Res Rev* 2009; 15; 284–94.

[283] Ross JL, Zeger MP, Kushner H, Zinn AR, Roeltgen DP. An extra X or Y chromosome: contrasting the cognitive and motor phenotypes in childhood in boys with 47,XYY syndrome or 47,XXY Klinefelter syndrome. *Dev Disabil Res Rev* 2009; 15; 309–17.

Inflammatory, immune-mediated, and systemic disorders

6.1 Multiple sclerosis (MS)

Multiple sclerosis (MS) is a common inflammatory, demyelinating disorder of central nervous system (CNS) white matter, the most common cause of neurological disability in young adults. Ultimately, it results from immune-mediated attack on the myelin–oligodendrocyte complex, although many features of pathogenesis remain unclear [1,2]. Viral infections may be a sufficient but not necessary triggering or exacerbating factor [3–5]. Natural history studies indicate that the disease may follow a variable course, permitting classification into a number of groups, which are helpful in defining cohorts for study: relapsing-remitting disease (RRMS), when acute exacerbations resolve over time with no permanent disability, is common at disease onset, but this may evolve into secondary progressive disease (SPMS) when disability accrues between or in the absence of acute exacerbations; rarely, disease is relentlessly progressive from the onset, the primary progressive pattern (PPMS). Benign variants are also recognized. Diagnostic criteria for MS encompass the clinical, neuroradiological, and laboratory findings [6].

Although MS is most commonly envisaged as a cause of physical disability, cognitive impairment is also a frequent occurrence. This was recognized by Charcot in his *Lectures on the Diseases of the Nervous System* delivered at the Salpetriere in 1877, but it has only been in the last two decades that a large literature on the subject has developed [7–10].

Community and clinical samples have suggested consistently that around 45%–60% of MS patients have some degree of cognitive impairment [11], although severe dementia is uncommon. Etiologically, cognitive dysfunction in MS is currently viewed as a multiple disconnection syndrome (Section 1.3.4).

This high frequency of cognitive deficits, with implications for quality of life and vocational status, has prompted recommendations that cognitive impairment be actively sought in MS, using instruments sensitive to the most commonly affected domains. Because, typically for a white matter disorder, these deficits may be regarded as subcortical [12], commonly used bedside neuropsychological tests such as the Mini-Mental State Examination (MMSE) may be insensitive, particularly to early changes [13]. Screening tests suggested to be both valid and relevant include the Symbol–Digit Modalities (or Substitution) Test (SDMT), Paced Auditory Serial Addition Test (PASAT) and its visual equivalent (PVSAT), the Clock Drawing Test (CDT), backward Digit Span, the learning stage of the California Verbal Learning Test (CVLT), and verbal fluency [7,14–16]. Test batteries designed for use in MS also exist, such as the Brief Repeatable Battery of Neuropsychological Tests (BRB-N; [11]), the MS Inventory of Cognition (MUSIC; [17]), the Minimal Assessment of Cognitive Function in MS (MACFIMS; [18]), and the MS Neuropsychological Questionnaire (MSNQ; [19]). Concurrent neurological and psychiatric features may contribute to cognitive morbidity, including depression, fatigue, primary sensory abnormalities of vision or hearing, dominant hand dysfunction, or medication use, factors which need to be considered when assessing subjective memory complaints in MS patients [10].

Neuropsychological profile (Table 6.1)

The cognitive profile in MS is heterogeneous, as for the neurological findings, so only a general picture can be given. Domains most frequently affected include verbal and nonverbal memory, with impaired attention, reduced speed of information processing, abstract reasoning and verbal fluency deficits, with or without mild visuospatial impairments. As deficits typical of cortical dementia, such as aphasia, agnosia, and apraxia, seldom occur, the cognitive impairment in MS has been classified as a subcortical dementia [12].

Attention

Although simple tests of attention such as Digit Span may be normal in MS, analysis of the more demanding backward component of this task demonstrates more impairment in MS patients than in controls [11]. More stringent tests of attention, such as the PASAT and PVSAT [20], may be abnormal even in early disease [21]. The capacity to store and access information held in working memory seems intact, although it may become impaired in disease exacerbations [22] or if the disease course becomes progressive [23].

These results may reflect an inability to devote sufficient attentional resources to process simultaneously the multiple components of these tasks. These are also tests of speed of information

Table 6.1. Typical neuropsychological deficits in multiple sclerosis

Attention	Impaired processing speed, working memory (backward digit span, PASAT)
General intelligence	↓ FSIQ vs. premorbid IQ; PIQ typically more impaired than VIQ
Memory	Impaired verbal and spatial learning, acquisition +/− encoding; semantic and implicit memory relatively preserved
Language	Aphasia rare
Perception	Visuospatial and visuoperceptual deficits may occur
Praxis	Praxis difficult to assess with concurrent motor deficits but apraxia may occur
Executive function	Dysexecutive syndrome common: impaired abstract reasoning, concept formation, and problem solving

processing, as well as of arithmetical ability and short-term memory, such that fatigue is a potential confounder. In support of a defect in cognitive speed, slowed scanning of working memory (Reed–Sternberg paradigm) has been demonstrated [24], as has slowed information processing in both auditory and visual tasks when controlling for accuracy of task performance. On the basis of these findings, it has been suggested that impaired speed of information processing may be a key deficit in MS, with implications for rehabilitation strategies [25,26]; for example, avoidance of "multitasking" (switching between two or more tasks). Slowed cognitive processing in MS may be related to atrophy in the thalamus and putamen [27].

General intelligence (IQ)

Measures of general intelligence in MS, virtually all using the National Adult Reading Test (NART) to predict premorbid IQ, have consistently found a fall in IQ, but this is mainly related to measures on the performance scales, impairments in which may be related to sensorimotor dysfunction. Verbal IQ scores generally remain stable.

Memory

Although impairments in "short-term memory" are present in MS (considered under *Attention*), deficits specifically of long-term (secondary) memory are probably the most common type of memory impairment in MS, affecting both verbal and nonverbal

categories [11,22,28]. As deficits are more apparent on tests of recall than recognition, a greater defect of retrieval rather than of encoding has been postulated, although there is also evidence of impaired acquisition or encoding of new information [29]. As regards remote (retrograde) memory, deficits in famous faces recognition tests have been reported by some authors [23] but not others [11], although the patient case mix in these two studies was not comparable. Impairments in verbal fluency also suggest a retrograde memory loss [11]. Implicit (procedural) memory seems relatively intact in MS [30]. Mesial temporal lobe including hippocampal atrophy correlates with memory impairment in MS [31,32].

A relatively isolated acute amnesic syndrome is rarely encountered in MS [33,34], although a "cortical variant" of MS, which presents with progressive dementia with prominent amnesia, has been described [35].

Language

Although disorders of speech (dysarthria) are common in MS, disorders of language (aphasia) have been considered rare [36]. However, careful assessment of language function may reveal abnormalities in patients with onset of cognitive decline [37]. Verbal fluency impairments have already been mentioned [11]. Aphasia, alexia, and agraphia may be present in the "cortical variant" of MS [35].

A study of 2700 patients from three centers in France found 22 cases (0.81%) of acute aphasia in MS, rarely occurring as a monosymptomatic presentation [38] or as an acute exacerbation in established disease associated with new left hemisphere white matter lesions on magnetic resonance imaging (MRI) of the brain [39]. However, etiologies other than acute inflammation need to be considered in MS patients with acute aphasia, including nonconvulsive "aphasic" status epilepticus [40] or a second pathology [41]. It has also been suggested that aphasic presentations of MS may, in fact, be cases of acute disseminated encephalomyelitis (ADEM; Section 6.2) [42].

Perception

Assessment of visuospatial and visuoconstructive functions is problematic in MS because of concurrent peripheral visual impairments (optic/retrobulbar neuritis); motor deficits may also contribute to testing difficulties. Impairments in tests reliant on complex spatial stimuli, such as Raven's Progressive Matrices, have been detected by some authors [11] but not others [43]. Visual-form agnosia has been reported [44]. A neuropsychological study in which 31 tasks assessing visuoperceptual abilities were given to 49 MS patients found that about one-quarter of patients failed four or more tasks, particularly color discrimination, the Müller–Lyer illusion, and two tests of object recognition [45].

Praxis

Motor deficits including weakness and spasticity may confound any assessment of praxis in MS patients. Apraxia has occasionally been mentioned as a symptom [44]. Callosal disconnection syndromes seem to be rare in MS [46], notwithstanding the predilection for corpus callosum involvement evident on brain MRI. A more recent study documented apraxia in about one-quarter of patients examined, in progressive more than

relapsing-remitting disease, and found that this contributed to disability [47].

Executive function

Tests of planning, problem solving, concept formation, utilization of feedback, and abstract reasoning, all of which may be subsumed under the heading of "executive function" or cognitive flexibility (even though different skills and neuroanatomical substrates may be implicated), have often been found to be impaired in MS patients.

On the Wisconsin Card Sorting Test (WCST), MS patients may show poor performance sufficient to differentiate them from healthy controls, perhaps more so in chronic progressive disease. Problem solving with Raven's Progressive Matrices is also impaired, although this similarly tests visuospatial skills. Tests of verbal fluency, such as the Controlled Oral Word Association Test (COWAT), are affected [11]. WCST performance has been associated with frontal white matter demyelinating lesions [48], although in other studies, poor performance on executive tasks could not be attributed solely to frontal lobe MR changes, suggesting that there was a general effect of cerebral dysfunction on tasks such as WCST [49]. Because of the links between frontal cortex and subcortical structures (thalamus, basal ganglia), remote lesions might account for these symptoms; for example, through undercutting of frontosubcortical circuits by white matter lesions.

Etiology: relationship of MS cognitive impairment to natural history of disease

The relationship of cognitive impairment to the natural history of MS has been investigated extensively. Cognitive impairment is not predicted by disease duration. It may be an early feature of MS, but may be absent even after many years of disease. IQ decline and auditory attention deficits were found in one study of patients with clinically isolated syndromes of the kind that often evolve to MS (optic neuritis, brainstem and partial spinal cord syndromes) with a mean duration of symptoms of over two years [50]. Even in patients with symptoms of only a few days duration, impaired PASAT and PVSAT performance has been recorded, particularly in patients with neuroradiological evidence of brain lesions [21].

Disease course is also poorly predictive of cognitive impairment. A review of cross-sectional and longitudinal studies came to the conclusion that cognitive dysfunction was more frequent in SPMS than in PPMS and RRMS [51]. However, cognitive impairment may occur with any disease course, including mildly affected RRMS patients [52]. Longitudinal studies suggest that cognitive deterioration occurs in a minority of MS patients, with considerable individual variation over time. For example, follow-up of a cohort of patients with clinically isolated syndromes [50] found that at the group level only visual memory had deteriorated significantly, while patients who had developed a chronic progressive course were more impaired on tests of verbal memory and auditory attention [53]. Follow-up studies of patients with established MS have shown considerable individual variation, many patients not progressing, although new deficits may become apparent in others. Those with cognitive impairment at baseline seem more likely to develop progressive cognitive decline, whereas those who are cognitively normal may remain so [54]. A study of patients with primary progressive disease (PPMS) showed no change in mean cognitive scores over a two-year follow-up period, although one-third showed absolute cognitive decline on individual test scores, but only a weak relationship between cognitive and MRI measures was found [55]. It is unsurprising, therefore, that correlations between cognitive impairment and neurological dysfunction in MS are generally weak.

Etiology: relationship of MS cognitive impairment to neuroimaging correlates

The relationship of cognitive impairment to neuroimaging correlates has been investigated increasingly in recent years. Total lesion score in terms of area or volume on MRI has shown significant correlation with cognitive dysfunction [21,56] and longitudinal studies indicate that progression of brain pathology correlates with cognitive decline [53]. Stable MRI lesion scores seem to be associated with no cognitive decline. Brain atrophy may also be relevant. Rao et al. [56] showed an association between corpus callosum atrophy and reduced speed of information processing, and Zivadinov et al. [57] showed a correlation between cognitive deterioration and brain parenchymal volume atrophy in RRMS, suggesting that axonal loss was the key substrate for early disease development and progression. In a five-year prospective cohort study of RRMS, T_1 lesion volumes were predictive of future cognitive impairment, and IQ decline and memory impairment were more severe in those with higher atrophy scores [58]. Hence, both inflammatory and degenerative processes may contribute to cognitive dysfunction.

The appreciation of gray matter lesions [59] and ultrastructural injury in normal-appearing white matter in MS brains has prompted a multiple disconnection model of cognitive dysfunction in MS. MS lesions involving subcortical periventricular white matter fiber pathways effectively disconnect cortical and subcortical regions, with variable cognitive domains being functionally interrupted, and hence the heterogeneity of cognitive impairments encountered clinically [60].

Treatment of neuropsychological deficits

Currently, little is known about the optimal treatment of cognitive disorders in MS. Options include disease-modifying agents, symptomatic treatments, and cognitive rehabilitation techniques including cognitive behavioral therapy, and restorative and compensatory strategies [10]. Increasingly, cognitive measures are being included as endpoints in therapeutic trials.

Occasionally, acute focal cognitive deficits may resolve following administration of steroids [39,61], but generally deficits are more likely to accrue. Trials of "disease-modifying drugs" have sometimes suggested benefits in particular cognitive domains; for example, with the interferons beta-1a [62] and beta-1b [63,64], and the monoclonal antibody natilizumab [65], or stability (at best) of cognitive function over time with glatiramer acetate [66].

Cholinesterase inhibitors (ChEIs) and memantine, established agents· in the treatment of Alzheimer's disease (AD), have been suggested for use in MS, but few data have been published [67]. A small trial suggested that ChEIs might be helpful in MS patients with mild cognitive impairments [68]. A functional imaging study, which suggested that ChEIs may modulate functional adaptive neuroplasticity in the MS brain [69], lent some support to the rationale for ChEI use in MS. However, changes in brain activation patterns observed on fMRI during cognitive testing in MS patients compared with controls may be interpreted as compensatory, adaptive responses, reflecting inherent brain neuroplasticity [70]. Such changes may need to be taken into account when assessing whether MS disease-modifying drugs or ChEIs have any effect on cognitive function. Trials of memantine in MS patients have been negative, and sometimes associated with worsening of neurological symptoms [71,72].

6.2 Acute disseminated encephalomyelitis (ADEM)

Acute disseminated encephalomyelitis (ADEM) is an inflammatory CNS disorder of presumed autoimmune etiology. ADEM affects children mainly, sometimes following infection or immunization, but is also well recognized in adults, usually as a monophasic illness although multiphasic and recurrent variants have occasionally been described, making it difficult to differentiate ADEM from a first episode of MS. Suggested operational diagnostic criteria [73] may be confounded in clinical practice [74].

The clinical picture is heterogeneous, with encephalopathy, focal neurological signs, and even psychosis being the presenting features. Aphasia has been reported as a presenting feature with hemiplegia, hemisensory deficit, and facial palsy, prompting the suggestion that acute aphasic presentations of MS may, in fact, be cases of ADEM [42].

Follow-up of ADEM patients has reported cognitive impairment in children affected before the age of five years [75], but no account of such problems in adult-onset ADEM has been identified.

6.3 Neuromyelitis optica (NMO)

Neuromyelitis optica (NMO), sometimes known as Devic's disease (but probably described by others before Devic, including most notably Allbutt in 1870 [76]), is an inflammatory demyelinating disorder of the CNS associated with antibodies to aquaporin-4 and amenable to immunosuppressant treatment with agents such as azathioprine, mycophenolate, and rituximab to prevent relapses [77]. The pathology was initially conceived to be limited to the optic nerves and the spinal cord, hence the name, with sparing of brain parenchyma, but it has become evident that the brain may be involved clinically in NMO spectrum disorders, with homonymous hemianopia, aphasia, hemiparesis, and cognitive impairment [78]. In a group of 30 NMO patients, performance was impaired on tests of attention and verbal fluency, akin to deficits in MS patients [79]. Cognitive impairment in NMO patients may be correlated with a decrease in global and focal white matter brain volume [80].

6.4 Neurosarcoidosis

Sarcoidosis is a systemic immunologically mediated disorder of uncertain etiology characterized pathologically by noncaseating epithelioid cell granulomata. The organs most commonly affected are the lymph nodes, lungs, liver, spleen, skin, and eyes. Neurosarcoidosis as one feature of systemic sarcoidosis is relatively rare (5%–15% of cases), isolated intracranial disease even more so, the most common neurological features being hypothalamic involvement and cranial nerve palsy [81].

In a series of 68 patients with or without systemic sarcoidosis, cognitive decline was reported to be the clinical presentation of neurosarcoidosis in seven (10%) patients [82]. Flowers *et al.* [83] reported five patients with biopsy-confirmed neurosarcoidosis with dementia. The index case presented at the age of 29 years with short-term and spatial memory difficulties. Neuropsychological assessment showed impairments in mental tracking, concentration, cognitive speed, and memory retrieval, as well as subtle expressive language difficulties. Improvement was reported following immunosuppressive treatment, prompting the authors to suggest that sarcoidosis is a treatable cause of cognitive impairment. A prior review of dementia as a presenting manifestation of neurosarcoidosis identified only 10 cases, in which frontosubcortical deficits were evident, including apathy, bradyphrenia, verbal perseveration, impaired speech fluency, as well as memory difficulties, with associated paratonia, grasp reflex, and motor perseveration. All patients had abnormal cerebrospinal fluid (CSF) indices (raised protein, white cell count) where these were tested. The importance of obtaining tissue confirmation of diagnosis prior to commencement of steroid therapy and exclusion of CNS tuberculosis was emphasized. These patients were noted to be older at age of onset (>50 yr) than expected for systemic sarcoidosis (median, 35 yr) [84]. In this context, it should be remembered that chance concurrence of dementia and sarcoidosis may occur; a patient with relatively indolent pulmonary sarcoidosis who developed AD has been seen in the author's clinic.

Neurosarcoidosis causing an isolated amnesic syndrome has been reported [85], but without neuropsychological assessment and with diagnosis based on histological appearances of a skin lesion. Focal cognitive deficits related to the rare presentation of neurosarcoidosis as a cerebral mass lesion ("sarcoid tumor" [86]) or as cerebral hemorrhage related to thrombocytopenia [87] might also be anticipated.

6.5 Systemic lupus erythematosus (SLE)

Systemic lupus erythematosus (SLE) is a multisystem autoimmune disorder of the collagen–vascular disease group, seldom associated with true vasculitis, with systemic, dermatological, rheumatological, renal, pulmonary, cardiac, and hematological, as well as neurological complications. Neurological features may affect both the central (delirium, psychosis, headache, cerebrovascular disease, myelopathy, movement disorder, demyelination, epileptic seizures, aseptic meningitis) and peripheral nervous systems (cranial neuropathy, polyneuropathy, plexopathy, mononeuropathy/multiplex, Guillain–Barré syndrome, autonomic neuropathy, myasthenia gravis) [88]. Because of the frequency of neuropsychiatric complications, nervous system involvement is sometimes referred to as "NP-SLE". What contribution antiphospholipid antibodies, found in around 30% of SLE cases, make to these clinical features is uncertain (see Hughes' syndrome, Section 3.5.6).

Cognitive deficits observed in SLE patients involve attention, information processing, memory, and executive function domains with relative sparing of language, but no dominant pattern has emerged and it is likely that there is no single syndrome of cognitive dysfunction in SLE. Deficits may be subclinical, fluctuating, and only a minority of patients progress [89]. Confounding factors such as pain, depression, and fatigue need to be taken into account when assessing cognitive function in SLE. Up to 66% of adult SLE patients without a history of NP-SLE have "mild cognitive impairment" and many patients with a previous history of NP-SLE have significant cognitive dysfunction that may progress to dementia, possibly due to active CNS disease, "burned-out" NP-SLE, and/or multiple infarcts [90–93].

One longitudinal study found cognitive impairment in around one-third of SLE patients in "stable neurological condition" with or without neuropsychiatric symptoms, deficits which remained at retest (mean interval between assessments, 21.5 months), suggesting that cognitive impairment is a persistent finding in SLE with CNS involvement. No relationship with neuropsychiatric disorder, neuroradiological findings, disease activity, or use of immunosuppressive therapy was found in this study. The most sensitive tests were those examining visuospatial reasoning and visuoconstructive function [94]. Another study found cognitive impairments in SLE patients included attentional skills, psychomotor speed, and abstract problem solving; in other words, executive function. This was felt to be largely due to cerebral infarction, and hence potentially amenable to prevention with anticoagulation [95]. Focal, cortical-type deficits may also occur in SLE. A case of Gerstmann syndrome (finger agnosia, right–left confusion, agraphia, acalculia) with an appropriately placed white matter lesion (left parieto-occipital, underlying the angular gyrus) due to SLE has been reported [96]. Likewise, amnesia associated with hippocampal damage has been presented [97], as has an amnesic syndrome mimicking limbic encephalitis (Section 6.12) [98].

The etiology of cognitive deficits in SLE is uncertain but thought to be related to damage to white matter tracts; the profile of impairment is similar to that in MS [99]. There is no linkage to markers of disease activity other than an association between persistent elevation of antiphospholipid antibodies and cognitive decline. An observational study suggested that regular aspirin use may be associated with better cognitive performance [100]. One small double-blind placebo-controlled study reported improved cognition in a trial of daily prednisolone, but no long-term outcome was reported [101].

6.6 Sjögren's syndrome

Sjögren's syndrome is a chronic autoimmune disorder of the exocrine glands associated with lymphocytic infiltrates, occurring either alone (primary Sjögren's syndrome) or in the presence of another autoimmune disorder such as rheumatoid arthritis, SLE, or progressive systemic sclerosis (secondary or associated Sjögren's syndrome). Extraglandular manifestations may occur in the skin, lungs, heart, kidneys, and nervous system, both central and peripheral [102]. Diagnostic criteria [103] include ocular and oral symptoms, objective evidence of dry eyes and salivary gland involvement, and laboratory abnormalities (at least one of anti-SS-A [anti-Ro] or SS-B [anti-La], ANA, IgM rheumatoid factor). Neurological manifestations occur in about 20% of patients and include CNS involvement, cranial nerve palsies, myelopathy, peripheral neuropathy (especially sensory, including a ganglionopathy) and a MS-like syndrome [104].

Cognitive impairment has been described in Sjögren's syndrome. The pattern of neuropsychological impairment in one series of patients was fairly homogeneous, with either subcorticofrontal or corticosubcortical dysfunction. In the former group, there was normal IQ, memory, and visuoconstructional skills but impaired attention control, abstraction, response-inhibition and set-shifting abilities, thus a dysexecutive-frontal type pattern; in the latter group there was additional intellectual decline and poor visuoconstructional abilities, associated with overt signs of CNS involvement (spastic tetraparesis, pseudobulbar syndrome, cerebellar syndrome). Brain MRI was normal or showed only nonspecific punctate periventricular white matter high signal intensities on T_2-weighted scans, with normal findings in CSF or only mild protein elevation [105]. Another series reported cognitive impairment with reduced speed of processing and executive dysfunction in all 11 patients [106]. Abnormalities on neuropsychological tests, particularly of frontal lobe function and memory, have been reported, which correlate with defects on functional imaging with single-photon emission computed tomography (SPECT) when MRI is normal; hence, it has been argued that neuropsychological testing is the most sensitive test for CNS involvement in Sjögren's [107]. However, others have detected similar functional imaging deficits in patients with or without "psychoneurological" symptoms [108]. Pain and depression may be confounders when assessing cognitive function in Sjögren's syndrome, particularly executive functions, but a recent study suggested that impairment of verbal reasoning ability compared to controls could not be ascribed to these factors [109].

Occasional cases mimicking AD have also been reported, but retrospectively, certain features were identified arguing against AD, including no disproportionate loss of memory or anomia, and presence of cognitive fluctuation, psychotic features, and somatic symptoms, and signs such as tremor, hyperreflexia and gait ataxia [110]. Likewise, three cases of rapidly progressive dementia, manifesting as intellectual decline over months with bradyphrenia and impaired executive function in previously undiagnosed Sjögren's syndrome, have been reported, two of whom showed marked improvement with (unspecified) immunosuppression [111]. A patient with a 20-year history of poor memory, impaired speech, and apathy provisionally diagnosed as frontotemporal dementia underwent diagnostic revision to Sjögren's syndrome when a positive Schirmer test and Ro and La antibodies were found [112].

6.7 Neuro-Behçet's disease

Behçet's disease is a recurrent systemic inflammatory disorder of unknown etiology, diagnostic criteria for which include recurrent aphthous ulceration plus any two of genital ulceration, skin lesions (such as erythema nodosum), eye involvement (anterior or posterior uveitis, or retinal vasculitis), and a positive pathergy test (skin hypersensitivity to pin-prick) [113]. Neuro-Behçet's disease, confined almost entirely to the central rather than the peripheral nervous system, occurs in about 5% of cases. Involvement may be defined as either parenchymal or nonparenchymal, the former affecting particularly the brainstem with ataxia, dysarthria,

hemiparesis, and pyramidal signs, with accompanying or preceding cognitive and neuropsychiatric changes. Nonparenchymal involvement usually takes the form of intracranial hypertension due to dural sinus thrombosis, wherein cognitive evaluation is usually normal [114–117].

Cognitive impairments may be common in neuro-Behçet's disease if specifically sought. For example, of 74 patients tested in a cohort of 200, 65 were cognitively abnormal, the most common impairments being in memory (verbal and visual), attention, and frontal lobe functions, with relative sparing of orientation, language, arithmetic, and visuospatial function [114]. In a more detailed analysis of 12 patients with neuro-Behçet's disease, memory deficit was the most common finding, particularly delayed recall of both verbal and visual material, suggesting a retrieval deficit, although acquisition and storage were also affected. Attention and executive function deficits also occurred while language and visuospatial function were largely spared. Neuropsychological deficits were evident before there were detectable changes on structural brain imaging, and insidious deterioration was observed independent of neurological relapses [118]. Cases presenting with amnesia [119] or resembling herpes simplex encephalitis [120] have been reported. Another case series noted cognitive and/or behavioral features in 16% of patients, a frequency less common than headache, upper motor neuron type weakness, and brainstem and cerebellar signs [121]. Cognitive deficits may also be common in Behçet's patients without overt neurological involvement: Monastero *et al.* [122] found deficits in almost half of a cohort of 26 patients, memory being the domain most often affected although visuospatial skills were also impaired relative to controls. High disease activity and high prednisolone dosage were independently associated with cognitive impairment after adjustment for demographic variables. Contrariwise, Ozisik *et al.* [123] found no difference in neuropsychological tests between controls and 20 patients without neurological involvement. Reports of dementia in neuro-Behçet's disease are rare [124].

6.8 Rheumatoid arthritis (RhA)

CNS involvement is rare in rheumatoid arthritis (RhA), although meningeal or parenchymal nodules and vasculitis may occur. RhA with cerebral vasculitis causing Gerstmann syndrome and dementia has been reported [125]. There may be an increased risk of atrial fibrillation and stroke in RhA [126], but whether this might increase the risk of vascular cognitive impairment and vascular dementia in RhA is not established currently. An inverse relation between RhA and AD was suggested, but this was based on a study of a highly selected population of geriatric in-patients [127].

Because of the rarity of CNS involvement in RhA, these patients have sometimes been used as a control group (chronic, inflammatory, but non-CNS disease) in studies of cognitive deficits in other disorders. However, in a study of the prevalence of cognitive impairment in MS, in a group of RhA patients included to control for any possible effects of depression related to chronic illness, 12% of the group were found to be impaired [128]. A more recent study in a cohort of RhA patients suggested that almost one-third had cognitive impairment, defined as scoring one standard deviation below age-based population norms on at least four of 16 indices. Oral glucocorticoid use and presence of vascular risk factors were more likely in the impaired patients [129].

6.9 Systemic sclerosis, scleroderma

Systemic sclerosis is characterized by excess collagen deposition in blood vessels affecting the skin particularly; CNS involvement is rare. Nevertheless, cognitive impairment typical of a dysexecutive syndrome has been documented in individuals without overt neurological involvement, perhaps related to cerebral hypoperfusion [130]. A vasospastic mechanism was postulated in a patient with scleroderma and Raynaud's phenomenon who suffered two episodes of transient global amnesia [131].

6.10 Relapsing polychondritis

This rare disorder is characterized by recurrent episodes of inflammation of the cartilage of the ear, nose, trachea, and larynx, as enshrined in proposed clinical diagnostic criteria [132]. It may be complicated by systemic and cerebral vasculitis, with clinical presentations including aseptic meningitis, encephalopathy, epileptic seizures, stroke, and transient ischemic attacks. Cases with cognitive impairment, sometimes amounting to dementia, have been reported, probably due to nonparaneoplastic limbic encephalitis [133–136].

6.11 Cerebral vasculitides

The vasculitides are inflammatory disorders of blood vessels, probably of autoimmune origin. Vasculitis may be exclusive to the CNS, as in primary or isolated angiitis of the CNS (PACNS), also known as intracranial vasculitis or, in older texts, granulomatous angiitis [137], but more commonly CNS involvement is part of a systemic disorder [138]. The vasculitides include polyarteritis nodosa, Churg–Strauss syndrome, Wegener's granulomatosis, giant cell (temporal) arteritis, and Takayasu's arteritis. Connective tissue disorders may also be complicated by vasculitis, including RhA, SLE (rarely), Sjögren's syndrome, progressive systemic sclerosis, and dermatomyositis/polymyositis. Vasculitis is also recognized secondary to certain infections, neoplasias, and toxins/drugs [139].

6.11.1 Primary angiitis of the CNS (PACNS)

Our understanding of PACNS has developed greatly over recent years [140], although diagnostic criteria were suggested over 20 years ago [141]. In a series of over 100 patients, altered cognition was noted in about 50% [142]. Dementia may be a feature of pathologically confirmed PACNS [143,144] and is occasionally the neuropathological substrate for dementia of unknown cause submitted to brain biopsy [145]. "Rapidly progressive dementia" as the presentation of primary (isolated) angiitis of the CNS has been reported [146], although it is possible that this was a disease-related encephalopathy, as intermittent confusion, and behavioral and psychiatric symptoms are not uncommon in PACNS. Dementia evolving in a patient with biopsy-proven but quiescent angiitis may reflect a second pathology such as AD [147].

Cognitive problems are reported to be prominent in the rare syndrome of amyloid β-related angiitis (ABRA), a granulomatous angiitis resembling PACNS with additional sporadic amyloid β-peptide-related cerebral amyloid angiopathy. Alterations in mental status were common in ABRA and, although not systematically examined, were said to include confusion, poor memory, and concentration, sometimes progressing to frank dementia, which was sometimes diagnosed premortem as AD [148].

6.11.2 Systemic vasculitides

The systemic vasculitides may be classified according to the size of the affected blood vessels [149]:

- Large arteries: giant cell (temporal) arteritis; Takayasu's arteritis;
- Medium arteries: Kawasaki disease; classical polyarteritis nodosa;
- Small vessels and medium arteries: Wegener's granulomatosis; Churg–Strauss syndrome; microscopic polyangiitis;
- Small vessels: Henoch–Schonlein purpura; essential cryoglobulinemia; cutaneous leukocytoclastic vasculitis.

Some of these systemic vasculitides may be accompanied by autoantibodies directed against constituents of the neutrophil azurophilic granules (anti-neutrophil cytoplasmic antibodies, ANCA); cytoplasmic ANCA (c-ANCA) is associated with Wegener's granulomatosis with approximately 95% specificity; perinuclear ANCA (p-ANCA) directed at myeloperoxidase is found in microscopic polyangiitis and Churg–Strauss syndrome with lesser specificity. A distinction may be drawn between primary

disorders and vasculitides occurring secondary to infection (e.g., hepatitis B, syphilis, HIV), drugs (e.g., sulfonamides, cocaine), or other connective tissue disorders (e.g., RhA, SLE, Sjögren's syndrome). ANCA assays are sometimes positive in SLE [150].

Neurological presentations of systemic vasculitis are very diverse, but those affecting the CNS generally manifest as an acute or subacute encephalopathy, or as an "MS-like" relapsing-remitting disorder with features atypical for MS, such as epileptic seizures and headache, or as a rapidly progressive space-occupying lesion [151]. Cognitive disorders are unusual, but occasionally described.

Occasional reports of dementia as a symptom, sometimes the presentation, of giant cell arteritis (GCA) have appeared, the dementia presumed to reflect multiple infarctions, sometimes in association with bilateral carotid artery occlusion, but without brain pathology to confirm the supposition [152]. This must be a rare scenario as GCA typically affects the extracranial carotid arteries and stroke is an uncommon vasculitic complication that usually involves the posterior intracranial circulation. Moreover, most patients with GCA are over 50 years of age so there may be other, confounding factors that might contribute to cognitive decline. CNS involvement in Takayasu's arteritis is due to carotid stenosis, cerebral hypoperfusion, and subclavian steal syndrome.

In polyarteritis nodosa, dementia has been reported in the context of lymphocytic meningitis and encephalitis, reversing after immunosuppressive treatment [153]. In Churg–Strauss syndrome, encephalopathy and stroke-like episodes may occur, although peripheral nervous system involvement is more common. Rapid onset dementia with microscopic polyangiitis, ascribed to CNS small vessel disease but without pathological proof and also causing peripheral neuropathy, has been described, with some patients improving cognitively following institution of immunosuppressive therapy [154]. In RhA, cerebral vasculitis has been reported as a cause of Gerstmann syndrome and dementia [125]. Cerebral vasculitis causing severe autobiographical amnesia but with preserved semantic memory has also been documented [155]. In a group of nondemented patients with ANCA-associated small vessel vasculitides (Wegener's granulomatosis, Churg–Strauss syndrome, microscopic polyangiitis), neuropsychological testing revealed subclinical deficits in abstract reasoning, speed of information processing, and visual memory in just under a third of patients, the suggestion being that small vessel vasculitis may mediate subcortical brain damage [156].

6.12 Limbic encephalitides

Limbic encephalitis is a syndrome of subacute onset characterized by cognitive decline, particularly memory impairment, due to limbic system involvement, with or without additional epileptic seizures of temporal lobe origin and MRI evidence of signal change in the limbic system, particularly the hippocampus. Initially described as a remote effect of occult neoplasia (paraneoplasia), a similar picture may also result from infective and autoimmune pathologies.

6.12.1 Paraneoplastic limbic encephalitis (PNLE)

Paraneoplastic limbic encephalitis (PNLE) was first described as such in the 1960s [157]. The syndrome is most often associated with lung tumors but also with breast and testicular neoplasms, and a variety of onconeural antibodies may be found, including anti-Hu (ANNA1), anti-Ma2, and ANNA-3, although their absence does not exclude the diagnosis [158,159]. Whole body positron emission tomography (PET) scanning may identify an occult tumor when other imaging modalities have been negative [160].

Detailed reports of neuropsychological assessment in PNLE are relatively few, perhaps because of concurrent confusion, altered consciousness, and psychiatric features precluding assessment. Martin *et al.* [161] found severe anterograde amnesia for both verbal and visual information but preserved visual perception and construction, language, speed

of information processing, and verbal abstract reasoning, all consistent with pathology confined to the mesial temporal lobes. A case with topographical disorientation as well as amnesia in association with anti-Hu antibodies has been reported, with MR signal change not only in the anteromedial temporal lobes bilaterally but also in the right retrosplenial region and inferior precuneus [162]. More widespread deficits and imaging changes may have prognostic implications. Bak *et al.* [163] reported two patients with PNLE, one with pure anterograde amnesia and a normal MRI, who recovered completely with tumor remission, the other with dense anterograde and extensive retrograde amnesia with anomia and executive impairments, and atrophy of the hippocampus and amygdala on MRI and frontotemporal hypoperfusion on SPECT, who showed no cognitive recovery following tumor regression. Progressive atrophy after transient cognitive improvement following tumor resection has also been recorded [164].

6.12.2 Nonparaneoplastic limbic encephalitis (NPLE): LGI1, NMDA-R

Non-paraneoplastic limbic encephalitis (NPLE) is a syndrome of limbic encephalitis associated with antibodies directed against cell membrane antigens, including LGI1 (previously attributed to voltage-gated potassium channels, VGKC [165]), and receptors for NMDA (often associated with ovarian teratoma in young women [166]), GABA(B), and AMPA, among others.

Probably the best defined among these NPLE syndromes is LGI1-associated NPLE, a subacute amnesic syndrome with associated behavioral features, epileptic seizures, and sometimes hyponatremia due to the syndrome of inappropriate antidiuretic hormone (ADH) secretion. The neuropsychological profile, when it can be tested, shows prominent episodic memory impairment with frontotemporal dysfunction but with relative sparing of parietal lobe function. Treatment with immunosuppressive agents (high dose steroids, IVIg, plasma exchange) may ameliorate many of the symptoms if commenced early, but memory problems may persist particularly if there is associated medial temporal lobe atrophy (possibly associated with high initial antibody titers) [167]. Early treatment has also been reported to be associated with better outcomes in anti-NMDA receptor encephalitis [168].

Cases resembling limbic encephalitis have occasionally been reported in association with connective tissue disorders such as SLE (Section 6.5) [98], Behçet's disease (Section 6.7) [120], and relapsing polychondritis (Section 6.10). Of the infective causes of limbic encephalitis, herpes simplex encephalitis is the most common (Section 9.1.1), but other pathogens include herpes simplex type 2 (Section 9.1.5) and human herpes viruses 6 and 7 (Section 9.1.6), particularly in immunocompromised patients, and neurosyphilis (Section 9.4.1) [169].

6.13 Hashimoto's encephalopathy (HE)

This entity, first reported in the 1960s [170], consists of a clinical syndrome of encephalopathy associated with stroke-like episodes, epileptic seizures, and psychosis in association with high serum titers of antithyroid autoantibodies (microsomal, thyroglobulin). Thyroid function may vary from overt hypothyroidism to overt hyperthyroidism, but most commonly there is subclinical hypothyroidism. Females are more commonly affected (4:1). The course may be relapsing-remitting in around half of the patients, for which reason some authors envisage Hashimoto's encephalopathy as a form of recurrent acute disseminated encephalomyelitis (Section 6.2) [171]. CSF protein is often elevated and electroencephalogram (EEG) abnormalities (diffuse slowing) are almost ubiquitous. The condition is usually (96%) responsive to steroids [172]. The antithyroid autoantibodies are probably epiphenomenal, unrelated to disease pathogenesis; α-enolase antibodies may be a better marker. It has been suggested by some authors that the name Hashimoto's encephalopathy be abandoned because of uncertainty about nosology, "steroid-responsive encephalopathy"

being one proposed alternative name. Differential diagnosis encompasses mitochondrial disease, vasculitides, nonparaneoplastic limbic encephalitis due to voltage-gated potassium channel antibodies, and Creutzfeldt–Jakob disease (CJD) [173].

Cognitive dysfunction ranging from subtle executive and linguistic disturbance [174] to rapidly progressive dementia [175–177] has been reported in HE, the clinical phenotype often closely resembling sporadic CJD (Section 2.5.1) [178]. Indeed, cases of pathologically confirmed CJD resembling HE have been reported [173]. Although rare, HE is an important diagnosis to consider, especially in rapidly progressive dementia with epileptic seizures and psychiatric features, as the condition may be reversed with steroid treatment.

6.14 Sydenham's chorea; pediatric autoimmune neuropsychiatric disorders associated with streptococcal infections (PANDAS)

Sydenham's chorea is a movement disorder of childhood and early adulthood related to infection with group A streptococci, now regarded as an example of postinfectious (post-streptococcal) movement and neuropsychiatric disorders of autoimmune origin (PANDAS). The neuropsychiatric features usually reported have been those of obsessive-compulsive disorder (Section 12.4.1). Basal ganglia (striatal) involvement may be observed on structural and functional imaging (hyperperfusion and hypermetabolism).

Neuropsychological deficits do not seem to be a clinical feature of these conditions, although dementia associated with striatal hypermetabolism and the detection of antistriatal antibodies that reversed with steroids has been reported [179]. Cases clinically resembling Sydenham's chorea but with additional dementia and associated with antiphospholipid antibodies have also been described [180]. Patients with childhood Sydenham's chorea examined in adulthood have been found to have reduced performance in attention, information processing speed, executive functions, and working memory, suggesting persistent dysfunction in basal ganglia circuits [181].

6.15 Histiocytosis

The histiocytoses or histiocytic disorders are a diverse group in which proliferation of phagocytic or antigen-presenting dendritic cells may occur. Typical patterns of CNS involvement include infiltrative parenchymal disease (especially involving the hypothalamopituitary axis), meningeal infiltration, and a neurodegenerative pattern that may include cognitive decline. Langerhans cell histiocytosis and Erdheim–Chester disease are examples of dendritic cell-related disorders, and Rosai–Dorfman disease (also known as sinus histiocytosis with massive lymphadenopathy; sometimes confused with meningioma; Section 7.1.2) is a macrophage-related disorder [182].

6.15.1 Neurodegenerative Langerhans cell histiocytosis (ND-LCH)

Patients with Langerhans cell histiocytosis (LCH), a rare granulomatous disorder of broad phenotype, may develop neurodegeneration in addition to hypothalamic-hypophyseal axis involvement. Low IQ, problems with perceptual tasks, and verbal and visuospatial working memory dysfunction were recorded in one series of patients [183].

6.15.2 Erdheim–Chester disease

Erdheim–Chester disease is a rare, sporadic, non-Langerhans cell histiocytosis, which may affect multiple organs, including the CNS [184]. Proposed diagnostic criteria require typical histological findings of foamy histiocytes nested among polymorphic granuloma and fibrosis or xanthogranulomatosis with CD68-positive and CD1a-negative immunohistochemical staining, with typical skeletal findings of bilateral symmetrical cortical osteosclerosis and/or increased labeling of the distal ends of the lower limb long bones on

^{99}Tc bone scintigraphy [185]. In addition to skeletal involvement, common findings are diabetes insipidus, and retroperitoneal, orbital, cutaneous, and cardiac involvement. In a review of over 200 cases, Lachenal *et al.* [186] found neurological features in about one-third of patients, most often cerebellar and/or pyramidal signs, but in six cases there was dementia, cognitive impairment, or amnesia.

6.16 Bilateral vestibulopathy

The syndrome of bilateral peripheral loss of vestibular function is characterized by oscillopsia during walking and head movements, and unsteadiness of gait in the dark and on uneven ground. Although often idiopathic, some cases are associated with autoantibodies to inner ear structures. Deficits of spatial memory and navigation associated with bilateral hippocampal atrophy have been reported in bilateral vestibulopathy associated with neurofibromatosis type 2 [187].

6.17 Chronic inflammatory demyelinating polyneuropathy (CIDP)

There has been a report that cognitive impairment may be present in up to 50% of CIDP patients, manifested as slowed speed of information processing and executive dysfunction on the Brief Repeatable Battery of Neuropsychological Tests, changes the authors claim are comparable to those in MS [188].

REFERENCES

[1] Compston A, Confavreux C, Lassmann H, *et al.* *McAlpine's Multiple Sclerosis* (4th edn.). London: Churchill Livingstone, 2006.

[2] Compston A, Coles A. Multiple sclerosis. *Lancet* 2008; 372: 1502–17.

[3] Larner AJ. Aetiological role of viruses in multiple sclerosis: a review. *J R Soc Med* 1986; 79: 412–17.

[4] Kennedy PGE, Steiner I. On the possible viral aetiology of multiple sclerosis. *Q J Med* 1994; 87: 523–8.

[5] Dalgleish AG. Viruses and multiple sclerosis. *Acta Neurol Scand* 1997; 169: S8–15.

[6] Polman CH, Reingold SC, Banwell B, *et al.* Diagnostic criteria for multiple sclerosis: 2010 revisions to the McDonald criteria. *Ann Neurol* 2011; 69: 292–302.

[7] Rogers JM, Panegyres PK. Cognitive impairment in multiple sclerosis: evidence-based analysis and recommendations. *J Clin Neurosci* 2007; 14: 919–27.

[8] Chiaravalloti ND, DeLuca J. Cognitive impairment in multiple sclerosis. *Lancet Neurol* 2008; 7: 1139–51.

[9] Langdon DW. Cognition in multiple sclerosis. *Curr Opin Neurol* 2011; 24: 244–9.

[10] LaRocca NG. Cognitive impairment and mood disturbances. In: Giesser B (ed.). *Primer on Multiple Sclerosis*. Oxford: Oxford University Press, 2011; 241–62.

[11] Rao SM, Leo GJ, Bernadin L, Unversagt F. Cognitive dysfunction in multiple sclerosis. I. Frequency, patterns and predictions. *Neurology* 1991; 41: 685–91.

[12] Rao SM. White matter disease and dementia. *Brain Cogn* 1996; 31: 250–68.

[13] Swirsky-Sacchetti T, Field HL, Mitchell DR, *et al.* The sensitivity of the Mini-Mental State Examination in the white matter dementia of multiple sclerosis. *J Clin Psychol* 1992; 48: 779–86.

[14] Lensch E, Matzke M, Peteriet H-F, *et al.* Identification and management of cognitive disorders in multiple sclerosis – a consensus approach. *J Neurol* 2006; 253(Suppl 1): 29–31.

[15] Sartori E, Edan G. Assessment of cognitive dysfunction in multiple sclerosis. *J Neurol Sci* 2006; 245: 169–75.

[16] Connick P, Kolappan M, Bak TH, Chandran S. Verbal fluency as a rapid screening test for cognitive impairment in progressive multiple sclerosis. *J Neurol Neurosurg Psychiatry* 2012; 83: 346–7.

[17] Calabrese P. Neuropsychology of multiple sclerosis: an overview. *J Neurol* 2006; 253(Suppl 1): 10–15.

[18] Benedict RHB, Fischer JS, Archibald CJ, *et al.* Minimal neuropsychological assessment of MS patients: a consensus approach. *Clin Neuropsychol* 2002; 16: 381–97.

[19] Benedict RHB, Cox D, Thompson LL, *et al.* Reliable screening for neuropsychological impairment in multiple sclerosis. *Mult Scler* 2004; 10: 675–8.

[20] Feinstein A, Youl B, Ron M. Acute optic neuritis. A cognitive and magnetic resonance imaging study. *Brain* 1992; 115: 1403–15.

[21] Schulz D, Kopp B, Kunkel A, Faiss JH. Cognition in the early stage of multiple sclerosis. *J Neurol* 2006; 253: 1002–10.

[22] Grant I, McDonald WI, Trimble MR, Smith E, Reed R. Deficient learning and memory in early and middle phases of multiple sclerosis. *J Neurol Neurosurg Psychiatry* 1984; 47: 250–5.

[23] Beatty WW, Goodkin DE, Monson N, Beatty PA, Hertsgaard D. Anterograde and retrograde amnesia in patients with chronic progressive multiple sclerosis. *Arch Neurol* 1988; 45: 611–19.

[24] Rao SM, St Aubin-Faubert P, Leo GJ. Information processing speed in patients with multiple sclerosis. *J Clin Exp Neuropsychol* 1989; 11: 471–7.

[25] Demaree HA, DeLuca J, Gaudino EA, Diamond BJ. Speed of information processing as a key deficit in multiple sclerosis: implications for rehabilitation. *J Neurol Neurosurg Psychiatry* 1999; 67: 661–3.

[26] Macniven JA, Davis C, Ho MY, *et al.* Stroop performance in multiple sclerosis: information processing, selective attention, or executive functioning? *J Int Neuropsychol Soc* 2008; 14: 805–14.

[27] Batista S, Ziavadinov R, Hoogs M, *et al.* Basal ganglia, thalamus and neocortical atrophy predicting slowed cognitive processing in multiple sclerosis. *J Neurol* 2012; 259: 139–46.

[28] Rao SM, Leo GJ, St Aubin-Faubert P. On the nature of memory disturbance in multiple sclerosis. *J Clin Exp Neuropsychol* 1989; 11: 699–712.

[29] DeLuca J, Gaudino E, Diamond BJ, Christodoulou C, Engel RA. Acquistion and storage deficits in multiple sclerosis. *J Clin Exp Neuropsychol* 1998; 20: 376–90.

[30] Grafman J, Rao S, Bernardin L, Leo GJ. Automatic memory processes in patients with multiple sclerosis. *Arch Neurol* 1991; 48: 1072–5.

[31] Sicotte NL, Kern KC, Giesser BS, *et al.* Regional hippocampal atrophy in multiple sclerosis. *Brain* 2008; 131: 1134–41.

[32] Benedict RH, Ramasamy D, Munschauer F, Weinstock-Guttman B, Zivadinov R. Memory impairment in multiple sclerosis: correlation with deep grey matter and mesial temporal atrophy. *J Neurol Neurosurg Psychiatry* 2009; 80: 201–6.

[33] Vighetto A, Charles N, Salzmann M, Confavreux C, Aimard G. Korsakoff's syndrome as the initial presentation of multiple sclerosis. *J Neurol* 1991; 238: 351–4.

[34] Larner AJ, Young CA. Acute amnesia in multiple sclerosis revisited. *Int MS J* 2009; 16: 102–4.

[35] Zarei M, Chandran S, Compston A, Hodges J. Cognitive presentation of multiple sclerosis: evidence for a cortical variant. *J Neurol Neurosurg Psychiatry* 2003; 74: 872–7.

[36] Murdoch B, Theodoros D (eds.). *Speech and Language Disorders in Multiple Sclerosis.* London: Whurr, 2000.

[37] Kujala P, Portin R, Ruutiainen J. Language functions in incipient cognitive decline in multiple sclerosis. *J Neurol Sci* 1996; 141: 79–86.

[38] Lacour A, De Seze J, Revenco E, *et al.* Acute aphasia in multiple sclerosis: a multicenter study of 22 patients. *Neurology* 2004; 62: 974–7.

[39] Devere TR, Trotter JL, Cross AH. Acute aphasia in multiple sclerosis. *Arch Neurol* 2000; 57: 1207–9.

[40] Trinka E, Unterberger I, Luef G, *et al.* Acute aphasia in multiple sclerosis. *Arch Neurol* 2001; 58: 133–4.

[41] Larner AJ, Lecky BRF. Acute aphasia in multiple sclerosis revisited. *Int MS J* 2007; 14: 76–7.

[42] Brinar VV, Poser CM, Basic S, Petelin Z. Sudden onset aphasic hemiplegia: an unusual manifestation of disseminated encephalomyelitis. *Clin Neurol Neurosurg* 2004; 106: 187–96.

[43] Jennekens-Schinkel A, Laboyrie PM, Lanser JB, van der Velde EA. Cognition in patients with multiple sclerosis. After four years. *J Neurol Sci* 1990; 99: 229–47.

[44] Okuda B, Tanaka H, Tachibana H, *et al.* Visual form agnosia in multiple sclerosis. *Acta Neurol Scand* 1996; 94: 38–44.

[45] Vleugels L, Lafosse C, van Nunen A, *et al.* Visuoperceptual impairment in multiple sclerosis patients diagnosed with neuropsychological tasks. *Mult Scler* 2000; 6: 241–54.

[46] Schnider A, Benson F, Rosner LJ. Callosal disconnection in multiple sclerosis. *Neurology* 1993; 43: 1243–5.

[47] Kamm CP, Heldner MR, Vanbellingen T, *et al.* Limb apraxia in multiple sclerosis: prevalence and impact on manual dexterity and activities of daily living. *Arch Phys Med Rehabil* 2012; 93: 1081–5.

[48] Arnett PA, Rao SM, Bernardin L, *et al.* Relationship between frontal lobe lesions and Wisconsin Card Sorting Test performance in patients with multiple sclerosis. *Neurology* 1994; 44: 420–5.

[49] Foong J, Rozewicz L, Quaghebeur G, *et al.* Executive function in multiple sclerosis. The role of frontal lobe pathology. *Brain* 1997; 120: 15–26.

[50] Callanan M, Logsdail SJ, Ron MA, Warrington EK. Cognitive impairment in patients with clinically isolated lesions of the type seen in multiple sclerosis. A psychometric and MRI study. *Brain* 1989; 112: 361–74.

[51] Amato MP, Zipoli V, Portaccio E. Multiple sclerosis-related cognitive changes: a review of cross-sectional and longitudinal studies. *J Neurol Sci* 2006; 245: 41–6.

[52] Amato MP, Zipoli V, Goretti B, *et al.* Benign multiple sclerosis: cognitive, psychological and social aspects in a clinical cohort. *J Neurol* 2006; 253: 1054–9.

[53] Feinstein A, Kartsounis L, Miller D, Youl B, Ron M. Clinically isolated lesions of the type seen in multiple sclerosis: a cognitive, psychiatric and MRI follow-up study. *J Neurol Neurosurg Psychiatry* 1992; 55: 869–76.

[54] Kujala P, Portin R, Ruutiainen J. The progress of cognitive decline in multiple sclerosis. A controlled 3-year follow-up. *Brain* 1997; 120: 289–97.

[55] Camp SJ, Stevenson VL, Thompson AJ *et al.* A longitudinal study of cognition in primary progressive multiple sclerosis. *Brain* 2005; 128: 2891–8.

[56] Rao SM, Leo GJ, Haughton VM, St Aubin-Faubert P, Bernadin L. Correlation of magnetic resonance imaging with neuropsychological testing in multiple sclerosis. *Neurology* 1989; 39: 161–6.

[57] Zivadinov R, Sepcic J, Nasuelli D, *et al.* A longitudinal study of brain atrophy and cognitive disturbances in the early phase of relapsing-remitting multiple sclerosis. *J Neurol Neurosurg Psychiatry* 2001; 70: 773–80.

[58] Summers MM, Fisniku LK, Anderson VM, *et al.* Cognitive impairment in relapsing-remitting multiple sclerosis can be predicted by imaging performed several years earlier. *Mult Scler* 2008; 14: 197–204.

[59] Kidd D, Barkhof F, McConnell R, *et al.* Cortical lesions in multiple sclerosis. *Brain* 1999; 122: 17–26.

[60] Dineen RA, Vilisaar J, Hlinka L, *et al.* Disconnection as a mechanism for cognitive dysfunction in multiple sclerosis. *Brain* 2009; 132: 239–49.

[61] Rozewicz L, Langdon DW, Davie CA, Thompson AJ, Ron MA. Resolution of left hemisphere cognitive dysfunction in multiple sclerosis with magnetic resonance correlates: a case report. *Cogn Neuropsychiatry* 1996; 1: 17–25.

[62] Fischer JS, Priore RL, Jacobs LD, *et al.* Neuropsychological effects of interferon beta-1a in relapsing multiple sclerosis. Multiple Sclerosis Collaborative Research Group. *Ann Neurol* 2000; 48: 885–92.

[63] Pliskin NH, Hamer DP, Goldstein DS, *et al.* Improved delayed visual reproduction test performance in

multiple sclerosis patients receiving interferon beta-1b. *Neurology* 1996; 47: 1463–8.

[64] Barak Y, Achiron A. Effect of interferon-beta-1b on cognitive functions in multiple sclerosis. *Eur Neurol* 2002; 47: 11–14.

[65] Iaffaldano P, Viterbo RG, Paolicelli D, *et al.* Impact of natilizumab on cognitive performances and fatigue in relapsing multiple sclerosis: a prospective, open-label, two years observational study. *PLoS One* 2012; 7: e35843.

[66] Weinstein A, Schwid SI, Schiffer RB, *et al.* Neuro-psychologic status in multiple sclerosis after treatment with glatiramer. *Arch Neurol* 1999; 56: 319–24.

[67] Larner AJ. Cholinesterase inhibitors – beyond Alzheimer's disease. *Expert Rev Neurother* 2010; 10: 1699–705.

[68] Krupp LB, Christodoulou C, Melville P, *et al.* Donepezil improved memory in multiple sclerosis in a randomized clinical trial. *Neurology* 2004; 63: 1579–85.

[69] Parry AMM, Scott RB, Palace J, Smith S, Matthews PM. Potentially adaptive functional changes in cognitive processing for patients with multiple sclerosis and their acute modulation by rivastigmine. *Brain* 2003; 126: 2750–60.

[70] Staffen W, Mair A, Zauner H, *et al.* Cognitive function and fMRI in patients with multiple sclerosis: evidence for compensatory cortical activation during an attention task. *Brain* 2002; 125: 1275–82.

[71] Villoslada P, Arrondo G, Sepulcre J, Alegre M, Artieda J. Memantine induces reversible neurologic impairment in patients with MS. *Neurology* 2009; 72: 1630–3.

[72] Lovera JF, Frohman E, Brown TR, *et al.* Memantine for cognitive impairment in multiple sclerosis: a randomized placebo-controlled trial. *Mult Scler* 2010; 16: 715–23.

[73] Schwarz S, Mohr A, Knauth M, Wildemann B, Storch-Hagenlocher B. Acute disseminated encephalomyelitis: a follow-up study of 40 adult patients. *Neurology* 2001; 56: 1313–18.

[74] John L, Khaleeli AA, Larner AJ. Acute disseminated encephalomyelitis: a riddle wrapped in a mystery inside an enigma. *Int J Clin Pract* 2003; 57: 235–7.

[75] Jacobs RK, Anderson VA, Neale JL, Shield LK, Kornberg AJ. Neuropsychological outcome after acute disseminated encephalomyelitis: impact of age at illness onset. *Pediatr Neurol* 2004; 31: 191–7.

[76] Jacob A, Larner AJ. Clifford Allbutt (1836–1925). *J Neurol* 2013; 260: 346–7.

[77] Jacob A. Neuromyelitis optica–an update: 2007–2009. *Ann Indian Acad Neurol* 2009; 12: 231–7.

[78] Chan KH, Tse CT, Chung CP, *et al.* Brain involvement in neuromyelitis optica spectrum disorders. *Arch Neurol* 2011; 68: 1432–9.

[79] Blanc F, Zephir H, Lebrun C, *et al.* Cognitive functions in neuromyelitis optica. *Arch Neurol* 2008; 65: 84–8.

[80] Blanc F, Noblet V, Jung B, *et al.* White matter atrophy and cognitive dysfunctions in neuromyelitis optica. *PloS One* 2012; 7: e33878.

[81] Hoitsma E, Faber CG, Drent M, Sharma OP. Neuro-sarcoidosis: a clinical dilemma. *Lancet Neurol* 2004; 3: 397–403.

[82] Zajicek JP, Scolding NJ, Foster O, *et al.* Central nervous system sarcoidosis–diagnosis and management. *Q J Med* 1999; 92: 103–17.

[83] Flowers JM, Omer SM, Wren DW, Al-Memar AY. Neurosarcoidosis presenting with cognitive impairment: a series of five cases. *J Neurol Neurosurg Psychiatry* 2006; 77: 128 (abstract 010).

[84] Schielke E, Nolte C, Muller W, Bruck W. Sarcoidosis presenting as a rapidly progressive dementia: clinical and neuropathological evaluation. *J Neurol* 2001; 248: 522–4.

[85] Willigers P, Kohler P. Amnesic syndrome caused by neurosarcoidosis. *Clin Neurol Neurosurg* 1993; 95: 131–5.

[86] Larner AJ, Ball JA, Howard RS. Sarcoid tumour: continuing diagnostic problems in the MRI era. *J Neurol Neurosurg Psychiatry* 1999; 66: 510–12.

[87] Larner AJ. Life-threatening thrombocytopenia in sarcoidosis. *BMJ* 1990; 300: 317–9.

[88] Joseph FG, Scolding NJ. Neurolupus. *Pract Neurol* 2010; 10: 4–15.

[89] Kozora E, Hanly JG, Lapteva L, Filley CM. Cognitive dysfunction in systemic lupus erythematosus. Past, present, and future. *Arthritis Rheum* 2008; 58: 3286–98.

[90] Carbotte RM, Denburg SD, Denburg JA. Prevalence of cognitive impairment in systemic lupus erythematosus. *J Nerv Ment Dis* 1986; 174: 357–64.

[91] Hanly JG, Fisk JD, Sherwood G, *et al.* Cognitive impairment in patients with systemic lupus erythematosus. *J Rheumatol* 1992; 19: 562–7.

[92] Kozora E, Thompson L, West S, *et al.* Analysis of cognitive and psychological deficits in systemic lupus

erythematosus patients without overt central nervous system disease. *Arthritis Rheum* 1996; 39: 2035–45.

[93] Denburg SD, Carbotte RM, Denburg JA. Psychological aspects of systemic lupus erythematosus: cognitive function, mood, and self-report. *J Rheumatol* 1997; 24: 998–1003.

[94] Carlomagno S, Migliaresi S, Ambrosone L, *et al.* Cognitive impairment in systemic lupus erythematosus: a follow-up study. *J Neurol* 2000; 247: 273–9.

[95] Waterloo K, Omdal R, Sjoholm H, *et al.* Neuropsychological dysfunction in systemic lupus erythematosus is not associated with changes in cerebral blood flow. *J Neurol* 2001; 248: 595–602.

[96] Jung RE, Yeo RA, Sibbitt WL Jr, *et al.* Gerstmann syndrome in systemic lupus erythematosus: neuropsychological, neuroimaging and spectroscopic findings. *Neurocase* 2001; 7: 515–21.

[97] Schnider A, Bassetti C, Schnider A, Gutbrod K, Ozdoba C. Very severe amnesia with acute onset after isolated hippocampal damage due to systemic lupus erythematosus. *J Neurol Neurosurg Psychiatry* 1995; 59: 644–6.

[98] Stubgen JP. Nervous system lupus mimics limbic encephalitis. *Lupus* 1998; 7: 557–60.

[99] Benedict RH, Shucard JL, Zivadinov R, Shucard DW. Neuropsychological impairment in systemic lupus erythematosus: a comparison with multiple sclerosis. *Neuropsychol Rev* 2008; 18: 149–66.

[100] McLaurin EY, Holliday SL, Williams P, Brey RL. Predictors of cognitive dysfunction in patients with systemic lupus erythematosus. *Neurology* 2005; 64: 297–303.

[101] Denburg SD, Carbotte RM, Denburg JA. Corticosteroids and neuropsychological functioning in patients with systemic lupus erythematosus. *Arthritis Rheum* 1994; 37: 1311–20.

[102] Fox RI. Sjögren's syndrome. *Lancet* 2005; 366: 321–31.

[103] Vitali C. Classification criteria for Sjögren's syndrome. *Ann Rheum Dis* 2003; 62: 94–5.

[104] Delalande S, de Seze J, Fauchais AL, *et al.* Neurologic manifestations in primary Sjögren's syndrome: a study of 82 patients. *Medicine (Baltimore)* 2004; 83: 280–91.

[105] Lafitte C, Amoura Z, Cacoub P, *et al.* Neurological complications of primary Sjögren's syndrome. *J Neurol* 2001; 248: 577–84.

[106] Blanc F, Kleitz C, Longato N, *et al.* Cognitive dysfunctions in primary Sjögren's syndrome. *Neurodegen Dis* 2009; 6(Suppl 1): 1994.

[107] Belin C, Moroni C, Caillat-Vigneron N, *et al.* Central nervous system involvement in Sjögren's syndrome: evidence from neuropsychological testing and HMPAO-SPECT. *Ann Med Interne Paris* 1999; 150: 598–604.

[108] Lass P, Krajka-Lauer J, Homziak M, *et al.* Cerebral blood flow in Sjögren's syndrome using 99Tcm-HMPAO brain SPET. *Nucl Med Commun* 2000; 21: 31–5.

[109] Segal BM, Pogatchnik B, Holker E, *et al.* Primary Sjögren's syndrome: cognitive symptoms, mood, and cognitive performance. *Acta Neurol Scand* 2012; 125: 272–8.

[110] Caselli RJ, Scheithauer BW, O'Duffy JD, *et al.* Chronic inflammatory meningoencephalitis should not be mistaken for Alzheimer's disease. *Mayo Clin Proc* 1993; 68: 846–53.

[111] Jarman PR, Ward N, Bradbury P, Swash M. Primary Sjögren's syndrome: a reversible cause of dementia. *J Neurol Neurosurg Psychiatry* 2001; 70: 274 (abstract).

[112] Xiromerisiou G, Tegos T, Tichalas A, *et al.* Severe dementia associated with Sjögren syndrome. *Neurodegen Dis* 2009; 6(Suppl 1): 1076.

[113] International Study Group for Behçet's Disease. Criteria for the diagnosis of Behçet's disease. *Lancet* 1990; 335: 1078–80.

[114] Akman-Demir G, Serdaroglu P, Tasçi B and the Neuro-Behçet Study Group. Clinical patterns of neurological involvement in Behçet's disease: evaluation of 200 patients. *Brain* 1999; 122: 2171–81.

[115] Kidd D, Steuer A, Denman AM, Rudge P. Neurological complications in Behçet's syndrome. *Brain* 1999; 122: 2183–94.

[116] Akman-Demir G, Serdaroglu P. Neuro-Behçet's disease: a practical approach to diagnosis and treatment. *Pract Neurol* 2002; 2: 340–7.

[117] Al-Araji A, Kidd DP. Neuro-Behcet's disease: epidemiology, clinical characteristics, and management. *Lancet Neurol* 2009; 8: 192–204.

[118] Oktem-Tanör O, Baykan-Kurt B, Gurvit IH, Akman-Demir G, Serdaroglu P. Neuropsychological follow-up of 12 patients with neuro-Behçet disease. *J Neurol* 1999; 246: 113–19.

[119] Mimura M, Kato M, Kashima H. Neuro-Behcet's disease presenting with amnesia and frontal dysfunction. *Clin Neurol Neurosurg* 2009; 111: 889–92.

[120] Hasegawa T, Kanno S, Kato M, *et al.* Neuro-Behçet's disease presenting initially as mesiotemporal lesions mimicking herpes simplex encephalitis. *Eur J Neurol* 2005; 12: 661–2.

[121] Siva A, Kantarci OH, Saip Ş, *et al.* Behçet's disease: diagnostic and prognostic aspects of neurological involvement. *J Neurol* 2001; 248: 95–103.

[122] Monastero R, Camarda C, Pipia C, *et al.* Cognitive impairment in Behçet's disease patients without overt neurological involvement. *J Neurol Sci* 2004; 220: 99–104.

[123] Ozisik HI, Karlidag R, Hazneci E, Kizkin S, Ozcan C. Cognitive event-related potential and neuropsychological findings in Behcet's disease without neurological manifestations. *Tohoku J Exp Med* 2005; 206: 15–22.

[124] Warren JE, Sandhu A, Thompson PD, Blumbergs PC. Dementia in a case of Behcet's disease. *Intern Med J* 2006; 36: 611–16.

[125] Ramos M, Mandybur TI. Cerebral vasculitis and rheumatoid arthritis. *Arch Neurol* 1975; 32: 271–5.

[126] Lindhardsen J, Ahlehoff O, Gislason GH, *et al.* Risk of atrial fibrillation and stroke in rheumatoid arthritis: Danish nationwide cohort study. *BMJ* 2012; 344: e1257.

[127] Jenkinson ML, Bliss MR, Brain AT, Scott DL. Rheumatoid arthritis and senile dementia of the Alzheimer's type. *Br J Rheumatol* 1989; 28: 86–8.

[128] McIntosh-Michaelis SA, Wilkinson SM, Diamond ID, *et al.* The prevalence of cognitive impairment in a community survey of multiple sclerosis. *Br J Clin Psychol* 1991; 30: 333–48.

[129] Shin SY, Katz P, Wallhagen M, Julian L. Cognitive impairment in persons with rheumatoid arthritis. *Arthritis Care Res (Hoboken)* 2012; 64: 1144–50.

[130] Yilmaz N, Mollahasanoglu A, Gurvit H, *et al.* Dysexecutive syndrome: a specific pattern of cognitive impairment in systemic sclerosis. *Cogn Behav Neurol* 2012; 25: 57–62.

[131] Nishida A, Kaiya H, Uematsu M, *et al.* Transient global amnesia and Raynaud's phenomenon in scleroderma. *Acta Neurol Scand* 1990; 81: 550–2.

[132] McAdam LP, O'Hanlan MA, Bluestone R, Pearson CM. Relapsing polychondritis: prospective study of 23 patients and a review of the literature. *Medicine (Baltimore)* 1976; 55: 193–215.

[133] Fujiki F, Tsuboi Y, Hashimoto K, *et al.* Non-herpetic limbic encephalitis associated with relapsing polychondritis. *J Neurol Neurosurg Psychiatry* 2004; 75: 1646–7.

[134] Ohta Y, Nagano I, Niiya D, *et al.* Nonparaneoplastic limbic encephalitis with relapsing polychondritis. *J Neurol Sci* 2004; 220: 85–8.

[135] Irani SR, Soni A, Beynon H, Athwal BS. Relapsing "encephalo" polychondritis. *Pract Neurol* 2006; 6: 372–5.

[136] Erten-Lyons D, Oken B, Woltjer RL, Quinn J. Relapsing polychondritis: an uncommon cause of dementia. *J Neurol Neurosurg Psychiatry* 2008; 79: 609–10.

[137] Schmidley JW. *Central Nervous System Angiitis.* Boston, MA: Butterworth Heinemann, 2000.

[138] Younger DS. Vasculitis of the nervous system. *Curr Opin Neurol* 2004; 17: 317–36.

[139] Moore PM, Richardson B. Neurology of the vasculitides and connective tissue diseases. *J Neurol Neurosurg Psychiatry* 1998; 65: 10–22.

[140] Hajj-Ali RA, Singhal AB, Benseler S, Molloy E, Calabrese LH. Primary angiitis of the CNS. *Lancet Neurol* 2011; 10: 561–72.

[141] Calabrese LH, Furlan AJ, Gragg LA, Ropos TJ. Primary angiitis of the central nervous system: diagnostic criteria and clinical approach. *Cleve Clin J Med* 1992; 59: 293–306.

[142] Salvarani C, Brown RD Jr, Calamia KT, *et al.* Primary central nervous system vasculitis: analysis of 101 patients. *Ann Neurol* 2007; 62: 442–51.

[143] Koo EH, Massey EW. Granulomatous angiitis of the central nervous system: protean manifestations and response to treatment. *J Neurol Neurosurg Psychiatry* 1988; 51: 1126–33.

[144] Chu CT, Gray L, Goldstein LB, Hulette CM. Diagnosis of intracranial vasculitis: a multi-disciplinary approach. *J Neuropathol Exp Neurol* 1998; 57: 30–8.

[145] Warren JD, Schott JM, Fox NC, *et al.* Brain biopsy in dementia. *Brain* 2005; 128: 2016–25.

[146] Castelnovo G, Bouly S, Vladut M, Marty-Double C, Labauge P. Rapidly progressive dementia disclosing primary angiitis of the central nervous system [in French]. *Ann Med Interne Paris* 2001; 152: 273–5.

[147] Brotman DJ, Eberhart CG, Burger PC, McArthur JC, Hellmann DB. Primary angiitis of the central nervous system and Alzheimer's disease: clinically and pathologically evident in a single patient. *J Rheumatol* 2000; 27: 2935–7.

[148] Scolding NJ, Joseph F, Kirby PA, *et al.* Aβ-related angiitis: primary angiitis of the central nervous system

associated with cerebral amyloid angiopathy. *Brain* 2005; 128: 500–15.

[149] Siva A. Vasculitis of the nervous system. *J Neurol* 2001; 248: 451–68.

[150] Joseph FG, Scolding NJ. Cerebral vasculitis: a practical approach. *Pract Neurol* 2002; 2: 80–93.

[151] Scolding NJ, Jayne DRW, Zajicek JP, *et al.* Cerebral vasculitis–recognition, diagnosis and management. *Q J Med* 1997; 90: 61–73.

[152] Caselli RJ. Giant cell (temporal) arteritis: a treatable cause of multi-infarct dementia. *Neurology* 1990; 40: 753–5.

[153] Harlé JR, Disdier P, Ali Cherif A, *et al.* Curable dementia and panarteritis nodosa [in French]. *Rev Neurol Paris* 1991; 147: 148–50.

[154] Capra R, Gregorini G, Mattioli F, Santostefano M, Galluzzi S. Rapid onset dementia in patients with microscopic polyangiitis. *J Neurol* 1998; 245: 397 (abstract P64).

[155] Evans JJ, Breen EK, Antoun N, Hodges JR. Focal retrograde amnesia for autobiographical events following cerebral vasculitis: a connectionist account. *Neurocase* 1996; 2: 1–12.

[156] Mattioli F, Capra R, Rovaris M, *et al.* Frequency and patterns of subclinical cognitive impairment in patients with ANCA-associated small vessel vasculitides. *J Neurol Sci* 2002; 195: 161–6.

[157] Corsellis JA, Goldberg GJ, Norton AR. "Limbic encephalitis" and its association with carcinoma. *Brain* 1968; 91: 481–96.

[158] Gultekin SH, Rosenfeld MR, Voltz R, *et al.* Paraneoplastic limbic encephalitis: neurological symptoms, immunological findings and tumour association in 50 patients. *Brain* 2000; 123: 1481–94.

[159] Lawn ND, Westmoreland BF, Kiely MJ, *et al.* Clinical, magnetic resonance imaging, and electroencephalographic findings in paraneoplastic limbic encephalitis. *Mayo Clin Proc* 2003; 78: 1363–8.

[160] Rees JH, Hain SF, Johnson MR, *et al.* The role of [18F]fluoro-2-deoxyglucose-PET scanning in the diagnosis of paraneoplastic neurological disorders. *Brain* 2001; 124: 2223–31.

[161] Martin RC, Haut MW, Goeta Kreisler K, Blumenthal D. Neuropsychological functioning in a patient with paraneoplastic limbic encephalitis. *J Int Neuropsychol Soc* 1996; 2: 460–6.

[162] Hirayama K, Taguchi Y, Sato M, Tsukamoto T. Limbic encephalitis presenting with topographical disorientation and amnesia. *J Neurol Neurosurg Psychiatry* 2003; 74: 110–12.

[163] Bak TH, Antoun N, Balan KK, Hodges JR. Memory lost, memory regained: neuropsychological findings and neuroimaging in two cases of paraneoplastic limbic encephalitis with radically different outcomes. *J Neurol Neurosurg Psychiatry* 2001; 71: 40–7.

[164] Benke T, Wagner M, Pallua AK, Muigg A, Stockhammer G. Long-term cognitive and MRI findings in a patient with paraneoplastic limbic encephalitis. *J Neurooncol* 2004; 66: 217–24.

[165] Lai M, Huijbers MG, Lancaster E, *et al.* Investigation of LGI1 as the antigen in limbic encephalitis previously attributed to potassium channels: a case series. *Lancet Neurol* 2010; 9: 776–85.

[166] Dalmau J, Gleichman AJ, Hughes EG, *et al.* Anti-NMDA-receptor encephalitis: case series and analysis of the effects of antibodies. *Lancet Neurol* 2008; 7: 1091–8.

[167] Wong SH, Saunders M, Larner AJ, Das K, Hart IK. An effective immunotherapy regimen for VGKC antibody-positive limbic encephalitis. *J Neurol Neurosurg Psychiatry* 2010; 81: 1167–9.

[168] Finke C, Kopp UA, Pruss H, *et al.* Cognitive deficits following anti-NMDA receptor encephalitis. *J Neurol Neurosurg Psychiatry* 2012; 83: 195–8.

[169] Schied R, Voltz R, Vetter T, *et al.* Neurosyphilis and paraneoplastic limbic encephalitis: important differential diagnoses. *J Neurol* 2005; 252: 1129–32.

[170] Brain L, Jellinek EH, Ball K. Hashimoto's disease and encephalopathy. *Lancet* 1966; 2: 512–14.

[171] Chaudhuri A, Behan PO. The clinical spectrum, diagnosis, pathogenesis and treatment of Hashimoto's encephalopathy (recurrent acute disseminated encephalomyelitis). *Curr Med Chem* 2003; 10: 1645–53.

[172] Chong JY, Rowland LP, Utiger RD. Hashimoto encephalopathy. Syndrome or myth? *Arch Neurol* 2003; 60: 164–71.

[173] Schott JM, Warren JD, Rossor MN. The uncertain nosology of Hashimoto encephalopathy. *Arch Neurol* 2003; 60: 1812.

[174] Garrard P, Hodges JR, De Vries PJ, *et al.* Hashimoto's encephalopathy presenting as "myxodematous madness". *J Neurol Neurosurg Psychiatry* 2000; 68: 102–3.

[175] Forchetti CM, Katsamakis G, Garron DC. Autoimmune thyroiditis and a rapidly progressive dementia: global hypoperfusion on SPECT scanning suggests a possible mechanism. *Neurology* 1997; 49: 623–6.

[176] Seipelt M, Zerr I, Nau R, *et al.* Hashimoto's encephalitis as a differential diagnosis of Creutzfeldt–Jakob disease. *J Neurol Neurosurg Psychiatry* 1999; 66: 172–6.

[177] Spiegel J, Hellwig D, Becker G, Müller M. Progressive dementia caused by Hashimoto's encephalopathy–report of two cases. *Eur J Neurol* 2004; 11: 711–13.

[178] Creutzfeldt CJ, Haberl RL. Hashimoto encephalopathy: a do-not-miss in the differential diagnosis of dementia. *J Neurol* 2005; 252: 1285–7.

[179] Léger GC, Johnson N, Horowitz SW, *et al.* Dementia-like presentation of striatal hypermetabolic state with anti-striatal antibodies responsive to steroids. *Arch Neurol* 2004; 61: 754–7.

[180] Van Horn G, Arnett FC, Dimachkie MM. Reversible dementia and chorea in a young woman with the lupus anticoagulant. *Neurology* 1996; 46: 1599–603.

[181] Cavalcanti A, Hilario MO, dos Santos FH, *et al.* Subtle cognitive deficits in adults with a previous history of Sydenham's chorea during childhood. *Arthritis Care Res (Hoboken)* 2010; 62: 1065–71.

[182] Selvarajah JR, Rodrigues MG, Ali S. Histiocytosis for the neurologist: a case of Erdheim–Chester disease. *Pract Neurol* 2012; 12: 319–23.

[183] Van't Hooft I, Gavhed D, Laurencikas E, Henter JI. Neuropsychological sequelae in patients with neurodegenerative Langerhans cell histiocytosis. *Pediatr Blood Cancer* 2008; 51: 669–74.

[184] Wright RA, Hermann RC, Parisi JE. Neurological manifestations of Erdheim–Chester disease. *J Neurol Neurosurg Psychiatry* 1999; 66: 72–5.

[185] Veyssier-Belot C, Cacoub P, Caparros-Lefebvre D, *et al.* Erdheim–Chester disease. Clinical and radiologic characteristics of 59 cases. *Medicine* 1996; 75: 757–69.

[186] Lachenal F, Cotton F, Desmurs-Clavel H, *et al.* Neurological manifestations and neuroradiological presentation of Erdheim–Chester disease: report of 6 cases and systematic review of the literature. *J Neurol* 2006; 253: 1267–77.

[187] Brandt T, Schautzer F, Hamilton D, *et al.* Vestibular loss causes hippocampal atrophy and impaired spatial memory in humans. *Brain* 2005; 128: 1579–89.

[188] Chanson JB, de Seze J, Echaniz A, Tranchant C, Blanc F. Cognitive functions in chronic inflammatory demyelinating polyneuropathy. *Neurodegen Dis* 2009; 6(Suppl 1): 1358.

Structural brain lesions

7.1 Brain tumors and their treatment

7.1.1 Brain tumors

Cognitive decline in patients with brain tumors may have many causes, including the tumor itself, concurrent tumor-related epileptic seizures, mood disorder, steroid therapy, and as a sequel of surgery, radiotherapy and chemotherapy for the tumor, or any combination thereof [1]. For impairment related to the tumor per se, both tumor type and tumor location may be relevant. For example, an amnesic syndrome may accompany tumors involving temporal-limbic structures while frontal tumors may cause a frontal lobe syndrome [2].

Cognitive decline may be more common with certain tumor types, such as central nervous system (CNS) lymphoma and gliomatosis cerebri, and with slowly rather than rapidly growing tumors. Dominant as opposed to nondominant hemisphere lesions may be associated with greater cognitive deficit, but the profile is more global than localized. Lesions located in specific, eloquent structures such as the hippocampus, frontal lobes, or fornix may produce specific deficits. In glioma patients with lesions in the temporal or frontal lobes examined before treatment initiation, 90% were found to have neurocognitive dysfunction, with executive impairments in 78% and memory and attention deficits in 60% of cases [3]. Longitudinal neuropsychological decline may be an early marker of tumor recurrence [4].

7.1.2 Meningioma

Meningiomas have a predilection for certain intracranial sites, including the olfactory groove, falx, parasagittal region, and sphenoid bone, in some of which there may be prominent cognitive as well as focal neurological signs.

Meningioma has long been recognized to be a potentially treatable cause of dementia, sometimes with dementia as the presenting feature [5–7]. Interhemispheric, parafalcine (subfrontal) meningiomas may grow to a huge size without producing neurological signs but with evidence of impaired executive function on neuropsychological testing [8]. Rare intraventricular meningiomas may also be associated with cognitive change [9]. Postoperative improvement in attention and working memory has been documented following resection of frontal meningiomas [10].

7.1.3 Glioma and gliomatosis cerebri

Cognitive impairment may be detected in some patients with low-grade glioma prior to treatment, especially with left frontal lobe tumors [11]. Another study found that mass effect, larger size, and higher grade were the tumor-related factors most likely to be associated with cognitive deficits, particularly in verbal and visual memory and verbal fluency [12].

Following treatment, cognitive deficits are common in survivors of low-grade glioma, whether they have or have not received radiotherapy, suggesting that the tumor per se, and/or other factors (e.g., antiepileptic drug therapy) may contribute to impairment [13,14]. In high-grade gliomas, survivors may have moderate to severe cognitive

deficits; although these may be treatment-related; nonetheless, there is evidence that the tumor itself may also contribute [15]. However, both cognitive improvement and worsening may be seen in glioma patients postoperatively [12]. In recurrent malignant glioma, cognitive test performance is a predictor of survival [16].

Gliomatosis cerebri is a neoplastic disorder in which malignant cells infiltrate the brain widely without forming mass lesions. Clinically, the condition most often presents with progressive headache, gait disorder, and epileptic seizures (partial, with or without secondary generalization), with signs of raised intracranial pressure (papilloedema, ophthalmoparesis), hemiparesis, and neurobehavioral changes [17]. Neuropsychological deficits reflecting affected brain regions may occur; for example, profound abulia with unilateral right hemisphere involvement [18] and executive dysfunction and verbal memory impairment with bifrontal and left temporal white matter involvement, progressing to a dementia of white matter type with bihemispheric white matter infiltration [19]. Progressive cognitive decline and parkinsonism said to resemble sporadic Creutzfeldt–Jakob disease has been reported [20], as has rapidly progressive dementia with parkinsonism [21].

7.1.4 Pituitary tumors

Tumors of the pituitary gland usually manifest with local effects of space occupation and compression of adjacent structures (e.g., the optic chiasm), or with endocrine effects.

Memory disturbance has been noted with massive pituitary tumors [22] and potentially reversible dementia has also been reported. For example, Brisman *et al.* presented a patient with personality change labeled as depression but unresponsive to antidepressant medication, with inappropriate and disinhibited behavior that evolved to apathy, and with memory loss (five-minute recall 0/3), who on imaging had a large pituitary tumor with suprasellar extension, which proved to be a macroprolactinoma. Within a month of starting treatment with a dopamine agonist (bromocriptine), the patient was subjectively normal. No detailed neuropsychological assessment was performed [23]. Decrements in both memory and attention in comparison to normative data were observed in patients with both treated pituitary Cushing's disease and nonfunctioning pituitary adenomas [24], perhaps reflecting an effect of pituitary tumors per se. A more recent study found memory impairment in patients with nonfunctioning pituitary adenomas compared to a reference sample, with no adverse effect in those receiving radiotherapy in addition to transphenoidal tumor resection [25]. This latter finding was in contrast to that of a retrospective study that concluded that treatment of pituitary tumors, either with surgery or radiotherapy, was culpable for associated memory disorders due to damage to diencephalic structures [26].

7.1.5 Craniopharyngioma

Memory disturbances may occur in association with craniopharyngiomas [22]. Cases of severe anterograde amnesia associated with third ventricle craniopharyngioma causing relatively selective damage to the mammillary bodies have been reported [27,28]. In one case, amnesia improved following tumor removal, although memory was still impaired, and brain MRI showed small atrophic mammillary bodies [27]. In another case in which the right hippocampus was involved as well as the mammillary bodies, albeit to a lesser extent, tumor removal was associated with complete recovery of memory function. Functional imaging (positron emission tomography, PET) showed no preoperative activity in memory-related structures, but improved perfusion of anterior thalamic nuclei postoperatively [28]. Relatively selective mammillary body damage thus may result in severe anterograde amnesia, which may be partially or completely reversible.

7.1.6 Primary CNS lymphoma (PCNSL) and lymphomatosis cerebri

Primary CNS lymphoma (PCNSL) is a rare highgrade non-Hodgkin's lymphoma that typically appears on MRI of the brain as homogeneously enhancing periventricular or subependymal mass lesions. However, diagnosis ultimately depends on histology, following which a variety of staging investigations are recommended to exclude systemic disease (around 10% of cases initially thought to be confined to the CNS are reported to have evidence of systemic involvement) and document the extent of CNS involvement [29]. Transient clinical and radiological response to steroids is well attested, but optimal treatment involves methotrexate-based combination chemotherapy followed by radiotherapy, despite which survival is around 10 to 20 months.

The risk of developing dementia in PCNSL survivors has been high, possibly related to the patient's age and to treatment-related neurocognitive toxicity. Cognitive impairment in the domains of memory and executive function was noted to be more pronounced following whole brain radiotherapy with or without chemotherapy, and correlated with the extent of white matter disease [30]. Whether tumor-related factors render these patients more susceptible to cognitive impairment, such as the tendency to seed by cerebrospinal fluid (CSF) pathways [31] or to the adverse effects of treatment, is unknown.

Rarely, PCNSL presents as a diffuse infiltrating small cell B-cell lymphoma, lymphomatosis cerebri, without formation of the more common cohesive mass lesion(s). Lymphomatosis cerebri has been reported to present as a rapidly progressive dementia [32–34]. Differential diagnosis in this situation may include subcortical vascular ischemic dementia, leukoencephalopathy or gliomatosis cerebri [33], or "white matter dementia" [32].

CNS lymphoma may also occur in the context of HIV infection (Section 9.3).

7.1.7 Splenial tumors

Tumors involving the splenium of the corpus callosum are reported to produce amnesia, thought to be related to damage to the fornix due to its anatomical propinquity to the splenium, and visual perceptual impairment due to hemispheric disconnection, while intellect is relatively preserved [35].

7.1.8 Radiotherapy and chemotherapy

The risk of cognitive deficits related to radiotherapy is a vexed question. The risk is known to increase with high radiation dose, large fraction, and field size (whole brain versus focal), but is also related to the patient's age and concurrent chemotherapy. Moreover, there are potential confounders, including the malignancy per se (e.g., disease progression), comorbid medical, neurological (e.g., epilepsy), or psychiatric conditions (e.g., depression), and surgical treatment [1,36–39]. Reviews of the literature have concluded that focal radiotherapy in patients with glioma is not the main reason for cognitive deficits [1] and that radiation effects on cognition are severe in only a minority of patients [36]. Impaired hippocampal neurogenesis following radiotherapy may contribute to neurocognitive impairment in cases without residual tumor [39].

Late delayed postradiation cognitive decline, occurring more than three years posttreatment, is a rare but feared complication of treatment, and of increasing importance as an outcome measure with improved survival from underlying malignancy. It is associated with diffuse white matter change (leukoencephalopathy) and cortical/subcortical atrophy on brain imaging, a subcortical pattern of cognitive deficits, with psychomotor slowing, executive and memory dysfunction, sometimes sufficiently severe to constitute dementia, and pathological changes of gliosis, demyelination, and thickening of small vessels [36,40,41]. In a series of patients with primary CNS lymphoma, five-year cumulative incidence of delayed neurotoxicity was

nearly 25% [41]. An annual incidence of 11% was noted in an older, retrospective series, in which relatively high doses of radiation were used [42].

Neurotoxicity from chemotherapeutic agents is more likely if they are given concomitantly with radiotherapy, or via intrathecal or intra-arterial routes as compared to systemically, all these factors increasing drug concentration in normal brain tissue by compromising or bypassing the blood–brain barrier.

7.2 Hydrocephalic dementias

The association of dementia with hydrocephalus may arise in a number of situations [43]. Hydrocephalus may be classified according to whether there is obstruction to the flow of CSF, and whether the ventricles are communicating. Obstructive noncommunicating hydrocephalus in the context of neoplasms, inflammation (ependymitis, arachnoiditis, pachymeningitis), and acquired aqueduct stenosis may present as a subacute dementia. Nonobstructive communicating hydrocephalus may result from ex vacuo brain atrophy, perhaps in the context of parenchymal brain disease or previous brain trauma, or extremely rarely, from CSF hypersecretion, as for example from a choroid plexus tumor.

Perhaps the most challenging clinical situation, both in terms of diagnosis and management, relates to cases of communicating hydrocephalus. These may be obstructive, secondary to subarachnoid hemorrhage, trauma, meningitis, or diffusely infiltrating tumor, or some other process (for example, Paget's disease of the skull; Section 7.2.4); or primary or idiopathic, the condition that has come to be known as normal pressure hydrocephalus (iNPH). Whether these latter cases represent some form of occult obstruction remains unclear. Because of the uncertainties about etiopathogenesis, retention of the term "occult hydrocephalus," as originally suggested by Adams *et al.* [44], or use of the term "chronic hydrocephalus" [45] may be theoretically preferable, although pragmatically neither is likely to supplant the entrenched usage of "normal pressure hydrocephalus."

7.2.1 Normal pressure hydrocephalus (NPH)

That normal pressure hydrocephalus (NPH) comprises the clinical triad of gait difficulties of parkinsonian type, urinary problems, and cognitive decline is a fact known to virtually every medical student, and a huge literature on the subject has developed since the condition was first described [44,46], much of it related to predicting which patients will respond to surgical shunting procedures [45,47]. The advent of widespread structural neuroimaging with computerized tomography (CT) has increased the frequency with which this disorder is considered; relative preservation of cortical gyri despite ventricular expansion is suggested to point to this diagnosis, and various radiological parameters (e.g., Evans ratio) have been suggested to be helpful in predicting shunt responsiveness.

Yet, despite this "evidence base," NPH remains in many ways obscure and perplexing, perhaps particularly for neurologists with an interest in cognitive disorders. Is it certain, for example, that at least some of these patients do not have an *ex vacuo* nonobstructive communicating hydrocephalus due to occult primary intraparenchymal pathology causing subcortical atrophy, a well-recognized correlate of Alzheimer's disease (AD)? Very few NPH patients come to pathological analysis, either biopsy or autopsy, and when they do, alternative pathologies may be found, such as AD [48,49], cerebrovascular disease [48], Parkinson's disease [50], or progressive supranuclear palsy [51], even when patients have proven to be temporarily "shunt-responsive." The presence of AD pathology in suspected iNPH patients has been associated with lack of response to shunting [49]. Patients shunted for presumed NPH without benefit and whose phenotype subsequently evolved to that of behavioral variant frontotemporal dementia (Section 2.2.1) have also been noted [52]. Secondary or symptomatic causes of NPH have been reported, such as neuroborreliosis (Section 9.4.2).

The CSF tap test, withdrawing 25–30 mL of CSF with pre- and posttest assessment of gait and cognitive function, has been advocated as a predictor of shunt responsiveness, but both false negatives and false positives may occur, the latter possibly due to the presence of alternative, primary neurodegenerative pathology [53].

With these diagnostic uncertainties, it might be anticipated that delineating the neuropsychological profile of iNPH would be difficult, yet there has been no shortage of attempts [54,55]. For example, Ogino *et al.* [56] found disproportionate impairment of frontal lobe functions (attention/concentration subtest of WMS-R; digit span, arithmetic, block design, and digit symbol substitution subtests of WAIS-R) in iNPH patients compared to AD patients but disproportionately mild memory impairment (general memory and delayed recall in WAIS-R). Impaired frontal lobe function as assessed by the Frontal Assessment Battery and verbal fluency tests was also reported by the same group [57]. The typical cognitive profile of frontal deficits in NPH (psychomotor slowing, impaired attention, working memory, verbal fluency and executive function) has prompted its classification as a subcortical dementia. However, in addition to frontal deficits, posterior (cortical) deficits have been reported in NPH such as visuospatial and visuoperceptual difficulties [58]. Indeed, in comparison with Binswanger's disease, a prototypical subcortical dementia (Section 3.1.2), impairment of memory and visuospatial attention may be more severe in NPH [55].

Amelioration of executive dysfunction is reported after shunting for NPH [58], whereas low verbal memory baseline scores were found to be predictors of poor response, the more so if there was concurrent visuoconstructional deficit or executive dysfunction [59]. It might be asked whether these more impaired patients may have been harboring primary neurodegenerative disease [49].

Hence, there are significant methodological difficulties in defining the cognitive profile of iNPH, perhaps related, at least in part, to etiological heterogeneity. Nonetheless, disruption of fronto-subcortical pathways would seem the most likely pathological substrate (for example, to account for the parkinsonian gait) with a corresponding neuropsychological profile dominated by, although not limited to, subcortical features. Efforts to exclude other pathologies, particularly AD, in suspected iNPH cases should be made before deciding on surgical treatment.

7.2.2 Aqueduct stenosis

Idiopathic stenosis of the aqueduct of Sylvius, or mesencephalic duct, which runs through the midbrain to connect the third and fourth ventricles, results in hydrocephalus. This is often thought to be congenital, but a late-onset idiopathic form has also been described, presenting with headache, gait disturbance, and cognitive deficits. The latter may be subtle, insufficient to interfere with occupation or everyday activities. A small study of adult patients submitted to third ventriculostomy found combined deficits of memory and frontal executive function, which resolved promptly and almost completely postoperatively [60].

7.2.3 Colloid cyst; fornix lesions

Colloid cysts are thought to arise from ependymal cells in the vestigial paraphysis in the anterior portion of the third ventricle, where they may block the third ventricle and cause obstructive hydrocephalus. Clinical presentation is either with intermittent obstruction causing severe bifrontal-bioccipital headache, unsteady gait, incontinence, visual impairment, and drop attacks without loss of consciousness, or with a picture resembling "NPH" (Section 7.2.1). Some cases are now found incidentally when patients undergo structural brain imaging for other reasons. Surgical resection of the cyst may be undertaken, although symptoms may sometimes be more easily controlled with shunting or stereotactic decompression.

Colloid cyst may present to the cognitive clinic with psychomotor slowing. Preoperative memory problems have also been noted [61]. However, postoperative cognitive problems as a consequence of damage to the fornix during surgery for colloid cyst are well described, specifically a persistent anterograde amnesia [62–66]. Bilateral fornix interruption was a predictor of poor memory performance in one study [64]; severity of damage to the left fornix was suggested to be the most important determinant of severity of impairment in verbal memory in another [63]. Recall may be less impaired than recognition [64]. Relative absence of retrograde amnesia was noted in some reports [62,65], but in others retrograde amnesia for autobiographical episodes and for semantic memory was recorded [66].

Fornix damage with subsequent neuropsychological deficits may also be seen as a consequence of surgery for other brain tumors [67–69], as well as with other pathologies such as focal or strategic stroke [70] (Section 3.2.2) and carbon monoxide poisoning [71] (Section 8.2.2.2).

7.2.4 Paget's disease of bone (osteitis deformans)

Paget's disease is a disorder of increased bone turnover with excessive osteoclastic resorption and disorganized new bone formation, with a predilection for involvement of the skull and vertebral column. Neurological complications are well recognized, particularly cranial nerve palsies due to foraminal entrapment, and extradural myelopathy due to disease in vertebral bodies [72]. Dementia as a consequence of basilar invagination is reported, producing a syndrome sometimes likened to NPH, although there has been debate as to whether the hydrocephalus is in some sense obstructive or non-communicating, and hence amenable to treatment with some form of ventricular shunting [73,74].

Paget's disease may rarely occur in association with an autosomal dominant frontotemporal dementia with or without inclusion body myopathy (IBMPFD) caused by mutations in the valosin-containing protein gene on chromosome 9 [75] (Section 2.2.5.2).

7.3 Other structural lesions

Subdural hematoma, arachnoid cyst, and spontaneous intracranial hypotension are considered here. Other potentially relevant structural brain lesions, such as arteriovenous malformations and fistulae are considered elsewhere (Section 3.4).

7.3.1 Subdural hematoma (SDH)

Cognitive sequelae associated with acute subdural hematoma (SDH) may be related to traumatic brain injury in the context of head injury, the most common cause of acute SDH; alcohol misuse may be a precipitating factor. Chronic SDH without a history of head trauma most commonly occurs in the elderly, where concurrent neurodegenerative disease (AD, dementia with Lewy bodies), with associated risk of repeated falls, may be present. Despite these possible confounding factors, SDH per se may be associated with cognitive deficits [76].

Chronic SDH most commonly presents with an alteration in mental state, with features of delirium or dementia, with or without fixed focal neurological deficit such as hemiparesis, or transient deficits such as aphasia, hemisensory loss, epileptic seizures, headache, and occasionally an akinetic-rigid syndrome. Recognized risk factors for the accumulation of blood and its liquefaction in the subdural space include increasing age, history of direct head trauma (although not invariably present), use of antiplatelet or anticoagulant drugs, and alcohol misuse. A history of falls may be a particular "red flag" [77]. The diagnosis may be overlooked, symptoms being attributed to other causes, such as a dementia syndrome, and structural brain imaging with CT may not be diagnostic if the collection is isodense rather than hyperdense (acute) or hypodense (>4 wk), or if bilateral collections cause no mass effect or midline shift. Surgical evacuation is often the treatment of choice.

Variable mental changes have been reported in chronic SDH, the most common being lethargy and poor concentration, withdrawal, confusion with aggressive outbursts, and failing memory and intelligence reminiscent of a dementia syndrome [78]. Slowed mental abilities with an akinetic-rigid syndrome but normal Abbreviated Mental Test Score have been reported [79], as has Gerstmann's syndrome [80].

Chronic subdural hematoma is often listed in textbooks as a cause of reversible dementia, but the published evidence base for this is slim [81]. Ishikawa *et al.* [82] reported that nearly 70% of a series of 26 patients operated on for chronic SDH (i.e., a highly selected cohort) were demented preoperatively on the basis of their performance on MMSE, with 50% (9 patients) making a good recovery. Younger patients with a higher preoperative MMSE showed better recovery, as did patients diagnosed and evacuated early.

7.3.2 Arachnoid cyst

Arachnoid cysts are not infrequent incidental findings on structural brain imaging, most commonly seen in the middle cranial fossa. Whether they have symptomatic effects related to space occupation (pressure, brain displacement, both, or other mechanisms) is debated. A literature search concluded that arachnoid cysts may be associated with cognitive impairments in various functions, including perception, memory, complex verbal tasks, visuospatial functions, and visual attention, with improvements noted after cyst surgery [83]. However, it remains uncertain what proportion of arachnoid cysts are symptomatic.

7.3.3 Spontaneous intracranial hypotension (SIH)

Spontaneous intracranial hypotension (SIH) is characterized by postural headache and low CSF opening pressure, thought to result from leakage of CSF, usually idiopathic. An epidural blood patch may help symptoms.

Cases of SIH associated with dementia, with features reported to be typical of frontotemporal dementia, and which remit following treatment with prednisolone, have been presented [84,85].

REFERENCES

[1] Taphoorn MJB, Klein M. Cognitive deficits in adult patients with brain tumours. *Lancet Neurol* 2004; 3: 159–68.

[2] Cappa SF, Cipolotti L. Cognitive and behavioural disorders associated with space-occupying lesions. In: Cappa SF, Abutalebi J, Démonet JF, Fletcher PC, Garrard P (eds.). *Cognitive Neurology: A Clinical Textbook*. Oxford: Oxford University Press, 2008: 161–82.

[3] Tucha O, Smely C, Preier M, Lange KW. Cognitive deficits before treatment among patients with brain tumors. *Neurosurgery* 2000; 47: 324–33.

[4] Armstrong CL, Goldstein B, Shera D, Ledakis GE, Tallent EM. The predictive value of longitudinal neuropsychological assessment in the early detection of brain tumor recurrence. *Cancer* 2003; 97: 649–56.

[5] Sachs E Jr. Meningiomas with dementia as the first and presenting feature. *J Ment Sci* 1950; 96: 998–1007.

[6] Erkinjuntti T, Sulkava R, Kovanen J, Palo J. Suspected dementia: evaluation of 323 consecutive referrals. *Acta Neurol Scand* 1987; 76: 359–64.

[7] Sahadevan S, Pang WS, Tan NJ, Choo GK, Tan CY. Neuroimaging guidelines in cognitive impairment: lessons from 3 cases of meningiomas presenting as isolated dementia. *Singapore Med J* 1997; 38: 339–43.

[8] Hanna MG, Papanastassiou V, Greenhall RCD. [Minerva]. *BMJ* 1996; 313: 502.

[9] Bertalanffy A, Roessler K, Koperek O, *et al.* Intraventricular meningiomas: a report of 16 cases. *Neurosurg Rev* 2006; 29: 30–5.

[10] Tucha O, Smely C, Preier M, *et al.* Preoperative and postoperative cognitive functioning in patients with frontal meningiomas. *J Neurosurg* 2003; 98: 21–31.

[11] Ek L, Almkvist O, Wiberg MK, Stragliotto G, Smits A. Early cognitive impairment in a subset of patients with presumed low-grade glioma. *Neurocase* 2010; 16: 503–11.

[12] Talacchi A, Santini B, Savazzi S, Gerosa M. Cognitive effects of tumour and surgical treatment in glioma patients. *J Neurooncol* 2011; 103: 541–9.

[13] Klein M, Heimans JJ, Aaronson MK, *et al.* Effect of radiotherapy and other treatment-related factors on mid-term to long-term cognitive sequelae in low-grade gliomas: a comparative study. *Lancet* 2002; 360: 1361–8.

[14] Torres IJ, Mundt AJ, Sweeney PJ, *et al.* A longitudinal neuropsychological study of partial brain radiation in adults with brain tumors. *Neurology* 2003; 60: 1113–18.

[15] Archibald YM, Lunn D, Ruttan LA, *et al.* Cognitive functioning in long-term survivors of high-grade glioma. *J Neurosurg* 1994; 80: 247–53.

[16] Meyers CA, Hess KR, Yung WK, Levin VA. Cognitive function as a predictor of survival in patients with recurrent malignant glioma. *J Clin Oncol* 2000; 18: 646–50.

[17] Herrlinger U. Gliomatosis cerebri. *Handb Clin Neurol* 2012; 105: 507–15.

[18] Muqit MM, Rakshi JS, Shakir RA, Larner AJ. Catatonia or abulia? A difficult differential diagnosis. *Mov Disord* 2001; 16: 360–2.

[19] Filley CM, Kleinschmidt-DeMasters BK, Lillehei KO, Damek DM, Harris JG. Gliomatosis cerebri: neurobehavioral and neuropathological observations. *Cogn Behav Neurol* 2003; 16: 149–59.

[20] Slee M, Pretorius P, Ansorge O, Stacey R, Butterworth R. Parkinsonism and dementia due to gliomatosis cerebri mimicking sporadic Creutzfeldt–Jakob disease (CJD). *J Neurol Neurosurg Psychiatry* 2006; 77: 283–4.

[21] Duron E, Lazareth A, Gaubert JY, *et al.* Gliomatosis cerebri presenting as rapidly progressive dementia and parkinsonism in an elderly woman: a case report. *J Med Case Reports* 2008; 2: 53.

[22] Williams M, Pennybacker J. Memory disturbance in third ventricle tumours. *J Neurol Neurosurg Psychiatry* 1954; 17: 115–23.

[23] Brisman MH, Fetell MR, Post KD. Reversible dementia due to macroprolactinoma. Case report. *J Neurosurg* 1993; 79: 135–7.

[24] Heald A, Parr C, Gibson C, O'Driscoll K, Fowler H. A cross-sectional study to investigate long-term cognitive function in people with treated pituitary Cushing's disease. *Exp Clin Endocrinol Diabetes* 2006; 114: 490–7.

[25] Brummelman P, Elderson MF, Dullaart RP, *et al.* Cognitive functioning in patients treated for non-functioning pituitary macroadenoma and the effects of pituitary radiotherapy. *Clin Endocrinol (Oxf)* 2011; 74: 481–7.

[26] Guinan EM, Lowy C, Stanhope N, Lewis PD, Kopelman MD. Cognitive effects of pituitary tumours and their treatments: two case studies and an investigation of 90 patients. *J Neurol Neurosurg Psychiatry* 1998; 65: 870–6.

[27] Tanaka Y, Miyazawa Y, Akaoka F, Yamada T. Amnesia following damage to the mammillary bodies. *Neurology* 1997; 48: 160–5.

[28] Kupers RC, Fortin A, Astrup J, Gjedde A, Ptito M. Recovery of anterograde amnesia in a case of craniopharyngioma. *Arch Neurol* 2004; 61: 1948–52.

[29] Abrey LE, Batchelor TT, Ferreri AJM, *et al.* Report of an international workshop to standardize baseline evaluation and response criteria for primary central nervous system lymphoma. *J Clin Oncol* 2005; 23: 5034–43.

[30] Correa DD, DeAngelis LM, Shi W, *et al.* Cognitive functions in survivors of primary central nervous system lymphoma. *Neurology* 2004; 62: 548–55.

[31] Larner AJ, D'Arrigo C, Scaravilli F, Howard RS. Bilateral symmetrical enhancing brainstem lesions: an unusual presentation of primary CNS lymphoma. *Eur J Neurol* 1999; 6: 721–3.

[32] Rollins KE, Kleinschmidt-DeMasters BK, Corboy JR, Damek DM, Filley CM. Lymphomatosis cerebri as a cause of white matter dementia. *Hum Pathol* 2005; 36: 282–90.

[33] Weaver JD, Vinters HV, Koretz B, *et al.* Lymphomatosis cerebri presenting as rapidly progressive dementia. *Neurologist* 2007; 13: 150–3.

[34] Leschziner G, Rudge P, Lucas S, Andrews T. Lymphomatosis cerebri presenting as a rapidly progressive dementia with a high methylmalonic acid. *J Neurol* 2011; 258: 1489–93.

[35] Rudge P, Warrington EK. Selective impairment of memory and visual perception in splenial tumours. *Brain* 1991; 114: 349–60.

[36] Armstrong CL, Gyato K, Awadalla AW, Lustig R, Tochner ZA. A critical review of the clinical effects of therapeutic irradiation damage to the brain: the roots of the controversy. *Neuropsychol Rev* 2004; 14: 65–86.

[37] Laack NN, Brown PD. Cognitive sequelae of brain radiation in adults. *Semin Oncol* 2004; 31: 702–13.

[38] Sarkissian V. The sequelae of cranial irradiation on human cognition. *Neurosci Lett* 2005; 382: 118–23.

[39] Byrne TN. Cognitive sequelae of brain tumour treatment. *Curr Opin Neurol* 2005; 18: 662–6.

[40] Crossen JR, Garwood D, Glatstein E, Neuwelt EA. Neurobehavioral sequelae of cranial irradiation in adults: a review of radiation-induced encephalopathy. *J Clin Oncol* 1994; 12: 627–42.

[41] Omuro AMP, Ben Porat LS, Panageas KS, *et al.* Delayed neurotoxicity in primary central nervous system lymphoma. *Arch Neurol* 2005; 62: 1595–600.

[42] DeAngelis LM, Delattre JY, Posner JB. Radiation-induced dementia in patients cured of brain metastases. *Neurology* 1989; 39: 789–96.

[43] Esiri MM, Rosenberg GA. Hydrocephalus and dementia. In: Esiri MM, Lee VM-Y, Trojanowski JQ (eds.). *The Neuropathology of Dementia* (2nd edn.). Cambridge: Cambridge University Press, 2004; 442–56.

[44] Adams RD, Fisher CM, Hakim S, *et al.* Symptomatic occult hydrocephalus with "normal" cerebrospinal fluid pressure. *N Engl J Med* 1965; 273: 117–26.

[45] Bret P, Guyotat J, Chazal J. Is normal pressure hydrocephalus a valid concept in 2002? A reappraisal in five questions and proposal for a new designation of the syndrome as "chronic hydrocephalus." *J Neurol Neurosurg Psychiatry* 2002; 73: 9–12.

[46] Hakim S, Adams RD. The special clinical problem of symptomatic hydrocephalus with normal cerebrospinal fluid pressure. Observations on cerebrospinal fluid hydrodynamics. *J Neurol Sci* 1965; 2: 307–27.

[47] Malm J, Eklund A. Idiopathic normal pressure hydrocephalus. *Pract Neurol* 2006; 6: 14–27.

[48] Bech-Azeddine R, Høgh P, Juhler M, Gjerris F, Waldemar G. Idiopathic normal-pressure hydrocephalus: clinical comorbidity correlated with cerebral biopsy findings and outcome of cerebrospinal fluid shunting. *J Neurol Neurosurg Psychiatry* 2007; 78: 157–61.

[49] Hamilton R, Patel S, Lee EB, *et al.* Lack of shunt response in suspected idiopathic normal pressure hydrocephalus with Alzheimer disease pathology. *Ann Neurol* 2010; 68: 535–40.

[50] Krauss JK, Regel JP, Droste DW, *et al.* Movement disorders in adult hydrocephalus. *Mov Disord* 1997; 12: 53–60.

[51] Schott JM, Williams DR, Butterworth R, *et al.* Shunt responsive progressive supranuclear palsy. *Mov Disord* 2007; 22: 902–3.

[52] Davies M, Larner AJ. Frontotemporal dementias: development of an integrated care pathway through an experiential survey of patients and carers. *Int J Care Pathways* 2010; 14: 65–9.

[53] Larner MJ, Larner AJ. Normal pressure hydrocephalus: false positives. *Pract Neurol* 2006; 6: 264.

[54] Devito EE, Pickard JD, Salmond CH, *et al.* The neuropsychology of normal pressure hydrocephalus. *Br J Neurosurg* 2005; 19: 217–24.

[55] Kazui H. Cognitive impairment in patients with idiopathic normal pressure hydrocephalus [in Japanese]. *Brain Nerve* 2008; 60: 225–31.

[56] Ogino A, Kazui H, Miyoshi N, *et al.* Cognitive impairment in patients with idiopathic normal pressure hydrocephalus. *Dement Geriatr Cogn Disord* 2006; 21: 113–19.

[57] Miyoshi N, Kazui H, Ogino A, *et al.* Association between cognitive impairment and gait disturbance in patients with idiopathic normal pressure hydrocephalus. *Dement Geriatr Cogn Disord* 2005; 20: 71–6.

[58] Saito M, Nishio Y, Kanno S, *et al.* Cognitive profile of idiopathic normal pressure hydrocephalus. *Dement Geriatr Cogn Dis Extra* 2011; 1: 202–11.

[59] Thomas G, McGirt MJ, Woodworth G, *et al.* Baseline neuropsychological profile and cognitive response to cerebrospinal fluid shunting for idiopathic normal pressure hydrocephalus. *Dement Geriatr Cogn Disord* 2005; 20: 163–8.

[60] Burtshcer J, Bartha L, Twerdy K, Eisner W, Benke T. Effect of endoscopic third ventriculostomy on neuropsychological outcome in late onset idiopathic aqueduct stenosis: a prospective study. *J Neurol Neurosurg Psychiatry* 2003; 74: 222–5.

[61] Sampath R, Vannemreddy P, Nanda A. Microsurgical excision of colloid cyst with favourable cognitive outcomes and short operative time and hospital stay: operative techniques and analyses of outcomes with review of previous studies. *Neurosurgery* 2010; 66: 368–74.

[62] Hodges JR, Carpenter K. Anterograde amnesia with fornix damage following removal of a third ventricle colloid cyst. *J Neurol Neurosurg Psychiatry* 1991; 54: 633–8.

[63] McMackin D, Cockburn J, Anslow P, Gaffan D. Correlation of fornix damage with memory impairment in six cases of colloid cyst removal. *Acta Neurochir Wien* 1995; 135: 12–18.

[64] Aggleton JP, McMackin D, Carpenter K, *et al.* Differential cognitive effects of colloid cysts in the third ventricle that spare or compromise the fornix. *Brain* 2000; 123: 800–15.

[65] Spiers HJ, Maguire EA, Burgess N. Hippocampal amnesia. *Neurocase* 2001; 7: 357–82.

[66] Poreh A, Winocour G, Moscovitch M, *et al.* Anterograde and retrograde amnesia in a person with bilateral fornix lesions following removal of a colloid cyst. *Neuropsychologia* 2006; 44: 2241–8.

[67] Calabrese P, Markowitsch HJ, Harders AG, Scholz M, Gehlen W. Fornix damage and memory. A case report. *Cortex* 1995; 31: 555–64.

[68] Yasuno F, Hirata M, Takimoto H, *et al.* Retrograde temporal order amnesia resulting from damage to the fornix. *J Neurol Neurosurg Psychiatry* 1999; 67: 102–5.

[69] Ibrahim I, Young CA, Larner AJ. Fornix damage from solitary subependymal giant cell astrocytoma causing postoperative amnesic syndrome. *Br J Hosp Med* 2009; 70: 478–9.

[70] Moudgil SS, Azzouz M, Al-Azzaz A, Haut M, Gutmann L. Amnesia due to fornix infarction. *Stroke* 2000; 31: 1418–19.

[71] Kesler SR, Hopkins RO, Blatter DD, Edge Booth H, Bigler ED. Verbal memory deficits associated with fornix atrophy in carbon monoxide poisoning. *J Int Neuropsychol Soc* 2001; 7: 640–6.

[72] Poncelet A. The neurologic complications of Paget's disease. *J Bone Miner Res* 1999; 14: S88–91.

[73] Chan YP, Shui KK, Lewis RR, Kinirons MT. Reversible dementia in Paget's disease. *J R Soc Med* 2000; 93: 595–6.

[74] Fereydoon R, Mann D, Kula RW. Surgical management of hydrocephalic dementia in Paget's disease of bone: the 6-year outcome of ventriculo-peritoneal shunting. *Clin Neurol Neurosurg* 2005; 107: 325–8.

[75] Watts GDJ, Wymer J, Kovach MJ, *et al.* Inclusion body myopathy associated with Paget disease of bone and frontotemporal dementia is caused by mutant valosin-containing protein. *Nat Genet* 2004; 36: 377–81.

[76] Machulda MM, Haut MW. Clinical features of chronic subdural hematoma: neuropsychiatric and neuropsychologic changes in patients with chronic subdural hematoma. *Neurosurg Clin N Am* 2000; 11: 473–7.

[77] Adhiyaman V, Asghar M, Ganeshram KN, Bhowmick BK. Chronic subdural haematoma in the elderly. *Postgrad Med J* 2002; 78: 71–5.

[78] Schebesch KM, Woertgen C, Rothoerl RD, Ullrich OW, Brawanski AT. Cognitive decline as an important sign for an operable cause of dementia: chronic subdural haematoma. *Zentralbl Neurochir* 2008; 69: 61–4.

[79] Abdulla AJJ, Pearce VR. Reversible akinetic-rigid syndrome due to bilateral subdural haematomas. *Age Ageing* 1999; 28: 582–3.

[80] Maeshima S, Okumura Y, Nakai K, Itakura T, Komai N. Gerstmann's syndrome associated with chronic subdural haematoma: a case report. *Brain Inj* 1998; 12: 697–701.

[81] Allison RS. *The Senile Brain. A Clinical Study*. London: Edward Arnold, 1962; 261–2.

[82] Ishikawa E, Yanaka K, Sugimoto K, Ayuzawa S, Nose T. Reversible dementia in patients with chronic subdural haematomas. *J Neurosurg* 2002; 96: 680–3.

[83] Wester K. Intracranial arachnoid cysts–do they impair mental functions? *J Neurol* 2008; 255: 1113–20.

[84] Hong M, Shah GV, Adams KM, Turner RS, Foster NL. Spontaneous intracranial hypotension causing reversible frontotemporal dementia. *Neurology* 2002; 58; 1285–7.

[85] Walker L, DeMeulemeester C. Spontaneous intracranial hypotension masquerading as frontotemporal dementia. *Clin Neuropsychol* 2008; 22: 1035–53.

Endocrine, metabolic, and toxin-related disorders

8.1 Endocrine disorders

8.1.1 Diabetes mellitus

The relationship between diabetes mellitus and cognitive function is an area of significant current research interest, in particular because of the increasing prevalence of type 2 diabetes [1]. Cognitive dysfunction may be one of the chronic complications of diabetes, but the pathophysiology is uncertain. Possible mediating and modulating factors may include the effects of glycemic control: hyperglycemia, insulin resistance (hyperinsulinemia), and treatment-induced hypoglycemia.

8.1.1.1 Impaired glucose tolerance; hyperglycemia

A link between diabetes mellitus per se and cognitive decline may be obscured by comorbid cerebrovascular disease (both microvascular and macrovascular), hypertension, or depression [2], as these conditions may confound any assessment of cognitive performance. Nonetheless, a systematic literature search that analyzed 23 studies examining glucose tolerance and cognitive function found that poor glucose tolerance was associated with cognitive impairment, particularly in verbal memory [3]. A meta-analysis of studies of cognitive performance in type 1 diabetes found evidence for slowing of mental speed and diminished mental flexibility with sparing of learning and memory [4]. Observational studies suggest that acute hyperglycemia is associated with a slowing of cognitive performance in some subjects with either type 1 or type 2 diabetes, with a possible threshold around 15 mmol/L [5]. Whether this is a consequence of hyperglycemia per se or of underlying insulin resistance is not certain; hyperinsulinemia has been reported in epidemiological studies to be a risk factor for the development of dementia and memory decline [6].

Systematic reviews have shown a greater risk and rate of cognitive functional decline [7] and of dementia [8] in diabetes, with processing speed and verbal memory the most affected cognitive domains [2]. Epidemiological studies provide some evidence that cognition may be impaired in the early stages of type 2 diabetes. In the Whitehall II study, a prospective study of the incidence of diabetes, an association was noted between diabetes and poor performance on a test of inductive reasoning (Alice Heim 4) in stroke-free patients, but verbal memory, verbal meaning, and verbal fluency tests were not affected. The study suggested that effects of diabetes on cognitive performance might be evident within five years of diagnosis [9].

Diabetes does not appear to be a risk factor for the development of Alzheimer's disease (AD) overall, but might increase relative risk in certain subgroups [10]. Whether AD may be characterized as "type 3 diabetes" because of a potential pathogenic role for brain insulin resistance remains a topic of debate [11].

8.1.1.2 Hypoglycemia

A management strategy of strict glycemic control in diabetes mellitus may exacerbate the risk of episodes of treatment-induced hypoglycemia, which potentially might contribute to cognitive impairment. Hypoglycemia is recognized to cause acute neuropsychiatric features as a consequence of neuroglycopenia, with or without concurrent features of autonomic activation.

Severe hypoglycemia is a recognized cause of acute amnesia [12]. An amnesic syndrome has been reported in patients with diabetes following hypoglycemic coma [13], or as a consequence of intensive insulin treatment using a subcutaneous pump causing profound hypoglycemia [14,15]. Bilateral high signal intensity hippocampal lesions on magnetic resonance imaging (MRI) of the brain have been noted in some patients [14] but are not invariably found [15]. Prognosis is variable: the amnesia may be completely [14] or partially reversible [15], or irreversible [13], presumably a reflection of the extent of hippocampal vulnerability to the effects of neuroglycopenia.

Whether repeated episodes of hypoglycemia cause persistent cognitive deficits in diabetes remains an open question. Small studies initially suggested that adults with a history of severe hypoglycemia (i.e., episodes requiring assistance from another person to be reversed) scored lower on some neuropsychological tests than those who had never experienced severe hypoglycemia [16,17], and cohort studies also suggested a modest association between reported frequency of severe hypoglycemia, lower IQ, and slowed and more variable reaction times [18,19]. In contrast, some longitudinal studies have failed to find any deleterious cognitive effects of repeated severe hypoglycemia [20,21], but a large study in type 2 diabetics (n = 16667) with prolonged follow-up (27 years) found that hypoglycemia severe enough to require emergency room attendance or hospitalization was a risk factor for dementia [22]. It is possible that this association may result from an effect of hypoglycemia on age-related cognitive decline [23].

8.1.2 Thyroid disorders

The focus here is on under- and over-active thyroid states. Thyroid dysfunction may also be seen in association with cognitive disorder in Hashimoto's encephalopathy (Section 6.13). A high prevalence of thyroid dysfunction has been noted in a memory clinic population, although the clinical relevance of these findings is uncertain [24].

8.1.2.1 Hypothyroidism

Neuropsychiatric features complicating hypothyroidism are well recognized, popularized by Richard Asher in his 1949 paper as "myxoedematous madness." Interestingly, a number of Asher's cases were stated to have dementia (cases 4, 6, 13), one was initially referred with a suspected diagnosis of AD, and others were mentally slow, becoming more alert with treatment [25], these symptoms perhaps reflecting neuropsychological deficits in addition to neuropsychiatric features.

Hypothyroidism features ubiquitously in the textbook rubric of "reversible dementia," and few patients presenting with memory complaints do not have thyroid function tests checked. An examination of the evidence base, however, discloses rather few convincing cases. In a literature search of studies on the etiology of dementia, Clarnette and Patterson [26] found only a single case due to hypothyroidism in 2781 cases of reversible dementia. Dugbartey [27] noted that hypothyroidism has been associated with deficits in general intelligence, complex attention and concentration, memory, perceptual and visuoperceptual function, expressive and receptive language, and executive/frontal functions. A study of thyroid cancer patients on and off thyroxine suggested that the memory defect in delayed recall of verbal information could not be solely attributed to reduced attentional resources [28]. Hypothyroid patients were found to have cognitive impairments that were predominantly mnemonic in nature, and not simply indicative of cognitive slowing, prompting the proposal that hippocampal structure and/or function is disrupted in hypothyroidism [29].

Subclinical hypothyroidism (SCH) is characterized by low levels of thyroid stimulating hormone (TSH) but with normal levels of T4, T3, free T4, and free T3, and may reflect incipient hypothyroidism. Some studies have found cognitive performance to be within the normal range in SCH [30] while others have found mnemonic deficits less marked than those in overt hypothyroidism [29,31]. A positive correlation between plasma thyroid hormone (T4) level and cognitive function as assessed with Mini-Mental State Examination (MMSE) has been noted in euthyroid older women [32].

Because the risk of hypothyroidism, like dementia, increases with age, the possibility that cognitive impairment is a comorbid rather than a causal relation in some cases cannot be ruled out. Mood may also need to be taken into account [30]. Currently, there seems little justification in performing thyroid function tests in all patients with cognitive complaints unless there are other somatic and/or neurological symptoms and signs pointing to the possibility of thyroid dysfunction. However, at the time of writing, TSH remained a mandatory test in the revised guidelines for dementia investigation promulgated by the European Federation of Neurological Societies [33].

8.1.2.2 Hyperthyroidism

Occasional reports of dementia associated with hyperthyroidism with reversal upon correction of thyroid status have appeared [34], but such cases must be exceptionally rare.

A case control study of patients with newly diagnosed thyrotoxicosis of Graves' type (a condition originally described by Caleb Hillier Parry [35]) found subjective reports of cognitive deficits in the toxic phase, but no impairment was found on comprehensive neuropsychological testing [36], contrasting with a case report of impairments of attention, memory, and constructive skills in a man with Graves' disease, whose symptoms and temporoparietal hypoperfusion on single-photon emission computed tomography (SPECT) scanning improved with a return to euthyroidism [37]. Cognitive dysfunction in a patient with sporadic periodic hypokalaemic paralysis and hyperthyroidism has been reported [38].

Epidemiological studies have suggested that subclinical hyperthyroidism is a risk factor for dementia and AD [39,40].

8.1.3 Parathyroid disorders

8.1.3.1 Hypoparathyroidism

Idiopathic hypoparathyroidism, probably an immune diathesis of the parathyroid glands, may result in a variety of systemic and neurological disorders, the latter including epileptic seizures, extrapyramidal signs, altered mental state, signs of raised intracranial pressure including papilledema, neuromuscular hyperactivity (carpopedal spasm, muscle cramps, Chvostek's and Trousseau's signs), as well as dementia. Many of these clinical features may be explained by the accompanying hypocalcemia, and reverse with its correction.

Dementia has been reported as the presenting sign of hypoparathyroidism [41–43], as well as a postsurgical phenomenon [44], and in association with other neurological features [45]. Dementia in hypoparathyroidism, which reverses with 1,25-dihydroxycholecalciferol treatment, has been documented [46], including a case associated with normocalcemia [47].

8.1.3.2 Hyperparathyroidism

Occasional cases of cognitive impairment associated with hypercalcemia due to primary hyperparathyroidism have been reported, with reversal after parathyroidectomy [48,49].

8.1.4 Adrenal hormone disorders

8.1.4.1 Cushing's syndrome (hypercortisolism)

Most cases of Cushing's syndrome, due to hypercortisolemia, result from pituitary adenomas secreting adrenocorticotrophic hormone (ACTH; Cushing's disease), others from ectopic ACTH-producing tumors (usually in the lung), and adrenal cortex tumors. Exogenous steroid, most often given therapeutically for a wide variety of diseases, neurological and otherwise, can also result in cushingoid features. Complications include hypertension, impaired glucose tolerance or diabetes, osteoporosis, cushingoid habitus, cutaneous striae, myopathy, and neuropsychiatric features such as depression. Cognitive dysfunction may also occur; experimental animal studies have shown the hippocampus to be vulnerable to glucocorticoid excess.

The cognitive impairments identified in Cushing's syndrome patients have varied between studies; selective memory impairments were documented in one case-control study [50], whereas selective attention and visual spatial processing seemed most affected in another report [51]. Another study showed no differences in cognitive function between patients with pituitary Cushing's disease and a control group composed of patients with nonfunctioning pituitary adenomas, although the scores of both groups for memory and attention showed significant decrements compared to normative data [52], perhaps reflecting an effect of pituitary tumors per se (Section 7.1.4). A study comparing patients with Cushing's syndrome, age-matched healthy controls, and older subjects, suggested that the performance of the first and third groups was similar on a range of cognitive tests, and hence that hypercortisolism exacerbates cognitive aging [53].

Some studies have reported cognitive improvement after pituitary surgery for Cushing's disease [50], while others document little or no change in performance, suggesting long-lasting deleterious effects of hypercortisolism [54]. A follow-up study found that verbal fluency and recall improved after surgery, with an association noted between improved verbal recall and decreased cortisol levels and an increase in hippocampal volume assessed using serial MRI. Patient age was a significant factor in recovery, with younger patients regaining and sustaining cognitive improvement more quickly than older patients [55], an observation which may support the notion of enhanced cognitive aging in Cushing's syndrome [53]. Although cognitive improvement may occur up to 18 months postsurgery [55], persistent subtle cognitive deficits in the domains of memory and executive function have been noted following cure of Cushing's disease in comparison with patients with nonfunctioning pituitary macroadenomas [56].

8.1.4.2 Addison's disease (hypocortisolism)

Addison's disease may be associated with cognitive impairment in the context of cerebral forms of X-linked adrenoleukodystrophy (Section 5.5.2.2), but reports of cognitive impairment in isolated Addison's disease have not been identified.

8.1.4.3 Conn's syndrome (primary hyperaldosteronism)

Gudin *et al.* [57] reported a 64-year-old woman with a confusional state, disorientation, and apathy, with investigation findings of hypokalemia, metabolic alkalosis, raised aldosterone levels, and radiological evidence of a suprarenal adenoma. A seven-year history of decline in cognitive function had been noted two years earlier, ascribed to vascular dementia because of hypertension and CT evidence of cerebrovascular change. The patient's confusional state improved with ion replacement and spironolactone, and following surgical removal of the adenoma, the pre-existing cognitive decline also improved. The authors suggested Conn's syndrome is a treatable cause of dementia, albeit extremely rare.

8.2 Metabolic disorders

Discussed here are cognitive disorders related to gastrointestinal disease (certain vitamin deficiencies such as thiamine deficiency are covered elsewhere; see Section 8.3.1.1), respiratory disease, and renal and electrolyte-related problems.

8.2.1 Gastrointestinal disease

8.2.1.1 Cobalamin (vitamin B_{12}) deficiency

Addison's original description of pernicious anemia in 1853 included the clinical observation that "the mind occasionally wanders." Cobalamin (vitamin B_{12}), deficiency of which is the cause of pernicious anemia, is a cofactor in several metabolic pathways. Deficiency may also be associated with dementia; indeed, this may be the sole manifestation, macrocytic anemia may be absent. The belief that vitamin B_{12} deficiency is a reversible cause of dementia became prevalent in the 1950s. Reversible dementias in general are increasingly uncommon [58], and convincing documentation of cognitive impairment associated with vitamin B_{12} deficiency with reversal on repletion is rare in the literature.

In a 17-year study of cobalamin deficiency, Healton *et al.* [59] recorded 18 cases of mental impairment in 143 cases, eight with global dementia and nine with recent memory loss; 11/18 recovered completely with repletion. Chiu [60] found 25 cases of dementia attributed to B_{12} deficiency reported between 1958 and 1995, 10 with marked improvement on repletion; all had some hematological abnormality (anemia, raised mean corpuscular volume [MCV], hypersegmented neutrophils) or neurological signs in addition to cognitive impairment.

Reports with careful and sequential neuropsychological assessment are also sparse. The case reported by Meadows *et al.* [61] was confounded by a history of alcohol misuse. Another patient, a health professional with marked clinical improvement after repletion therapy, declined a repeated neuropsychological assessment [62,63]. A report claiming a subcortical dementia pattern associated with vitamin B_{12} deficiency was based on clinical observations, unsubstantiated by neuropsychological assessment [64]. In a study that examined the cognitive profile in patients with vitamin B_{12} deficiency, those who improved with repletion were said to have more deficits in concentration, visuospatial performance, and executive functions (as well as more psychotic problems) than those who did not improve, who had language problems and ideomotor apraxia. The profile was said to be distinct from that in AD, although the study did not have an AD comparator group [65].

A low vitamin B_{12} is not an uncommon finding in patients with dementia or cognitive decline. For example, in 170 consecutive patients diagnosed with dementia, Teunisse *et al.* [66] found low vitamin B_{12} in 26 (15%), all but one of whom fulfilled the then current diagnostic criteria for AD. At the group level, no patient improved with vitamin B_{12} repletion, nor was there any evidence for slowing of AD progression. One patient with a sudden onset of cognitive decline after a respiratory tract infection did improve, but this may have been coincidental with recovery from the infection. Likewise, Eastley *et al.* [67] found low vitamin B_{12}

in 125 of 1432 consecutive clinic attendees (8.7%). No demented patient improved with vitamin B_{12} repletion, although patients with cognitive decline but without dementia did show improvement in verbal fluency with repletion at the group level, leading to the suggestion that vitamin B_{12} may improve frontal lobe and language function in patients with cognitive impairment. Hence, these studies would seem to suggest that, in most cases, a low vitamin B_{12} in a demented patient is a coexistent rather than a causal abnormality, perhaps related to prolonged dietary neglect and weight loss [68] (a common observation before AD diagnosis). A low vitamin B_{12} measurement has a low positive predictive value [60,69]. Vitamin B_{12} estimation is now said to be "often required" rather than mandatory in the investigation of suspected dementia [33]. However, using surrogate measures of vitamin B_{12} status, namely serum methylmalonic acid and holotranscobalamin, in nondemented elderly patients, likely vitamin B_{12} deficiency was found to be associated with lower cognitive function scores [70].

A separate issue is whether low vitamin B_{12} levels may be a risk factor for the development of dementia. Some studies have found low vitamin B_{12} and folate with elevated levels of total homocysteine in AD patients, independent of nutritional status [71,72], and some epidemiological studies have suggested that low vitamin B_{12} may increase the risk of developing AD [73]. The mechanism is not known, but a hypothesis has been proposed suggesting that functional vitamin B_{12} deficiency contributes to the pathogenesis of AD [74].

8.2.1.2 Cobalamin C disease

Cobalamin C disease, combined methylmalonic aciduria and homocystinuria, is an inborn error of cobalamin metabolism with an autosomal recessive mode of inheritance resulting from mutations in the MMACHC gene on chromosome 1p34 (OMIM#277400). Most cases have neonatal onset but occasional cases with adolescent or adult onset have been described [75,76]. The phenotype encompasses dementia, myelopathy, neuropsychiatric features, and thromboembolic phenomena. The dementia sometimes responds to intramuscular or intravenous hydroxycobalamin treatment; therefore, although this is a rare disorder, the diagnosis is worth considering in young adults with a suggestive phenotype.

8.2.1.3 Gluten sensitivity and celiac disease

The neurological associations of gluten sensitivity, with or without bowel disease (celiac disease), are protean, the most common being epilepsy, cerebellar ataxia, axonal neuropathy, myelopathy, myoclonus, intracerebral (especially occipital) calcification, migraine, and cerebral vasculitis with encephalopathy [77], as well as neurological sequelae following dissemination of enteropathy-type T-cell lymphoma, which may complicate the disease [78].

A presenile dementia of uncertain etiology has been reported in celiac disease, most patients failing to respond to a gluten-free diet [79]. Hu *et al.* [80] reported a series of 13 patients seen over a 35-year period with cognitive impairment coincident with gastrointestinal symptom-onset or exacerbation. A frontosubcortical pattern of cognitive impairment was said to be typical; many patients had concurrent ataxia or neuropathy. In three patients, cognitive function was reported to improve or stabilize on gluten withdrawal.

8.2.1.4 Pellagra

This condition, a deficiency of vitamins of the B group, including but not necessarily confined to niacin (nicotinic acid, nicotinamide), is sometimes remembered as the "3Ds": diarrhoea, dermatitis, dementia; or sometimes 4Ds (plus death). As far as can be ascertained, the nature of this dementia has not been described fully. A pellagra encephalopathy of alcoholic etiology has been described [81], but alcohol per se may contribute to any cognitive impairment irrespective of vitamin status (Section 8.3.1).

8.2.2 Respiratory disorders

In addition to the disorders considered here, respiratory compromise with hypoxemia may contribute to the cognitive dysfunction seen in obstructive sleep apnea–hypopnea syndrome (Section 11.1.1).

8.2.2.1 Chronic obstructive pulmonary disease (COPD)

A number of studies have examined neuropsychological function in patients with chronic obstructive pulmonary disease (COPD), and in general, have found impairments in comparison with control groups [82–85]. For example, a study of 36 patients with COPD reported that just under half had a specific pattern of cognitive deterioration characterized by impairments of verbal and visual memory tasks despite preserved visual attention, and with diffuse worsening of other functions. These changes were distinct from those seen in AD patients, and were correlated with age and duration of respiratory failure [86]. In a further study from the same group, decline of verbal memory was found to parallel that of overall cognitive function, due to impairment of both active recall and passive recognition of learned material. Poor adherence to medication was associated with abnormal delayed recall scores [87]. In a follow-up study, onset of depression was identified as a risk factor for cognitive decline [88].

Roehrs *et al.* [89] found deficits in complex reasoning and memory in COPD patients as well as motor skills, the latter sensitive to hypoxemia. One study found chronic oxygen therapy was associated with a small improvement in neuropsychological functioning, with a suggestion that continuous therapy was better than solely nocturnal treatment [83]. Another group reported MMSE abnormalities in COPD patients, affecting recent memory, construction, attention, language, and orientation, the cognitive abnormalities correlating with functional abnormalities; many were classified as questionable or mild dementia. These impairments could not be explained by depression [90]. However, a study by Kozora *et al.* [91] found that most COPD patients

studied were similar to controls on most cognitive tests, and easily distinguishable from mild AD, the exception being reduced letter fluency. The fact that three-quarters of the patients were receiving supplementary oxygen therapy may account for the preservation of cognitive function in this study.

In a community-based longitudinal study of cognitive impairment and dementia, COPD was noted to be more likely in patients with nonprogressive cognitive decline; that is, in those patients in whom an original diagnosis of dementia was not confirmed at follow-up [92].

8.2.2.2 Carbon monoxide poisoning

The French physiologist Claude Bernard (1813–1878) was the first to elucidate the mechanism of carbon monoxide (CO) poisoning. A delayed encephalopathy may develop a few days to weeks after CO poisoning, with or without a history of acute poisoning, sometimes with extrapyramidal or pyramidal signs and psychosis. MRI abnormalities occur in about 12% of patients, most typically widespread periventricular white matter changes, although basal ganglia involvement is also reported [93,94].

A prospective study of episodes of CO poisoning found cognitive deficits in 30% of patients [95]. Occasionally these deficits may be very focal, as for example in a renowned case of visual form agnosia [96], and a case of apparent visual motion blindness (akinetopsia) has been reported [97]. Delayed onset of cognitive (including memory) problems by up to 30 days after acute poisoning may occur, associated with extensive diffuse white matter change. Delayed atrophy of the fornix, correlating with decline on tests of verbal memory, has also been reported in patients poisoned with CO [98].

The complications of CO poisoning typically improve with time, but patients may sometimes be left with permanent neurological and/or neuropsychological sequelae [96]. Acute treatment with hyperbaric oxygen is indicated [99], and cholinesterase inhibitors have been used off-licence to try to ameliorate cognitive sequelae [100].

8.2.3 Renal and electrolyte disorders

8.2.3.1 Renal failure, dialysis

A relation between chronic kidney disease (CKD) and cognitive decline might be anticipated because of the prevalence of cardiovascular risk factors in CKD patients. However, a population-based cohort of nearly 8000 older adults followed up for seven years identified no increased risk of cognitive decline in those with a low estimated glomerular filtration rate (eGFR) at baseline. A rapid decline in eGFR was associated with global cognitive decline and incident vascular dementia, suggesting that the association between the two is probably mediated by vascular mechanisms [101]. Increasing severity of CKD is probably associated with progressive cognitive decline [102]. Cognitive impairment is common in patients receiving hemodialysis [103].

A syndrome of "dialysis dementia," now very rare, used to be seen in chronic dialysis patients and was thought to be related to aluminum in dialysate fluids; reduction of aluminum levels in these fluids was associated with a marked reduction in the incidence of this condition. Clinically, patients developed hesitant speech and even speech arrest, which progressed to cognitive decline with delusions, hallucinations, epileptic seizures, myoclonus, asterixis, and gait abnormalities. The electroencephalogram (EEG) showed slowing with multifocal bursts of more profound slowing and spikes. Patients typically died within six to 12 months [104]. Alzheimer-like changes in tau protein were demonstrated in the brains of patients on renal dialysis [105].

8.2.3.2 Central pontine (and extrapontine) myelinolysis; osmotic demyelination syndrome

Central pontine myelinolysis was first described as such by Adams *et al.* [106], as a relatively symmetrical destruction of myelin sheaths in the basal pons and sometimes extending beyond (hence "extrapontine myelinolysis"), often associated with hyponatremia or its treatment, and particularly but not exclusively seen in chronic alcoholics or other patients with chronic undernourishment. As change in serum osmolality is common to many of the recognized precipitating factors, the terms osmotic demyelination or osmotic myelinolysis are preferred by some authors [107]. Clinical presentations include quadriparesis, bulbar palsy, epileptic seizures, and locked-in syndrome.

Although some patients recover completely from profound neurological deficits without residual disability [108], postrecovery cognitive deficits have been documented. Odier *et al.* [109] noted subcortical/frontal dysfunction in survivors, which significantly limited return to normal activities. "Callosal dementia" (Section 1.3.4), a disconnection syndrome, has been described in association with central and extrapontine myelinolysis [110].

8.3 Toxin-related disorders

8.3.1 Alcohol-related disorders

Alcohol is probably the most widely available and socially tolerated neuroactive substance. A meta-analysis of prospective studies suggests moderate alcohol consumption is protective against dementia although the question of heavy drinking remains uncertain [111,112], some studies indicating that escalating alcohol dosage unequivocally increases the risk of late life dementia [113], an association perhaps related to genetic susceptibility (carriage of the apolipoprotein E epsilon-4 allele [114]). Changing drinking habits in the population, especially the binge culture among young people, has prompted the speculation that an epidemic of alcohol-related dementia may occur in the future [115]. Wernicke–Korsakoff syndrome is probably the best known of the syndromes of cognitive impairment related to alcohol misuse (amnesia in this context was described by Robert Lawson some years before Korsakoff [116]), although it can occur in the absence of a history of alcohol use. Other syndromes of cognitive impairment, which might also be encompassed under the rubric of "alcohol-related" as alcohol overuse is a risk factor for their development, include subdural hematoma (Section 7.3.1), pellagra (Section 8.2.1.4), and obstructive sleep apnea–hypopnea syndrome (Section 11.1.1).

8.3.1.1 Wernicke–Korsakoff syndrome (WKS)

The neurological and neuropsychological consequences of the Wernicke–Korsakoff syndrome (WKS) due to thiamine (vitamin B_1) deficiency have been studied extensively [117]. Although most cases relate to alcohol misuse with consequent undernutrition, WKS may also occur in the context of malnutrition from other causes, such as prolonged vomiting in pregnancy (hyperemesis gravidarum), parenteral nutrition with inadequate supplementation, hunger strike, bariatric surgery, or with other diencephalic lesions such as tumors or trauma [118].

WKS was classically described as a neurological disorder characterized by nystagmus, ophthalmoplegia, and ataxia, and a neuropsychological syndrome of selective anterograde amnesia with relative preservation of intelligence, sometimes complicated by confabulations [119]. For this reason, Korsakoff patients have often been used in group studies to compare their cognitive profile with that seen in other cognitive disorders such as AD and Huntington's disease [120]. However, with the development of new WKS diagnostic criteria [121], the phenotypic spectrum broadened to include patients without the classical neurological signs. In this broader group, there is evidence for generalized cognitive impairment or dementia ("thiamine dementia") rather than solely selective ("diencephalic") amnesia [122].

Neuropathologically, WKS is characterized by shrinkage of the mammillary bodies, structures around the third and fourth ventricles (i.e., the diencephalon), and the medial thalamus. Which of these is the substrate of the cognitive impairments has been argued, but generally the mammillary bodies are not thought to be relevant [123], with better correlations for the medial thalamus, although the exact nuclei involved (mediodorsal, centromedial, anterior) may vary [124–126]. There may be loss of hippocampal volume but without

neuronal loss [127], but this does not necessarily imply normal hippocampal function; functional imaging studies have suggested loss of hippocampal memory encoding in WKS patients, possibly as a consequence of hippocampal-thalamic involvement [128].

Alcohol cessation must be the first step in management of any alcohol-related cognitive problem. Because of the potential reversibility of the cognitive deficits of WKS with thiamine repletion, and the fact that many cases were previously overlooked on clinical grounds, there is a strong case for making a presumptive diagnosis of WKS in any patient with a history suggestive of nutritional deficiency, with or without alcohol dependence, albeit that both the definitive dosage and route of thiamine treatment remain unknown [118]. Other options have only been mentioned anecdotally. The selective noradrenaline reuptake inhibitor reboxetine has been reported to produce cognitive improvements in WKS [129]. Rodent models of WKS show loss of cholinergic innervation and reduced acetylcholine release, and loss of neurons in the nucleus basalis of Meynert might also be relevant to WKS pathogenesis, observations which may justify use of cholinesterase inhibitors for the memory defect in WKS [130].

8.3.1.2 Alcohol-related dementia, alcohol-induced dementia

Whether alcohol (i.e., ethanol) per se is neurotoxic and may cause cognitive decline independent of thiamine deficiency remains a subject of debate [122,131]. Although provisional diagnostic criteria for alcohol-related dementia have been proposed [132], this syndrome may be better conceptualized as a multifactorial "alcohol-induced dementia," related to comorbidities including nutritional deficiency (perhaps causing prior episodes of WKS); damage to other organs, particularly the liver, with repeated episodes of hepatic encephalopathy; head injury; subdural hematoma; epileptic seizures; hydrocephalus; Marchiafava–Bignami disease (Section 8.3.1.3); obstructive sleep apnea

(Section 11.1.1); and pre-existing cognitive status. Concurrent morbidity such as cerebrovascular disease and/or AD might also contribute to cognitive decline. Many patients conforming to the proposed criteria might also conform to the criteria for WKS [121]. An important differential diagnosis is behavioral variant frontotemporal dementia (Section 2.2.1), in which disinhibition and hyperorality may include alcohol overconsumption.

Neuroradiological studies of alcoholics with no obvious history of nutritional deficiency show volume loss, particularly in prefrontal cortex white matter [133]. Neuropathological studies have shown cerebral atrophy due to white matter loss, and neuronal and synaptic losses in some areas such as the frontal association cortex [134], changes likened by some authors to those seen in frontotemporal dementia [135], but no specific form of neuropathology has been identified [122]. There is relative sparing of other areas including the hippocampus [127]. In keeping with these observations, frontal type cognitive deficits are often seen (planning, organization, problem solving, lack of insight, disinhibition, perseveration), along with visuospatial impairments [136], but again no specific profile has emerged. It is argued that, with appropriate assessment, most aspects of cognition will be found affected, but with considerable heterogeneity between patients, related at least in part to current alcohol consumption. Cognitive improvement with alcohol abstinence is recognized. It is possible that cases of "alcohol-related dementia" are, in fact, cases of "atypical" or, more plausibly, unrecognized WKS [122]. Donepezil treatment for alcohol-related dementia has been reported [137].

8.3.1.3 Marchiafava–Bignami disease

Marchiafava–Bignami disease is a rare alcohol-associated disorder characterized by demyelination and necrosis of the corpus callosum; lesions may also occur in the putamen. Clinically, a distinction may be drawn between those cases in which impaired consciousness occurs, with a poorer prognosis, and those in which consciousness is preserved. Cognitive impairment may occur in both the prodrome and recovery phase of the former, as may interhemispheric disconnection syndromes (Section 1.3.4) [138,139]. The latter may include combinations of apraxia, agraphia, and Balint's syndrome, along with neurobehavioral features [140], a syndrome which has been labeled "callosal dementia" [110].

8.3.1.4 Acquired (non-Wilsonian) hepatocerebral degeneration (ANWHCD)

Acquired (non-Wilsonian) hepatocerebral degeneration (ANWHCD) has been characterized as a syndrome of fixed or progressive neurological deficits, including dementia, dysarthria, gait ataxia, intention tremor, parkinsonism, spastic paraparesis, and choreoathetosis, as a consequence of cerebral degeneration in the context of repeated episodes of hepatic encephalopathy, the liver damage usually following alcohol misuse. It is argued that, individually, such episodes of hepatic encephalopathy may be reversible, but that, cumulatively, there is a degenerative effect on neural tissue, with microcavitary changes in layers V and VI of the cortex, underlying white matter, basal ganglia, and cerebellum [141,142]. Others have doubted whether this condition exists as a separate entity. Cases with features overlapping those of extrapontine myelinolysis (Section 8.2.3.2) have been reported [143]. Structural MRI of the brain shows high signal intensity on T_1-weighted images in the internal pallidum, and sometimes in the putamen, caudate nucleus, internal capsule, mesencephalon, and cerebellum, changes which are thought to reflect accumulation of manganese [142]. Manganese poisoning or manganism, first described in miners of manganese ore, is a recognized cause of a parkinsonian syndrome with neuropsychiatric features. Although the movement disorder of ANWHCD may sometimes be helped (with levodopa, branched-chain amino acid therapy, trientine, liver transplantation), no report of cognitive improvement has been identified.

8.3.2 Solvent exposure

Long and intense occupational exposure to certain organic solvents may cause chronic organic solvent neurotoxicity (e.g., painter's encephalopathy), manifested as neuropsychiatric symptoms and cognitive decline, particularly slowed information processing and reaction time, easy fatigue, and impairments on tests of frontal lobe function and memory for new material [144–146]. Individuals with lower levels of education may be at greater risk of poor cognition after solvent exposure [147].

Recreational solvent inhalation ("glue sniffing") may produce impairments in memory, attention and concentration, and nonverbal intelligence in the long-term [148], as well as neuropsychiatric symptoms.

8.3.3 Domoic acid poisoning (amnesic shellfish poisoning)

In Prince Edward Island, Canada, an outbreak of food poisoning following ingestion of mussels occurred in 1987. Patients presented within hours of eating mussels with diarrhea, vomiting, abdominal cramps, with or without headaches. Other features included delirium, epileptic seizures, myoclonus, ataxia, alternating hemiparesis, and complete external ophthalmoplegia. In the acute stages, EEG showed slowing and positron emission tomography (PET) scanning showed hypometabolism of the amygdala and hippocampus. Gradual and spontaneous recovery occurred over three months but some patients were left with residual anterograde amnesia, temporal lobe epilepsy, and motor neuronopathy or sensorimotor axonal neuropathy. Autopsy studies of nonsurvivors showed cell loss and astrocytosis in the amygdala and hippocampus. The syndrome of amnesic shellfish poisoning was shown to be due to production of domoic acid, an excitotoxin that binds to kainate-type glutamate receptors, produced in mussels infested with the phytoplankton *Nitzschia pungens*. The diagnosis can be made using a mouse bioassay for the toxin, although the condition is no longer seen in

Canada as shellfish are now screened for the toxin [149].

REFERENCES

[1] McCrimmon RJ, Ryan CM, Frier BM. Diabetes and cognitive dysfunction. *Lancet* 2012; 379: 2991–9.
[2] Messier C. Impact of impaired glucose tolerance and type 2 diabetes on cognitive aging. *Neurobiol Aging* 2005; 26: S26–30.
[3] Lamport DJ, Lawton CL, Mansfield MW, Dye L. Impairments in glucose tolerance can have a negative impact on cognitive function: a systematic research review. *Neurosci Biobehav Rev* 2009; 33: 394–413.
[4] Brands AMA, Biessels GJ, De Haan EHF, Kappelle LJ, Kessels RPC. The effects of type 1 diabetes on cognitive performance. *Diabetes Care* 2005; 28: 726–35.
[5] Cox DJ, Kovatchev B, Gonder-Frederick LA, *et al.* Relationships between hyperglycemia and cognitive performance among adults with type 1 and type 2 diabetes. *Diabetes Care* 2005; 28: 71–7.
[6] Luchsinger JA, Tang-Ming X, Shea S, Mayeux R. Hyperinsulinemia and risk of Alzheimer disease. *Neurology* 2004; 63: 1187–92.
[7] Cukierman T, Gerstein HC, Williamson JD. Cognitive decline and dementia in diabetes–systematic overview of progressive observational studies. *Diabetologia* 2005; 48: 2460–9.
[8] Biessels GJ, Staekenborg S, Brunner E, Brayne C, Scheltens P. Risk of dementia in diabetes mellitus: a systematic review. *Lancet Neurol* 2006; 5: 64–74.
[9] Kumari M, Marmot M. Diabetes and cognitive function in a middle-aged cohort. Findings from the Whitehall II study. *Neurology* 2005; 65: 1597–603.
[10] Akomolafe A, Beiser A, Meigs JB, *et al.* Diabetes mellitus and risk of developing Alzheimer disease. Results from the Framingham Study. *Arch Neurol* 2006; 63: 1551–5.
[11] [No authors listed] Alzheimer research forum live discussion: is Alzheimer's a type 3 diabetes? *J Alzheimers Dis* 2006; 9: 349–53.
[12] Fisher CM. Unexplained sudden amnesia. *Arch Neurol* 2002; 59: 1310–13.
[13] Chalmers J, Risk MT, Kean DM, *et al.* Severe amnesia after hypoglycaemia. Clinical, psychometric, and magnetic resonance imaging correlations. *Diabetes Care* 1991; 14: 922–5.

[14] Holemans X, Dupuis M, Missan N, Vanderijst J-F. Reversible amnesia in a type 1 diabetic patient and bilateral hippocampal lesions on magnetic resonance imaging (MRI). *Diabet Med* 2001; 18: 761–3.

[15] Larner AJ, Moffat MA, Ghadiali E, *et al.* Amnesia following profound hypoglycaemia in a type 1 diabetic patient. *Eur J Neurol* 2003; 10(Suppl 1): 92 (abstract p. 1170).

[16] Wredling R, Levander S, Adamson U, Lins P. Permanent neuropsychological impairment after recurrent episodes of severe hypoglycaemia in man. *Diabetologia* 1990; 33: 152–7.

[17] Sachon C, Grimaldi A, Digy JP, *et al.* Cognitive function, insulin-dependent diabetes and hypoglycaemia. *J Intern Med* 1992; 231: 471–5.

[18] Langan SJ, Deary IJ, Hepburn DA, Frier BM. Cumulative cognitive impairment following severe hypoglycaemia in adult patients with insulin-treated diabetes mellitus. *Diabetologia* 1991; 34: 337–44.

[19] Lincoln NB, Faleiro RM, Kelly C, Kirk BA, Jeffcoate WJ. Effect of long-term glycemic control on cognitive function. *Diabetes Care* 1996; 19: 656–8.

[20] Reichard P, Pihl M. Mortality and treatment side effects during long-term intensified conventional insulin treatment in Stockholm Diabetes Intervention Study. *Diabetes* 1994; 43: 313–7.

[21] Diabetes Control and Complications Trial Research Group. Effects of intensive diabetes therapy on neuropsychological function in adults in the diabetes control and complications trial. *Ann Intern Med* 1996; 124: 379–88.

[22] Whitmer RA, Karter AJ, Yaffe K, Quesenberry CP, Selby JV. Hypoglycemic episodes and risk of dementia in older patients with type 2 diabetes mellitus. *JAMA* 2009; 301: 1565–72.

[23] Aung PP, Strachan MW, Frier BM, *et al.* Severe hypoglycaemia and late-life cognitive ability in older people with Type 2 diabetes: the Edinburgh Type 2 Diabetes Study. *Diabet Med* 2012; 29: 328–36.

[24] Hejl AM, Phung K, Andersen BB, Feldt-Rasmussen U, Waldemar G. High prevalence of thyroid dysfunction in a mixed memory clinic population. *Eur J Neurol* 2007; 14(Suppl 1): 182 (abstract p. 2081).

[25] Asher R. Myxoedematous madness. In: Avery Jones F (ed.). *Richard Asher Talking Sense*. Edinburgh: Churchill Livingstone, 1986: 77–95.

[26] Clarnette RM, Patterson CJ. Hypothyroidism: does treatment cure dementia? *J Geriatr Psychiatry Neurol* 1994; 7: 23–7.

[27] Dugbartey AT. Neurocognitive aspects of hypothyroidism. *Arch Intern Med* 1998; 158: 1413–18.

[28] Burmeister LA, Ganguli M, Dodge HH, *et al.* Hypothyroidism and cognition: preliminary evidence for a specific defect in memory. *Thyroid* 2001; 11: 1177–85.

[29] Correia N, Mullally S, Cooke G, *et al.* Evidence for a specific defect in hippocampal memory in overt and subclinical hypothyroidism. *J Clin Endocrinol Metab* 2009; 94: 3789–97.

[30] Bono G, Fancellu R, Blandini F, Santoro G, Mauri M. Cognitive and affective status in mild hypothyroidism and interactions with L-thyroxine treatment. *Acta Neurol Scand* 2004; 110: 59–66.

[31] Zhu D-F, Wang Z-X, Zhang D-R, *et al.* fMRI revealed neural substrate for reversible working memory dysfunction in subclinical hypothyroidism. *Brain* 2006; 129: 2923–30.

[32] Volpato S, Guralnik JM, Fried LP, *et al.* Serum thyroxine level and cognitive decline in euthyroid older women. *Neurology* 2002; 58: 1055–61.

[33] Waldemar G, Dubois B, Emre M, *et al.* Recommendations for the diagnosis and management of Alzheimer's disease and other disorders associated with dementia. *Eur J Neurol* 2007; 14: e1–26.

[34] Bulens C. Neurological complications of hyperthyroidism: remission of spastic paraplegia, dementia, and optic neuropathy. *Arch Neurol* 1981; 38: 669–70.

[35] Larner AJ. Caleb Hillier Parry (1755–1822): clinician, scientist, friend of Edward Jenner (1749–1823). *J Med Biogr* 2005; 13: 189–94.

[36] Vogel A, Elberling TV, Hørding M, *et al.* Affective symptoms and cognitive functions in the acute phase of Graves' thyrotoxicosis. *Psychoneuroendocrinology* 2007; 32: 36–43.

[37] Fukui T, Hasegawa Y, Takenaka H. Hyperthyroid dementia: clinicoradiological findings and response to treatment. *J Neurol Sci* 2001; 184: 81–8.

[38] Joshi AN, Jain AP, Bhatt AD, Kumar S. A case of sporadic periodic hypokalemic paralysis with atypical features: recurrent differential right brachial weakness and cognitive dysfunction. *Neurol India* 2009; 57: 501.

[39] Kalmijn S, Mehta KM, Pols HA, *et al.* Subclinical hyperthyroidism and the risk of dementia. The Rotterdam study. *Clin Endocrinol (Oxf)* 2000; 53: 733–7.

[40] Bensenor IM, Lotufo PA, Menezes PR, Scazufca M. Subclinical hyperthyroidism and dementia: the Sao Paulo Ageing & Health Study (SPAH). *BMC Public Health* 2010; 10: 298.

[41] Robinson KC, Kallberg MH, Crowley MF. Idiopathic hypoparathyroidism presenting as dementia. *BMJ* 1954; 2: 1203–6.

[42] Eraut D. Idiopathic hypoparathyroidism presenting as dementia. *BMJ* 1974; 1: 429–30.

[43] Slyter H. Idiopathic hypoparathyroidism presenting as dementia. *Neurology* 1979; 29: 393–4.

[44] Adorni A, Lussignoli G, Geroldi C, Zanetti O. Extensive brain calcification and dementia in postsurgical hypoparathyroidism. *Neurology* 2005; 65: 1501.

[45] Galvez-Jimenez N, Hanson MR, Cabral J. Dopa-resistant parkinsonism, oculomotor disturbances, chorea, mirror movements, dyspraxia, and dementia: the expanding clinical spectrum of hypoparathyroidism. A case report. *Mov Disord* 2000; 15: 1273–6.

[46] Mateo D, Gimenez-Roldan S. Dementia in idiopathic hypoparathyroidism: rapid efficacy of alfacalcidol. *Arch Neurol* 1982; 39: 424–5.

[47] Stuerenburg HJ, Hansen HC, Thie A, Kunze K. Reversible dementia in idiopathic hypoparathyroidism associated with normocalcemia. *Neurology* 1996; 47: 474–6.

[48] Dennis M, Parker SG. Hyperthyroidism [sic] and dementia. *Postgrad Med J* 1997; 73: 755–7.

[49] Logullo F, Babbini MT, Di Bella P, Provinciali L. Reversible combined cognitive impairment and severe polyneuropathy resulting from primary hyperparathyroidism. *Ital J Neurol Sci* 1998; 19: 86–9.

[50] Mauri M, Sinforiani E, Bono G, *et al.* Memory impairment in Cushing's disease. *Acta Neurol Scand* 1993; 87: 52–5.

[51] Forget H, Lacroix A, Somma M, Cohen H. Cognitive decline in patients with Cushing's syndrome. *J Int Neuropsychol Soc* 2000; 6: 20–9.

[52] Heald A, Parr C, Gibson C, O'Driscoll K, Fowler H. A cross-sectional study to investigate long-term cognitive function in people with treated pituitary Cushing's disease. *Exp Clin Endocrinol Diabetes* 2006; 114: 490–7.

[53] Michaud K, Forget H, Cohen H. Chronic glucocorticoid hypersecretion in Cushing's syndrome exacerbates cognitive aging. *Brain Cogn* 2009; 71: 1–8.

[54] Forget H, Lacroix A, Cohen H. Persistent cognitive impairment following surgical treatment of Cushing's syndrome. *Psychoneuroendocrinology* 2002; 27: 367–83.

[55] Hook JN, Giordani B, Schteingart DE, *et al.* Patterns of cognitive change over time and relationship to age following successful treatment of Cushing's disease. *J Int Neuropsychol Soc* 2007; 13: 21–9.

[56] Tiemensma J, Kokshoorn NE, Biermasz NR, *et al.* Subtle cognitive impairments in patients with long-term cure of Cushing's disease. *J Clin Metab Endocrinol* 2010; 95: 2699–714.

[57] Gudin M, Sanabria C, Legido B, *et al.* Cognitive dysfunction related to hormonal and ionic levels in a patient diagnosed of Conn syndrome. *J Neurol* 2000; 247(Suppl 3): III/75 (abstract P275).

[58] Clarfield AM. The decreasing prevalence of reversible dementia: an updated meta-analysis. *Arch Intern Med* 2003; 163: 2219–29.

[59] Healton EB, Savage DG, Brust JCM, *et al.* Neurologic aspects of cobalamin deficiency. *Medicine (Baltimore)* 1991; 70: 229–45.

[60] Chiu HFK. Vitamin B_{12} deficiency and dementia. *Int J Geriatr Psychiatry* 1996; 11: 851–8.

[61] Meadows M-E, Kaplan RF, Bromfield EB. Cognitive recovery with vitamin B12 therapy: a longitudinal neuropsychiatric assessment. *Neurology* 1994; 44: 1764–5.

[62] Larner AJ, Janssen JC, Cipolotti L, Rossor MN. Cognitive profile in dementia associated with vitamin B12 deficiency due to pernicious anaemia. *J Neurol* 1999; 246: 317–19.

[63] Larner AJ, Rakshi JS. Vitamin B12 deficiency and dementia. *Eur J Neurol* 2001; 8: 730.

[64] Saracaceanu E, Tramoni AV, Henry JM. An association between subcortical dementia and pernicious anaemia: a psychiatric mask. *Compr Psychiatry* 1997; 38: 349–51.

[65] Osimani A, Berger A, Friedman J, Porat-Katz BS, Abarbanel JM. Neuropsychology of vitamin B12 deficiency in elderly dementia patients and control subjects. *J Geriatr Psychiatry Neurol* 2005; 18: 33–8.

[66] Teunisse S, Bollen AE, van Gool WA, Walstra GJM. Dementia and subnormal levels of vitamin B12: effects of replacement therapy on dementia. *J Neurol* 1996; 243: 522–9.

[67] Eastley R, Wilcock GK, Bucks RS. Vitamin B12 deficiency in dementia and cognitive impairment: the effects of treatment on neuropsychological function. *Int J Geriatr Psychiatry* 2000; 15: 226–33.

[68] Kim JM, Stewart R, Kim SW, *et al.* Changes in folate, vitamin B12 and homocysteine associated with incident dementia. *J Neurol Neurosurg Psychiatry* 2008; 79: 864–8.

[69] Connick P, Cooper S, Grosset D. Investigating B12 deficiency amongst neurological patients. *J Neurol Neurosurg Psychiatry* 2006; 77: 126 (abstract 002).

[70] McCracken C, Hudson P, Ellis R, *et al.* Methylmalonic acid and cognitive function in the Medical Research Council Cognitive Function and Ageing Study. *Am J Clin Nutr* 2006; 84: 1406–11.

[71] Clarke R, Smith AD, Jobst KA, *et al.* Folate, vitamin B12, and serum total homocysteine in confirmed Alzheimer disease. *Arch Neurol* 1998; 55: 1449–55.

[72] McCaddon A, Davies G, Hudson P, Tandy S, Cattell H. Total serum homocysteine in senile dementia of Alzheimer type. *Int J Geriatr Psychiatry* 1998; 13: 235–9.

[73] Wang H-X, Wahlin A, Basun H, *et al.* Vitamin B12 and folate in relation to the development of Alzheimer's disease. *Neurology* 2001; 56: 1188–94.

[74] McCaddon A, Regland B, Hudson P, Davies G. Functional vitamin B12 deficiency and Alzheimer disease. *Neurology* 2002; 58: 1395–9.

[75] Ben-Omran TI, Wong H, Blaser S, Feigenbaum A. Late-onset cobalamin-C disorder: a challenging diagnosis. *Am J Med Genet Part A* 2007; 143A: 979–84.

[76] Thauvin-Robinet C, Roze E, Couvreur G, *et al.* The adolescent and adult form of cobalamin C disease: clinical and molecular spectrum. *J Neurol Neurosurg Psychiatry* 2008; 79: 725–8.

[77] Freeman HJ. Neurological disorders in adult celiac disease. *Can J Gastoenterol* 2008; 22: 909–11.

[78] Doran M, du Plessis DG, Larner AJ. Disseminated enteropathy-type T-cell lymphoma: cauda equina syndrome complicating coeliac disease. *Clin Neurol Neurosurg* 2005; 107: 517–20.

[79] Collin P, Pirttilä T, Nurmikko T, Somer H, Erilä T, Keyriläinen O. Celiac disease, brain atrophy, and dementia. *Neurology* 1991; 41: 372–5.

[80] Hu WT, Murray JA, Greenaway MC, Parisi JE, Josephs KA. Cognitive impairment and celiac disease. *Arch Neurol* 2006; 63: 1440–6.

[81] Serdaru M, Hausser-Hauw C, Laplane D, *et al.* The clinical spectrum of alcoholic pellagra encephalopathy. *Brain* 1988; 111: 829–42.

[82] Grant I, Heaton RK, McSweeny AJ, Adams KM, Timms RM. Neuropsychologic findings in hypoxemic chronic obstructive pulmonary disease. *Arch Intern Med* 1982; 142: 1470–6.

[83] Heaton RK, Grant I, McSweeny AJ, Adams KM, Petty TL. Psychologic effects of continuous and nocturnal oxygen therapy in hypoxemic chronic obstructive pulmonary disease. *Arch Intern Med* 1983; 143: 1941–7.

[84] Grant I, Prigatano GP, Heaton RK, *et al.* Progressive neuropsychologic impairment and hypoxemia: Relationship in chronic obstructive pulmonary disease. *Arch Gen Psychiatry* 1987; 44: 999–1006.

[85] Favalli A, Miozzo A, Cossi S, Marengoni A. Differences in neuropsychological profile between healthy and COPD older persons. *Int J Geriatr Psychiatry* 2008; 23: 220–1.

[86] Incalzi RA, Gemma A, Marra C, *et al.* Chronic obstructive pulmonary disease. An original model of cognitive decline. *Am Rev Respir Dis* 1993; 148: 418–24.

[87] Incalzi RA, Gemma A, Marra C, *et al.* Verbal memory impairment in COPD: its mechanisms and clinical relevance. *Chest* 1997; 112: 1506–13.

[88] Incalzi RA, Chiappini F, Fuso L, *et al.* Predicting cognitive decline in patients with hypoxaemic COPD. *Respir Med* 1998; 92: 527–33.

[89] Roehrs T, Merrion M, Pedrosi B, *et al.* Neuropsychological function in obstructive sleep apnea syndrome (OSAS) compared to chronic obstructive pulmonary disease (COPD). *Sleep* 1995; 18: 382–8.

[90] Özge C, Özge A, Ünal O. Cognitive and functional deterioration in patients with severe COPD. *Behav Neurol* 2006; 17: 121–30.

[91] Kozora E, Filley CM, Julian LJ, Cullum CM. Cognitive functioning in patients with chronic obstructive pulmonary disease and mild hypoxemia compared with patients with mild Alzheimer disease and normal controls. *Neuropsychiatry Neuropsychol Behav Neurol* 1999; 12: 178–83.

[92] Schofield PW, Tang M, Marder K, *et al.* Consistency of clinical diagnosis in a community-based longitudinal study of dementia and Alzheimer's disease. *Neurology* 1995; 45: 2159–64.

[93] Ernst A, Zibrak JD. Carbon monoxide poisoning. *N Engl J Med* 1998; 339: 1603–8.

[94] Tapeantong T, Poungvarin N. Delayed encephalopathy and cognitive sequelae after acute carbon monoxide poisoning: report of a case and review of the literature. *J Med Assoc Thai* 2009; 92: 1374–9.

[95] Parkinson RB, Hopkins RO, Cleavinger HB, *et al.* White matter hyperintensities and neuropsychological outcome following carbon monoxide poisoning. *Neurology* 2002; 58: 1525–32.

[96] Goodale MA, Milner AD. *Sight Unseen: An Exploration of Conscious and Unconscious Vision.* Oxford: Oxford University Press, 2004.

[97] Larner AJ. Delayed motor and visual complications after attempted suicide. *Lancet* 2005; 366: 1826.

[98] Kesler SR, Hopkins RO, Blatter DD, *et al.* Verbal memory deficits associated with fornix atrophy in carbon monoxide poisoning. *J Int Neuropsychol Soc* 2001; 7: 640–6.

[99] Weaver LK, Valentine KJ, Hopkins RO. Carbon monoxide poisoning: risk factors for cognitive sequelae and the role of hyperbaric oxygen. *Am J Respir Crit Care Med* 2007; 176: 491–7.

[100] Wang P, Zeng T, Chi ZF. Recovery of cognitive dysfunction in a case of delayed encephalopathy of carbon monoxide poisoning after treatment with donepezil hydrochloride. *Neurol India* 2009; 57: 481–2.

[101] Helmer C, Stengel B, Metzger M, *et al.* Chronic kidney disease, cognitive decline, and incident dementia: the 3C Study. *Neurology* 2011; 77: 2043–51.

[102] Madan P, Kalra OP, Agarwal S, Tandon OP. Cognitive impairment in chronic kidney disease. *Nephrol Dial Transplant* 2007; 22: 440–4.

[103] Murray AM, Tupper De, Knopman DS, *et al.* Cognitive impairment in hemodialysis patients is common. *Neurology* 2006; 67: 216–23 [Erratum in: *Neurology* 2007; 69: 120].

[104] Chui HC, Damasio AR. Progressive dialysis encephalopathy ("dialysis dementia"). *J Neurol* 1980; 222: 145–57.

[105] Harrington CR, Wischik CM, McArthur FK, *et al.* Alzheimer's disease-like changes in tau protein processing: association with aluminium accumulation in brains of renal dialysis patients. *Lancet* 1994; 343: 993–7.

[106] Adams RD, Victor M, Mancall EL. Central pontine myelinolysis: a hitherto undescribed disease occurring in alcoholic and malnourished patients. *Arch Neurol Psychiatry Chicago* 1959; 81: 154–72.

[107] Sterns RH, Riggs JE, Schochet SS. Osmotic demyelination syndrome following correction of hyponatremia. *N Engl J Med* 1986; 314: 1535–42.

[108] Martin PJ, Young CA. Central pontine myelinolysis: clinical and MRI correlates. *Postgrad Med J* 1995; 71: 430–2.

[109] Odier C, Nguyen DK, Panisset M. Central pontine and extrapontine myelinolysis: from epileptic and other manifestations to cognitive prognosis. *J Neurol* 2010; 257: 1176–80.

[110] Ghika Schmid F, Ghika J, Assal G, Bogousslavsky J. Callosal dementia: behavioral disorders related to central and extrapontine myelinolysis [in French]. *Rev Neurol Paris* 1999; 155: 367–73.

[111] Anstey KJ, Mack HA, Cherbuin N. Alcohol consumption as a risk factor for dementia and cognitive decline: meta-analysis of prospective studies. *Am J Geriatr Psychiatry* 2009; 17: 542–55.

[112] Peters R, Peters J, Warner J, Beckett N, Bulpitt C. Alcohol, dementia and cognitive decline in the elderly: a systematic review. *Age Ageing* 2008; 37: 505–12.

[113] Saunders PA, Copeland JR, Dewey ME, *et al.* Heavy drinking as a risk factor for depression and dementia in elderly men. Findings from the Liverpool longitudinal community study. *Br J Psych* 1991; 159: 213–16.

[114] Anttila T, Helkala EL, Viitanen M, *et al.* Alcohol drinking in middle age and subsequent risk of mild cognitive impairment and dementia in old age: a prospective population based study. *BMJ* 2004; 329: 539.

[115] Gupta S, Warner J. Alcohol-related dementia: a 21st-century silent epidemic? *Br J Psychiatry* 2008; 193: 351–3.

[116] Larner AJ, Gardner-Thorpe C. Robert Lawson (?1846–1896). *J Neurol* 2012; 259: 792–3.

[117] Victor M, Adams RD, Collins GH. *The Wernicke–Korsakoff Syndrome and Related Neurologic Disorders due to Alcoholism and Malnutrition* (2nd edn.). Philadelphia, PA: Davis, 1989.

[118] Galvin R, Brathen G, Ivashynka I, *et al.* EFNS guidelines for diagnosis, therapy and prevention of Wernicke encephalopathy. *Eur J Neurol* 2010; 17: 1408–18.

[119] Butters N, Cermak LS. *Alcoholic Korsakoff's Syndrome: An Information-Processing Approach to Amnesia.* London: Academic Press, 1980.

[120] Butters N. The clinical aspects of memory disorders: contributions from experimental studies of amnesia and dementia. *J Clin Neuropsychol* 1984; 6: 17–36.

[121] Caine D, Halliday GM, Kril JJ, Harper CG. Operational criteria for the classification of chronic alcoholics: identification of Wernicke's encephalopathy. *J Neurol Neurosurg Psychiatry* 1997; 62: 51–60.

[122] Bowden SC. Alcohol-related dementia and Wernicke–Korsakoff syndrome. In: Ames D, Burns A, O'Brien J (eds.). *Dementia* (4th edn.). London: Hodder Arnold, 2010; 722–9.

[123] Victor M. The irrelevance of the mammillary body lesions in the causation of the Korsakoff amnesic state. *Int J Neurol* 1987; 21–22: 51–7.

[124] Mayes AR, Mendell PR, Mann D, Pickering A. Location of lesions in Korsakoff's syndrome: neuropsychological and neuropathological data on two patients. *Cortex* 1988; 24: 367–88.

[125] Halliday G, Cullen K, Harding A. Neuropathological correlates of memory dysfunction in the Wernicke–Korsakoff syndrome. *Alcohol Alcohol Suppl* 1994; 2: 245–51.

[126] Harding A, Halliday G, Caine D, Kril J. Degeneration of anterior thalamic nuclei differentiates alcoholics with amnesia. *Brain* 2000; 123: 141–54.

[127] Harper C, Scolyer RA. Alcoholism and dementia. In: Esiri MM, Lee VM-Y, Trojanowski JQ (eds.). *The Neuropathology of Dementia* (2nd edn.). Cambridge: Cambridge University Press, 2004; 427–41.

[128] Caulo M, Van Hecke J, Toma L, *et al.* Functional MRI study of diencephalic amnesia in Wernicke–Korsakoff syndrome. *Brain* 2005; 128: 1584–94.

[129] Reuster T, Buechler J, Winiecki P, Oehler J. Influence of reboxetine on salivary MHPG concentration and cognitive symptoms among patients with alcohol-related Korsakoff's syndrome. *Neuropsychopharmacology* 2003; 28: 974–8.

[130] Cochrane M, Cochrane A, Jauhar P, Ashton E. Acetylcholinesterase inhibitors for the treatment of Wernicke–Korsakoff syndrome–three further cases show response to donepezil. *Alcohol Alcohol* 2005; 40: 151–4.

[131] Moriyama Y, Mimura M, Kato M, Kashima H. Primary alcoholic dementia and alcohol-related dementia. *Psychogeriatrics* 2006; 6: 114–18.

[132] Oslin D, Atkinson RM, Smith DM, *et al.* Alcohol related dementia: proposed clinical criteria. *Int J Geriatr Psychiatry* 1998; 13: 203–12.

[133] Sullivan EV, Pfefferbaum A. Neurocircuitry in alcoholism: a substrate of disruption and repair. *Psychopharmacology (Berl)* 2005; 180: 583–94.

[134] Harper C. The neuropathology of alcohol-specific brain damage, or does alcohol damage the brain? *J Neuropathol Exp Neurol* 1998; 57: 101–10.

[135] Brun A, Andersson J. Frontal dysfunction and frontal cortical synapse loss in alcoholism–the main cause of alcohol dementia? *Dement Geriatr Cogn Disord* 2001; 12: 289–94.

[136] Bates ME, Bowden SC, Barry D. Neurocognitive impairment associated with alcohol use disorders: implications for treatment. *Exp Clin Psychopharmacol* 2002; 10: 193–212.

[137] Kim KY, Ke V, Adkins LM. Donepezil for alcohol-related dementia: a case report. *Pharmacotherapy* 2004; 24: 419–21.

[138] Kohler CG, Ances BM, Coleman AR, *et al.* Marchiafava–Bignami disease: literature review and case report. *Neuropsychiatry Neuropsychol Behav Neurol* 2000; 13: 67–76.

[139] Heinrich A, Runge U, Khaw AV. Clinicoradiologic subtypes of Marchiafava–Bignami disease. *J Neurol* 2004; 251: 1050–9.

[140] Kalckreuth W, Zimmermann P, Preilowski B, Wallesch CW. Incomplete split-brain syndrome in a patient with chronic Marchiafava–Bignami disease. *Behav Brain Res* 1994; 64: 219–28.

[141] Victor M, Adams RD, Cole M. The acquired (non-Wilsonian) type of chronic hepatocerebral degeneration. *Medicine (Baltimore)* 1965; 44: 345–95.

[142] Meissner W, Tison F. Acquired hepatocerebral degeneration. *Handb Clin Neurol* 2011; 100: 193–7.

[143] Kleinschmidt-DeMasters BK, Filley CM, Rojiani AM. Overlapping features of extrapontine myelinolysis and acquired chronic (non-Wilsonian) hepatocerebral degeneration. *Acta Neuropathol* 2006; 112: 605–16.

[144] Arlien-Soberg P, Bruhn P, Gyldensted C, Melgaard B. Chronic painters' syndrome: toxic encephalopathy in house painters. *Acta Neurol Scand* 1979; 60: 149–56.

[145] Ogden JA. The psychological and neuropsychological assessment of chronic occupational solvent neurotoxicity: a case series. *NZ J Psychol* 1993; 23: 83–94.

[146] Dryson E, Ogden JA. Organic solvent induced chronic toxic encephalopathy: extent of recovery and associated factors, following cessation of exposure. *Neurotoxicology* 2000; 21: 659–66.

[147] Sabbath EL, Glymour MM, Berr C, *et al.* Occupational solvent exposure and cognition: does the association vary by level of education? *Neurology* 2012; 78: 1754–60.

[148] Allison WM, Jerrom DW. Glue sniffing: a pilot study of the cognitive effects of long-term use. *Int J Addict* 1984; 19: 453–8.

[149] Perl TM, Bedard L, Kosatsky T, *et al.* An outbreak of toxic encephalopathy caused by eating mussels contaminated with domoic acid. *N Engl J Med* 1990; 322: 1775–80.

Infective disorders

The spectrum of infectious diseases causing cognitive impairment and dementia has changed over the past century. Whereas neurosyphilis was once common, now infection with human immunodeficiency virus (HIV) and herpes viruses, and diseases caused by prions (Section 2.5) are perhaps the most notable infectious causes of cognitive decline and dementia [1,2].

9.1 Encephalitides and meningoencephalitides

Infection of the brain parenchyma with or without involvement of the surrounding meninges may be caused by a wide variety of organisms, most usually viruses, but sometimes protozoa, rickettsiae, or fungi [3]. Despite intensive investigation, a causative organism is not always found and treatment may of necessity be empirical, covering the most likely candidate organisms.

Encephalitis is often a medical emergency, requiring intensive supportive care and control of epileptic seizures. With the advent of antiviral agents such as aciclovir, mortality has declined considerably, leaving increased numbers of survivors who may have neuropsychological sequelae.

Encephalitides and meningoencephalitides, covered elsewhere, include Rasmussen's syndrome of chronic encephalitis and epilepsy (Section 4.2.3), in which an infective etiology remains a possibility; and chronic inflammatory meningoencephalitis, a term sometimes used for Sjögren's syndrome (Section 6.6).

9.1.1 Herpes simplex encephalitis (HSE)

Herpes simplex virus type 1 (HSV) is the most common recognized cause of encephalitis, although it is more often clinically suspected than clinically proved [4], and there is a broad differential diagnosis including stroke, meningitis, subarachnoid hemorrhage, sinus thrombosis, and even central nervous system (CNS) tumor [5]. HSE produces acute necrotizing encephalitis of orbitofrontal and temporal lobes, sometimes involving insular and cingulate cortices, with overlying meningitis. Typically, the presentation is with fever and headache, sometimes with behavioral changes, which may progress to clouding of consciousness and coma, sometimes complicated by focal or secondarily generalized seizures [6]. However, presentation with isolated memory impairment has been described [7]. Magnetic resonance imaging (MRI) of the brain may show focal edema in the medial temporal lobes, orbital surface of the frontal lobes, insular and cingulate cortex, sometimes asymmetrically, with gadolinium enhancement. Cerebrospinal fluid (CSF) is typically under raised pressure with a lymphocytic pleocytosis (10–200 cells/mm^3) with a raised protein (0.6–6.0 g/L) but a normal glucose level. CSF polymerase chain reaction (PCR) for HSV is a highly sensitive and specific test for confirmation of the diagnosis, although false negatives may be encountered early (<48 hr) or late (>10 d) in the disease process. Electroencephalography (EEG) is invariably abnormal, showing nonspecific disorganized and slow background rhythm in the early stages, with epileptiform abnormalities such as high voltage periodic lateralizing epileptiform discharges (PLEDs) appearing later. Because early and appropriate treatment of HSE (e.g., aciclovir) has been shown to reduce mortality and morbidity significantly, brain biopsy may be considered to establish the diagnosis in atypical cases, or when a tumor in the temporal lobe is considered part of the differential diagnosis. The role of steroids remains uncertain, with no randomized study having yet been performed, although a retrospective study found a poorer outcome in patients who did not receive steroids [8].

Cognitive sequelae of HSE are well recognized [9–12], although cognitive recovery occurs in many patients [13]. The typical profile of cognitive impairment comprises deficits of new learning in both verbal and visual domains. In addition to amnesia, deficits in retrograde memory, executive functions, and language (with mild anomia) may be found, albeit less frequently. Semantic impairments akin to those seen in semantic dementia (Section 2.2.3) may occur as a consequence of temporal lobe damage [14]. Impaired autobiographical memory may occur in patients with bilateral damage [15].

Although persistent anterograde and retrograde (global) amnesia after HSE is well described in patients selected for symptoms of memory impairment, it seems to be an unusual complication, although the risk is greater (by 2–4 times) than in nonherpetic encephalitis. Greater deficits in verbal memory, verbal semantic functions, and visuoperceptual functions have been noted in herpetic as compared to nonherpetic encephalitis [16,17]. Executive deficits may also be seen following recovery from HSE, presumably reflecting orbitofrontal injury [12]. Duration of transient encephalitic amnesia correlates with neuropsychological outcome [13,18].

Amnesia may occur despite appropriate treatment of HSE with aciclovir, but shorter delay between symptom onset and treatment may be associated with better outcome.

The severity of the amnesic syndrome is related to the severity of damage, judged neuroradiologically, to medial limbic structures (hippocampus and amygdala). Intractable epilepsy and affective disorder may contribute to neuropsychological outcome.

9.1.2 Herpes zoster encephalitis

Varicella zoster virus (VZV), a herpes virus, may lay dormant for many years after a primary infection, to be reactivated as herpes zoster or shingles, which may sometimes be complicated by an encephalitis (herpes zoster encephalitis, HZE).

Neuropsychological sequelae of HZE were reported by Hokkanen *et al.* in nine immunocompetent patients. These included forgetfulness, slowing of thought processes, emotional and personality changes, and impaired cognitive ability, suggesting a subcortical type of impairment [19]. In contrast, a report of eight patients undergoing neuropsychological assessment four to 52 months after the onset of HZE found no significant differences between patients and controls [20]. The discrepancy in these studies may relate to the timing of assessment, which was carried out in most of the patients in the Hokkanen *et al.* study directly after they were able to cooperate adequately after the acute stage of infection [19].

Dementia has been reported following HZE, but it is not clear whether there was an etiological relationship or whether this was chance concurrence of a neurodegenerative dementia in an elderly individual [21].

9.1.3 Adenovirus encephalitis

Cases of adenovirus encephalitis with severe amnesia, resembling that seen in herpes simplex encephalitis, have been reported [16].

9.1.4 Coxsackie virus encephalitis

A possible case of subcortical type cognitive impairment has been described following encephalitis due to this RNA virus [22].

9.1.5 Herpes simplex type 2 encephalitis

Herpes simplex type 2 encephalitis is most commonly encountered in the neonatal period, but occasional adult cases have been described with mild widespread cognitive difficulties [23] or dementia [24], with CSF lymphocytic pleocytosis and low CSF glucose but with unremarkable brain imaging. Cognitive normalization following antiviral (acyclovir, valaciclovir) treatment was reported in one case [24].

9.1.6 Human herpes virus-6 infection

Infection with human herpes virus-6 (HHV-6) causes fever and a rash (exanthema subitum) in children; a benign, self-limiting condition. Seropositivity occurs in most children by the age of three years, with a decline after the age of 40 years. Symptomatic infection in adults is very rare, mostly occurring in the context of immunosuppression. Cases of persistent amnesia (anterograde and retrograde) have been reported as a consequence of HHV-6 infection [25]; for example, in the context of immunosuppression associated with lung transplantation [26], or bone marrow and stem cell transplantation [27–29]. High intensity signal change may be seen on brain MRI in the medial temporal lobe including the hippocampus; hence, this may be considered a form of nonparaneoplastic limbic encephalitis (Section 6.12.2). Response of amnesia to antiviral treatment is noted. Similar cases have been seen rarely with an HHV-7 infection [30].

9.1.7 Japanese encephalitis

Japanese encephalitis (formerly known as Japanese type B encephalitis) is caused by an RNA flavivirus, which has its reservoir in pigs, birds (heron, egrets), cows, and buffalo, and is spread by mosquitoes, most commonly *Culex* but also *Anopheles*, with humans a "dead-end" host. Japanese encephalitis is an example of the zoonotic arboviral encephalitides, and causes disease epidemics in the monsoon months in Asia [31]. According to one review, 20% of survivors have severe cognitive and language as well as motor impairment [32]. A follow-up study of more than 600 survivors in India reported higher cerebral dysfunction, especially memory and concentration, in more than half of the cases, with gradual improvement over time [33].

9.1.8 Rotavirus encephalitis

A case with cognitive impairment has been reported [16], although this is likely to be the exception rather than the rule.

9.1.9 Subacute sclerosing panencephalitis (SSPE)

Subacute sclerosing panencephalitis (SSPE) is usually a disorder of late childhood or early adolescence due to reactivation of the measles virus infection causing progressive inflammation and gliosis of the brain. The clinical phenotype is characterized by behavioral change, myoclonic jerks, epileptic seizures, abnormalities in vision often due to a necrotizing retinitis, and progressive dementia, followed by pyramidal signs, stupor, decorticate postures, and death. Characteristic investigation findings include antibodies against the measles virus and oligoclonal bands in CSF, a pathognomonic EEG signature with 2- to 3-per second periodic bursts of high voltage waves, and periventricular and subcortical white matter change on MRI. There is no effective treatment currently, although oral isoprinosine and intrathecal or intraventricular α-interferon may prolong survival [34].

Only occasional adult-onset cases have been reported [35,36], usually with the characteristic clinical picture, but one atypical case presenting with a "pure cortical dementia" without movement disorder has been presented [37]. The clinical description was of initial apathy, disorientation in time, psychomotor slowing, and depression, followed three years later by verbal perseverations, anomia, phonemic paraphasia, dysgraphia, dyslexia, ideomotor and ideational apraxia, with Mini-Mental State Examination score of 9.5/30. No more detailed neuropsychological assessment was presented. Serial brain MRI showed progressive generalized cerebral atrophy.

9.1.10 Tick-borne encephalitis

Cognitive impairment has been described as a long-term complication of tick-borne encephalitis, specifically deficits in memory, concentration, verbal fluency, and verbal learning [38]. A study from Poland has suggested that amnestic cognitive impairment may be a long-term sequel of the illness [39].

9.1.11 Postencephalitic parkinsonism, encephalitis lethargica, von Economo disease

The exact relationship of this condition, which occurred in epidemic proportions following the First World War, to brain infection remains uncertain; a suspected relationship to influenza infection has not been corroborated by examination of archival tissues. Basal ganglia autoimmunity may play a role in pathogenesis (as in Sydenham's chorea; Section 6.14). Occasional cases of encephalitis lethargica still occur, the clinical picture generally dominated by movement disorders (parkinsonism, dystonia, oculogyric crises, myoclonus) and neuropsychiatric features [40]. Neuropsychological features have been little studied, but in one case, a general cognitive decline was seen initially, particularly affecting memory and executive functions, which improved over time concurrent with cognitive rehabilitation strategies [41].

9.2 Meningitides

The meningitides are infections of the meningeal coverings of the brain (pia, arachnoid, dura mater), sometimes with involvement of the underlying brain parenchyma (meningoencephalitis; Section 9.1). Meningitis may be caused by a wide variety of organisms, including bacteria, viruses, fungi, and protozoa (see Section 9.4.3 for tuberculous meningitis) [42,43].

9.2.1 Bacterial meningitis

Although neurological recovery is now the norm when bacterial meningitis is promptly diagnosed and appropriately treated in adults, functional impairments precluding return to employment may persist, particularly in the cognitive domain.

One cohort study of adult patients found impairments in psychomotor performance, concentration, visuoconstructive capacity, and memory functions compared to healthy controls, a pattern said to resemble the subcortical type of cognitive impairment [44]. Deficits were found in 73% of patients in this study whereas in another study [45] only 27% of cases were impaired, although both suggested that pneumococcal meningitis had a worse cognitive outcome than meningococcal meningitis. This differential outcome according to infecting organism was not found in the study of Schmidt et al. [46], in which a history of alcoholism, a recognized predisposing cause for pneumococcal meningitis, was an exclusion criterion. This study found impairments in short-term and working memory and in executive tasks, with additional difficulties in language and visuoconstructive function. Reduced brain volume and increased ventricular volume were noted in neuroradiological studies, and white matter lesions correlated negatively with short-term and working memory performance. A pooled analysis found similar proportions with cognitive impairment after

pneumococcal and meningococcal meningitis, but the former group performed worse on memory tasks and tended to be cognitively slower, and impairment was stable over time [47]. A long-term follow-up study found normalization of cognitive function over a period of nine years [48].

9.2.2 Viral meningitis

Viral meningitis is generally considered a benign, self-limiting condition without cognitive sequelae. Mild cognitive impairment has been reported following viral meningitis due to enterovirus, myxovirus, and herpes virus infection [49], but follow-up studies to see whether such deficits progress, reverse, or remain static are awaited. Schmidt et al. found impairments in cognitive performance in viral meningitis patients in similar domains as in bacterial meningitis patients, but these were less severe and lacked the neuroradiological correlates found in bacterial meningitis patients [46].

9.2.3 Fungal meningitis

Meningitis due to the fungus *Cryptococcus neoformans* has been reported to mimic both vascular dementia [50] and Alzheimer's disease (AD) [51].

9.3 Human immunodeficiency virus (HIV) and related conditions

Human immunodeficiency virus (HIV; originally named human T-lymphotropic virus type III, HTLVIII) is the best known of the retroviruses and is the causative agent of the acquired immunodeficiency syndrome (AIDS) pandemic. In the body, HIV spreads hematogenously and is neurotropic, probably entering the brain within blood-derived macrophages. Neurological complications are prominent in HIV infection [52,53]. Pathogenesis is thought to be multifactorial, related to primary HIV infection, opportunistic CNS infection (e.g., with toxoplasmosis, cryptococcal meningitis, cytomegalovirus encephalitis, tuberculous meningitis, neurosyphilis, progressive multifocal leukoencephalopathy related to John Cunningham [JC] virus activation), or tumor formation (CNS lymphoma), sometimes resulting in dementia. Concurrent substance misuse and mood disorder may also contribute to cognitive impairment in some cases.

9.3.1 HIV dementia, AIDS dementia; HIV-associated neurocognitive disorder (HAND)

Cognitive impairment associated with HIV infection in the absence of mood disorder or opportunistic infection was recognized soon after the HIV epidemic was first defined, ranging from psychomotor slowing and mental dullness through to frank dementia [54]. Criteria for the diagnosis of HIV dementia and lesser degrees of cognitive impairment, HIV-associated neurocognitive disorder (HAND), have been proposed [55] and updated [56]. Assessment of cognition in the context of HIV infection may be confounded by other factors including drug and alcohol misuse, educational attainment, and head injury.

Dementia as the initial manifestation of HIV infection has been reported [57], with more rapid progression in association with advanced immunosuppression (CD4 count <200), and hence in parallel with progressive systemic disease. The neuropsychological profile of HIV dementia is characterized by psychomotor slowing, memory impairment (typically impaired free recall with relatively preserved recognition recall), and executive dysfunction, all suggestive of a subcortical pattern of dementia. There may be concurrent motor problems with gait and postural reflexes, and impaired reaction times. Neuropsychological deficits correlate with neuroradiological and neuropathological studies indicating frontostriatal involvement, although cortical areas may also be affected with disease evolution [58,59].

Treatment with antiretrovirals, and particularly combination highly active antiretroviral treatment (HAART), has resulted in a dramatic decline in the incidence of HIV dementia [60,61], but with increased patient survival, there has been an increase in the prevalence of HAND, with around 50% of patients in the CHARTER Study having neuropsychological impairments [62] with slowness, and difficulties in planning and concentration. In addition, there may also have been a change in disease phenotype, with more cortical features and a resemblance to AD [63]. Persistent neuroinflammation may lead to accelerated neurodegenerative changes and pathological overlap with AD, deposition of amyloid plaques being a common finding in HIV infection, possibly as a consequence of the action of antiretroviral medications on amyloid-β metabolism [64,65].

9.3.2 Progressive multifocal leukoencephalopathy (PML)

Progressive multifocal leukoencephalopathy (PML) is a white matter disorder related to JC virus activation. It was rarely seen other than in the context of HIV-induced immunosuppression, but cases related to treatment of multiple sclerosis with natalizumab have caused concern in recent years [66]. Hemiparesis, hemianopia, and dementia are common clinical features of PML. One series from the early years of the AIDS pandemic, which examined the initial symptoms of PML, found cognitive disorders in 36% and speech disturbance in 40% of cases [67]. With the advent of HAART for AIDS, the prognosis for PML has improved greatly (one-year survival of 50% vs. 10%) [68]. Mefloquine, an antimalarial agent with efficacy against JC virus, is being evaluated for use in PML [69].

9.3.3 HTLV-1

The retrovirus HTLV-1 classically causes a myelopathy (HTLV-1 associated myelopathy, HAM; or tropical spastic paraparesis, TSP), but other features have been described including cognitive decline and even subcortical dementia [70]. Silva *et al.* [71] reported psychomotor slowing, verbal and visual memory deficits, impaired attention, and visuomotor problems in both asymptomatic HTLV-1 carriers and patients with HAM/TSP, but there was no association with the degree of motor disability. MRI of white matter changes in HTLV-1 infected individuals may represent chronic perivascular inflammation causing cognitive deficits.

9.4 Other disorders of infective etiology

9.4.1 Neurosyphilis

Neurosyphilis has long been recognized to cause dementia; in the parenchymatous form as "general paresis [or paralysis] of the insane" (GPI), it was once a common cause of cognitive and behavioral decline [72–74]. Meningovascular syphilis may cause a vascular dementia. The advent of the antibiotic era saw a dramatic decline in cases, but a resurgence was seen in association with HIV infection and AIDS [75].

In a case series, in which neurosyphilis was defined by a positive CSF fluorescent treponemal antibody absorption test and very few cases had concurrent HIV positivity, the most common presentation (50%) was with "neuropsychiatric" disease (i.e., psychosis, delirium, dementia). Stroke, spinal cord disease (myelopathy), and epileptic seizures were the other typical presentations. No neuropsychological data were presented, and hence the pattern, if any, of cognitive deficits was not disclosed. Residual cognitive loss was reported in nearly 50% of patients for whom the outcome was known. The authors suggested that the term "syphilitic encephalitis" was preferable to GPI [76].

Syphilis has always been described as the great mimic of other conditions, and one important differential diagnosis is with limbic encephalitis [77]. Dementia related to meningovascular neurosyphilis in the context of HIV infection (Section 9.3) has been reported [78], as has a reversible amnestic syndrome [79].

9.4.2 Neuroborreliosis (Lyme disease)

Infection with the spirochate *Borrelia burgdorferi*, transmitted by the bite of infected *Ixodes* ticks, causes the zoonosis borreliosis or Lyme disease, which may produce multisystem disease with dermatological, cardiological, and neurological involvement. Features of neuroborreliosis may include aseptic meningitis with or without multiple radicular or peripheral nerve lesions, myelitis, cranial neuropathy especially involving the facial nerve, and meningoradiculitis of the cauda equina. Guidelines for the diagnosis and management (antibiotics) of neuroborreliosis have been published [80,81].

Cognitive complications may occur in late (Stage III) Lyme disease. Cases of dementia with *Borrelia spirochetes* found in the brain have been reported [74]. Lyme encephalopathy occurring years after the acute illness was reported, in one series, to produce defects in verbal memory, mental flexibility, verbal associative functions, and articulation, but with preserved intellectual and problem solving skills, sustained attention, visuoconstructive abilities, and mental speed [82]. Mental activation speed, as measured by response times, was found to be slower in Lyme patients but perceptual and motor speed was preserved [83]. Involvement primarily of frontal systems was the conclusion of one review of neuropsychological function in Lyme disease [84], and a case of rapidly progressive frontal-type dementia has been reported [85]. Occasional cases of borreliosis have been noted, presenting as "normal pressure hydrocephalus" (Section 7.2.1), cognitive impairments reversing after appropriate antibiotic treatment [86,87].

Although depression may complicate the presentation, memory impairment does seem to be associated with evidence of CNS involvement (CSF intrathecal antibodies to *B. burgdorferi*, elevated protein, or positive PCR for *B. burgdorferi* DNA) [88]. Few cases have come to autopsy; one showed evidence of spongiform change, neuronal loss, and microglial activation, along with silver-impregnated organisms strongly suggesting *B. burgdorferi* in both cortex and thalamus to account for the cognitive changes [89].

A study of 50 patients with Lyme neuroborreliosis, examined 30 months posttreatment, found lower scores in tests of processing speed, visual and verbal memory, and executive/attention functions when compared to matched controls, but these aggregate data concealed the fact that only a small subgroup of the patients (eight) had chronic and debilitating cognitive sequelae [90].

9.4.3 Tuberculosis and tuberculous meningitis

Infection with *Mycobacterium tuberculosis* can spread to intracranial contents, either as tuberculous meningitis or as focal tuberculomas. Although largely a disease of the past in developed countries, a resurgence in cases of tuberculosis as an opportunistic infection in the context of HIV infection has been noted, and is an infection which needs to be considered when assessing cognitive sequelae of tuberculosis. Studies from the Indian subcontinent list tuberculosis as a cause of dementia [91].

Disseminated brain tuberculomas may cause cognitive features [92], sometimes sufficient to mimic a primary dementia [93]. Dementia has been associated with a dorsal midbrain tuberculous granuloma [94]. A pure amnesic syndrome has been reported following recovery from probable tuberculous meningitis, with evidence of medial temporal lobe and mammillary body involvement [95].

9.4.4 Neurocysticercosis

Infection with the larval stage (cysticercus) of the helminth cestode *Taenia solium*, the pork tapeworm, usually results from eating undercooked pork. Various neurological syndromes may occur when cysticerci reach the CNS; intraparenchymal disease typically induces focal or generalized epilepsy, extraparenchymal disease causes mass effect and intracranial hypertension [96,97].

Cognitive impairment has been reported in neurocysticercosis. Cognitive evaluation of 40 treatment naïve patients found impairment of executive function, verbal and nonverbal memory, praxis, and verbal fluency to be ubiquitous compared to healthy controls, with 12.5% of patients being diagnosed with dementia. Comparison with patients with cryptogenic epilepsy suggested that seizure frequency and antiepileptic drug use could not account for the observed cognitive profile [98]. A study from Mexico City found 15% of patients with untreated neurocysticercosis fulfilled DSM-IV criteria for dementia, of whom more than three-quarters no longer fulfilled the criteria after treatment with albendazole and steroids, suggesting that neurocysticercosis is a reversible cause of dementia. Dementia was associated with the number of parasitic lesions seen in the frontal, temporal, and parietal lobes [99]. In a study from Brazil, patients with mesial temporal lobe epilepsy due to hippocampal sclerosis with incidental calcified neurocysticercosis had no greater cognitive deficits than those without, suggesting that these chronic lesions do not contribute to cognitive performance [100].

9.4.5 Whipple's disease

Although extremely rare, Whipple's disease is a diagnosis that is often considered by neurologists because of the possibility of reversing the movement and cognitive disorder that results from infection with the causative organism, *Tropheryma whippelii*. It is a multisystem granulomatous disorder, the clinical phenotype of which is pleomorphic, but neurological signs may occur in isolation from the more familiar gastrointestinal and systemic symptoms [101]. Diagnostic guidelines for neurological Whipple's have been published and it has been estimated that 11% of CNS Whipple's disease cases present with cognitive decline in the absence of other neurological symptoms and signs [102]. Cognitive features may be prominent in primary Whipple's disease of the brain along with other symptoms such as epileptic seizures and ataxia [103].

Detailed reports of the cognitive impairments in Whipple's disease are few. Manzel *et al.* [104]

reported a biopsy-confirmed case with impairments in sustained attention, memory, executive function, and constructional praxis, with behavioral disinhibition and confabulation, features which correlated with MRI changes in the mesial temporal lobe and basal forebrain. The cognitive picture was thought to resemble that seen after herpes simplex encephalitis or subarachnoid hemorrhage from a ruptured anterior communicating artery aneurysm. Reversible dementia has been reported [105], one case with a "frontotemporal-like dementia" [106]. A case of isolated limbic encephalitis due to Whipple's disease has been reported, in which anterograde amnesia and temporospatial disorientation improved after antibiotic treatment. MRI of the brain showed intense high signal in the amygdalae and hippocampi typical of limbic encephalitis [107].

REFERENCES

[1] Almeida OP, Lautenschlager NT. Dementia associated with infectious diseases. *Int Psychogeriatr* 2005; 17: S65–77.

[2] McGinnis SM. Infectious causes of rapidly progressive dementia. *Semin Neurol* 2011; 31: 266–85.

[3] Anderson M. Encephalitis and other brain infections. In: Donaghy M (ed.). *Brain's Diseases of the Nervous System* (11th edn.). Oxford: Oxford University Press, 2001: 1117–80.

[4] Bell DJ, Suckling R, Rothburn MM, *et al.* Management of suspected herpes simplex encephalitis in adults in a UK teaching hospital. *Clin Med* 2009; 9: 231–5.

[5] Smithson E, Larner AJ. Glioblastoma multiforme masquerading as herpes simplex encephalitis. *Br J Hosp Med* 2013; 74: 52–3.

[6] Kennedy PGE, Chaudhuri A. Herpes simplex encephalitis. *J Neurol Neurosurg Psychiatry* 2002; 73: 237–8.

[7] Young CA, Humphrey PR, Ghadiali EJ, Klapper PE, Cleator GM. Short-term memory impairment in an alert patient as a presentation of herpes simplex encephalitis. *Neurology* 1992; 42: 260–1.

[8] Kamei S, Sekizawa T, Shiota H, *et al.* Evaluation of combination therapy using aciclovir and corticosteroid in adult patients with herpes simplex virus encephalitis. *J Neurol Neurosurg Psychiatry* 2005; 76: 1544–9.

[9] Gordon B, Selnes OA, Hart J, Hanley DF, Whitley RJ. Long-term cognitive sequelae of acyclovir-treated herpes simplex encephalitis. *Arch Neurol* 1990; 47: 646–7.

[10] Kapur N, Barker S, Burrows EH, *et al.* Herpes simplex encephalitis: long-term magnetic resonance imaging and neuropsychological profile. *J Neurol Neurosurg Psychiatry* 1994; 57: 1334–42.

[11] Caparros-Lefebvre D, Girard-Buttoz I, Reboul S, *et al.* Cognitive and psychiatric impairment in herpes simplex virus encephalitis suggest involvement of the amygdalo-frontal pathways. *J Neurol* 1996; 243: 248–56.

[12] Utley TFM, Ogden JA, Gibb A, McGrath N, Anderson NE. The long-term neuropsychological outcome of herpes simplex encephalitis in a series of unselected survivors. *Neuropsychiatry Neuropsychol Behav Neurol* 1997; 10: 180–9.

[13] Hokkanen L, Launes J. Cognitive recovery instead of decline after acute encephalitis: a prospective follow up study. *J Neurol Neurosurg Psychiatry* 1997; 63: 222–7.

[14] Noppeney U, Patterson K, Tyler LK, *et al.* Temporal lobe lesions and semantic impairment: a comparison of herpes simplex virus encephalitis and semantic dementia. *Brain* 2007; 130: 1138–47.

[15] Eslinger PJ. Autobiographical memory after temporal and frontal lobe lesions. *Neurocase* 1998; 4: 481–95.

[16] Hokkanen L, Poutiainen E, Valanne L, *et al.* Cognitive impairment after acute encephalitis: comparison of herpes simplex and other aetiologies. *J Neurol Neurosurg Psychiatry* 1996; 61: 478–84.

[17] Hokkanen L, Salonen O, Launes J. Amnesia in acute herpetic and nonherpetic encephalitis. *Arch Neurol* 1996; 53: 972–8.

[18] Hokkanen L, Launes J. Duration of transient amnesia correlates with cognitive outcome in acute encephalitis. *Neuroreport* 1997; 8: 2721–5.

[19] Hokkanen L, Launes J, Poutiainen E, *et al.* Subcortical type cognitive impairment in herpes zoster encephalitis. *J Neurol* 1997; 244: 239–45.

[20] Wetzel K, Asholt I, Herrmann E, *et al.* Good cognitive outcome of patients with herpes zoster encephalitis: a follow-up study. *J Neurol* 2002; 249: 1612–14.

[21] Bangen KJ, Delano-Wood L, Wierenga CE, *et al.* Dementia following herpes zoster encephalitis. *Clin Neuropsychol* 2010; 24: 1193–203.

[22] Peatfield RC. Basal ganglia damage and subcortical dementia after possible insidious Coxsackie virus encephalitis. *Acta Neurol Scand* 1987; 76: 340–5.

[23] Harrison NA, MacDonald BK, Scott G, Kapoor R. Atypical herpes type 2 encephalitis associated with normal MRI imaging. *J Neurol Neurosurg Psychiatry* 2003; 74: 974–6.

[24] Urban PP, Johnck W, Pohlmann C, Marrakchi S, Bruning R. Reversible progressive cognitive decline due to herpes simplex type 2 encephalitis with normal MR imaging. *J Neurol* 2008; 255: 1975–7.

[25] Kapur N, Brooks DJ. Temporally specific retrograde amnesia in two cases of discrete bilateral hippocampal pathology. *Hippocampus* 1999; 9: 247–54.

[26] Bollen AE, Wartan AN, Krikke AP, Haaxma-Reiche H. Amnestic syndrome after lung transplantation by human herpes virus-6 encephalitis. *J Neurol* 2001; 248: 619–20.

[27] Wainwright MS, Martin PL, Morse RP, *et al.* Human herpesvirus 6 limbic encephalitis after stem cell transplantation. *Ann Neurol* 2001; 50: 612–19.

[28] Gorniak RJ, Young GS, Wiese DE, Marty FM, Schwartz RB. MR imaging of human herpesvirus-6-associated encephalitis in 4 patients with anterograde amnesia after allogeneic hematopoietic stem-cell transplantation. *AJNR Am J Neuroradiol* 2006; 27: 887–91.

[29] MacLean HJ, Douen AG. Severe amnesia associated with human herpesvirus 6 encephalitis after bone marrow transplantation. *Transplantation* 2002; 73: 1086–9.

[30] Dewhurst S. Human herpesvirus type 6 and human herpesvirus type 7 infections of the central nervous system. *Herpes* 2004; 11: 105A–11A.

[31] Solomon T. Flavivirus encephalitis. *N Engl J Med* 2004; 351: 370–8.

[32] Solomon T, Dung NM, Kneen R, *et al.* Japanese encephalitis. *J Neurol Neurosurg Psychiatry* 2000; 68: 405–15.

[33] Sarkari NBS, Thacker AK, Barthwal SP, *et al.* Japanese encephalitis (JE) part II: 14 years' follow-up of survivors. *J Neurol* 2012; 259: 58–69.

[34] Garg RK. Subacute sclerosing panencephalitis. *J Neurol* 2008; 255: 1861–71.

[35] Singer C, Lang AE, Suchowersky O. Adult-onset subacute sclerosing panencephalitis: case reports and review of the literature. *Mov Disord* 1997; 12: 342–53.

[36] Heath CA, Smith C, Davenport R, Donnan GA. Progressive cognitive decline and myoclonus in a young woman: clinicopathological conference at the Edinburgh Advanced Neurology Course, 2007. *Pract Neurol* 2008; 8: 296–302.

[37] Frings M, Blaeser I, Kastrup O. Adult-onset subacute sclerosing panencephalitis presenting as a degenerative dementia syndrome. *J Neurol* 2002; 249: 942–3.

[38] Günther G, Haglund M, Lindquist L, Forsgren M, Skoldenberg B. Tick-borne encephalitis in Sweden in relation to aseptic meningo-encephalitis of other etiology: a prospective study of clinical course and outcome. *J Neurol* 1997; 244: 230–8.

[39] Gustaw-Rothenberg K. Cognitive impairment after tick-borne encephalitis. *Dement Geriatr Cogn Disord* 2008; 26: 165–8.

[40] Vilensky JA (ed.). *Encephalitis Lethargica. During and After the Epidemic.* Oxford: Oxford University Press, 2011.

[41] Dewar BK, Wilson BA. Cognitive recovery from encephalitis lethargica. *Brain Inj* 2005; 19: 1285–91.

[42] Anderson M. Meningitis. In: Donaghy M (ed.). *Brain's Diseases of the Nervous System* (11th edn.). Oxford: Oxford University Press, 2001; 1097–116.

[43] Ginsberg L, Kidd D. Chronic and recurrent meningitis. *Pract Neurol* 2008; 8: 348–61.

[44] Merkelbach S, Sittinger H, Schweizer I, Müller M. Cognitive outcome after bacterial meningitis. *Acta Neurol Scand* 2000; 102: 118–23.

[45] Van de Beek D, Schmand B, de Gans J, *et al.* Cognitive impairment in adults with good recovery after bacterial meningitis. *J Infect Dis* 2002; 186: 1047–52.

[46] Schmidt H, Heimann B, Djukic M, *et al.* Neuropsychological sequelae of bacterial and viral meningitis. *Brain* 2006; 129: 333–45.

[47] Hoogman M, van de Beek D, Weisfelt M, de Gans J, Schmand B. Cognitive outcome in adults after bacterial meningitis. *J Neurol Neurosurg Psychiatry* 2007; 78: 1092–6.

[48] Schmand B, de Bruin E, de Gans J, van de Beek D. Cognitive functioning and quality of life nine years after bacterial meningitis. *J Infect* 2010; 61: 330–4.

[49] Sittinger H, Müller M, Schweizer I, Merkelbach S. Mild cognitive impairment after viral meningitis in adults. *J Neurol* 2002; 249: 554–60.

[50] Aharon-Peretz J, Kilot D, Finkelstein R, *et al.* Cryptococcal meningitis mimicking vascular dementia. *Neurology* 2004; 62: 2135.

[51] Hoffmann M, Muniz J, Carroll E, De Villasante J. Cryptococcal meningitis misdiagnosed as Alzheimer's disease: complete neurological and cognitive recovery with treatment. *J Alzheimers Dis* 2009; 16: 517–20.

[52] Gendelman HE, Grant I, Everall IP, Lipton SA, Swindells S (eds.). *The Neurology of AIDS* (2nd edn.). Oxford: Oxford University Press, 2005.

[53] McArthur JC, Brew BJ, Nath A. Neurological complications of HIV infection. *Lancet Neurol* 2005; 4: 543–55.

[54] Grant I, Sacktor N, McArthur J. HIV and neurocognitive disorders. In: Gendelman HE, Grant I, Everall IP, Lipton SA, Swindells S (eds.). *The Neurology of AIDS* (2nd edn.). Oxford: Oxford University Press, 2005: 357–73.

[55] Report of a Working Group of the American Academy of Neurology AIDS Task Force. Nomenclature and research case definitions for neurologic manifestations of human immunodeficiency virus-type 1 (HIV-1) infection. *Neurology* 1991; 41: 778–85.

[56] Antinori A, Arendt G, Becker JT, *et al.* Updated research nosology for HIV-associated neurocognitive disorders. *Neurology* 2007; 69: 1789–99.

[57] Navia BA, Jordan BD, Price RW. The AIDS dementia complex: I. Clinical features. *Ann Neurol* 1986; 19: 517–24.

[58] Oechsner M, Möller AA, Zaudig M. Cognitive impairment, dementia and psychological functioning in human immunodeficiency virus infection. A prospective study based on DSM-III-R and ICD-10. *Acta Psychiatr Scand* 1993; 87: 13–17.

[59] Power C, Johnson RT. HIV-1 associated dementia: clinical features and pathogenesis. *Can J Neurol Sci* 1995; 22: 92–100.

[60] Catalan J, Thornton S. Whatever happened to HIV dementia? *Int J STD AIDS* 1993; 4: 1–4.

[61] Sacktor N, McDermott MP, Marder K, *et al.* HIV-associated cognitive impairment before and after the advent of combination therapy. *J Neurovirol* 2002; 8: 136–42.

[62] Heaton RK, Clifford DB, Franklin DR Jr, *et al.* HIV-associated neurocognitive disorders persist in the era of potent antiretroviral therapy: CHARTER Study. *Neurology* 2010; 75: 2087–96.

[63] Brew BJ. Evidence for a change in AIDS dementia complex in the era of highly active retroviral therapy and the possibility of new forms of AIDS dementia complex. *AIDS* 2004; 18(Suppl 1): S75–8.

[64] Wang T, Rumbaugh JA, Nath A. Viruses and the brain: from inflammation to dementia. *Clin Sci (Lond)* 2006; 110: 393–407.

[65] Giunta B, Ehrhart J, Obregon DF, *et al.* Antiretroviral medications disrupt microglial phagocytosis of β-amyloid and increase its production by neurons: implications for HIV-associated neurocognitive disorders. *Mol Brain* 2011; 4: 23.

[66] Yousry TA, Major EO, Ryschkewitsch C, *et al.* Evaluation of patients treated with natalizumab for progressive multifocal leukoencephalopathy. *N Engl J Med* 2006; 354: 924–33.

[67] Berger JR, Pall L, Lanska D, Whiteman M. Progressive multifocal leukoencephalopathy in patients with HIV infection. *J Neurovirol* 1998; 4: 59–68.

[68] Lima MA, Bernal-Cano F, Clifford DB, Gandhi RT, Koralnik IJ. Clinical outcome of long-term survivors of progressive multifocal leukoencephalopathy. *J Neurol Neurosurg Psychiatry* 2010; 81: 1288–91.

[69] Gofton TE, Al-Khotani A, O'Farrell B, Ang LC, McLachlan RS. Mefloquine in the treatment of progressive multifocal leukoencephalopathy. *J Neurol Neurosurg Psychiatry* 2011; 82: 452–5.

[70] Araujo AQC, Silva MTT. The HTLV-1 neurological complex. *Lancet Neurol* 2006; 5: 1068–76.

[71] Silva MTT, Mattos P, Alfano A, Araújo AQ-C. Neuropsychological assessment in HTLV-1 infection: a comparative study among TSP/HAM, asymptomatic carriers and healthy controls. *J Neurol Neurosurg Psychiatry* 2003; 74: 1085–9.

[72] Dewhurst K. The neurosyphilis psychoses today: a survey of 91 cases. *Br J Psychiatry* 1969; 115: 31–8.

[73] Nieman EA. Neurosyphilis yesterday and today. *J R Coll Physicians Lond* 1991; 25: 321–4.

[74] Miklossy J. Biology and neuropathology of dementia in syphilis and Lyme disease. *Handb Clin Neurol* 2008; 89: 825–44.

[75] Carr J. Neurosyphilis. *Pract Neurol* 2003; 3: 328–41.

[76] Timmermans M, Carr J. Neurosyphilis in the modern era. *J Neurol Neurosurg Psychiatry* 2004; 75: 1727–30.

[77] Schied R, Voltz R, Vetter T, *et al.* Neurosyphilis and paraneoplastic limbic encephalitis: important differential diagnoses. *J Neurol* 2005; 252: 1129–32.

[78] Fox PA, Hawkins DA, Dawson S. Dementia following an acute presentation of meningovascular neurosyphilis in an HIV-1 positive patient. *AIDS* 2000; 14: 2062–3.

[79] Kearney H, Mallon P, Kavanagh P, *et al.* Amnestic syndrome due to meningovascular syphilis. *J Neurol* 2010; 257: 669–71.

[80] Report of the Quality Standards Subcommittee of the American Academy of Neurology. Practice parameter: diagnosis of patients with nervous system Lyme borreliosis (Lyme disease)–summary statement. *Neurology* 1996; 46: 881–2.

[81] Mygland A, Ljostad U, Fingerle V, *et al.* EFNS guidelines on the diagnosis and management of European Lyme neuroborreliosis. *Eur J Neurol* 2010; 17: 8–16.

[82] Benke T, Gasse T, Hittmair Delazer M, Schmutzhard E. Lyme encephalopathy: long-term neuropsychological deficits years after acute neuroborreliosis. *Acta Neurol Scand* 1995; 91: 353–7.

[83] Pollina DA, Sliwinski M, Squires NK, Krupp LB. Cognitive processing speed in Lyme disease. *Neuropsychiatry Neuropsychol Behav Neurol* 1999; 12: 72–8.

[84] Westervelt HJ, McCaffrey RJ. Neuropsychological functioning in chronic Lyme disease. *Neuropsychol Rev* 2002; 12: 153–77.

[85] Waniek C, Prohovnik I, Kaufman MA, Dwork AJ. Rapidly progressive frontal-type dementia associated with Lyme disease. *J Neuropsychiatry Clin Neurosci* 1995; 7: 345–7.

[86] Danek A, Uttner I, Yousry T, Pfister HW. Lyme neuroborreliosis disguised as normal pressure hydrocephalus. *Neurology* 1996; 46: 1743–5.

[87] Etienne M, Carvalho P, Fauchais AL, *et al.* Lyme neuroborreliosis revealed as a normal pressure hydrocephalus: a cause of reversible dementia. *J Am Geriatr Soc* 2003; 51: 579–80.

[88] Kaplan RF, Jones Woodward L, Workman K, *et al.* Neuropsychological deficits in Lyme disease patients with and without other evidence of central nervous system pathology. *Appl Neuropsychol* 1999; 6: 3–11.

[89] Kobayashi K, Mizukoshi C, Aoki T, *et al.* Borrelia burgdorferi-seropositive chronic encephalomyelopathy: Lyme neuroborreliosis? An autopsied report. *Dement Geriatr Cogn Disord* 1997; 8: 384–90.

[90] Eikeland R, Ljostad U, Mygland A, Herlofson K, Lohaugen GC. European neuroborreliosis: neuropsychological findings 30 months post-treatment. *Eur J Neurol* 2012; 19: 480–7.

[91] Jha S, Patel R. Some observations on the spectrum of dementia. *Neurol India* 2004; 52: 213–14.

[92] Akritidis N, Galiatsou E, Kakadellis J, Dimas K, Paparounas K. Brain tuberculomas due to miliary tuberculosis. *South Med J* 2005; 98: 111–13.

[93] Sethi NK, Sethi PK, Torgovnick J, Arsura E. Central nervous system tuberculosis masquerading as primary dementia: a case report. *Neurol Neurochir Pol* 2011; 45: 510–13.

[94] Meador KJ, Loring DW, Sethi KD, *et al.* Dementia associated with dorsal midbrain lesion. *J Int Neuropsychol Soc* 1996; 2: 359–67.

[95] Ceccaldi M, Belleville S, Royere ML, Poncet M. A pure reversible amnesic syndrome following tuberculous meningoencephalitis. *Eur Neurol* 1995; 35: 363–7.

[96] Garcia HH, Gonzalez AE, Tsang VCW, Gilman RH for the Cysticercosis Working Group in Peru. Neurocysticercosis: some of the essentials. *Pract Neurol* 2006; 6: 288–97.

[97] Sinha S, Sharma BS. Neurocysticercosis: a review of current status and management. *J Clin Neurosci* 2009; 16: 867–76.

[98] Ciampi de Andrade D, Rodrigues CL, Abraham R, *et al.* Cognitive impairment and dementia in neurocysticercosis: a cross-sectional controlled study. *Neurology* 2010; 74: 1288–95.

[99] Ramirez Bermudez J, Higuera J, Sosa AL, *et al.* Is dementia reversible in patients with neurocysticercosis? *J Neurol Neurosurg Psychiatry* 2005; 76: 1164–6.

[100] Terra Bustamente VC, Coimbra ER, Rezek KO, *et al.* Cognitive performance of patients with mesial temporal lobe epilepsy and incidental calcified neurocysticercosis. *J Neurol Neurosurg Psychiatry* 2005; 76: 1080–3.

[101] Anderson M. Neurology of Whipple's disease. *J Neurol Neurosurg Psychiatry* 2000; 68: 2–5.

[102] Louis ED, Lynch T, Kaufmann P, Fahn S, Odel J. Diagnostic guidelines in central nervous system Whipple's disease. *Ann Neurol* 1996; 40: 561–8.

[103] Panegyres PK, Edis R, Beaman M, Fallon M. Primary Whipple's disease of the brain: characterization of the syndrome and molecular diagnosis. *Q J Med* 2006; 99: 609–23.

[104] Manzel K, Tranel D, Cooper G. Cognitive and behavioral abnormalities in a case of central nervous system Whipple disease. *Arch Neurol* 2000; 57: 399–403.

[105] Rossi T, Haghighipour R, Haghighi M, Paolini S, Scarpino O. Cerebral Whipple's disease as a cause of reversible dementia. *Clin Neurol Neurosurg* 2005; 107: 258–61.

[106] Romero Munoz JP, Herrero A, Herreros J, *et al*. Isolated central nervous system Whipple's disease causing reversible frontotemporal-like dementia. *Eur J Neurol* 2008; 15(Suppl 3): 213 (abstract p. 1719).

[107] Blanc F, Ben Abdelghani K, Schramm F, *et al*. Whipple limbic encephalitis. *Arch Neurol* 2011; 68: 1471–3.

Neuromuscular disorders

It may seem odd that diseases of muscle or of the neuromuscular junction (NMJ), the most distal outposts of the nervous system, might be associated with dysfunction of higher cortical function. However, diseases manifesting with neuropathy or myopathy may, in fact, be multisystem disorders with a broad phenotype that also encompasses cognitive processes, sometimes related to expression of abnormal or dysfunctional proteins that are common to muscle/NMJ and brain [1]. Myotonic dystrophy type 1 is perhaps the classic example. Other neuropathic and myopathic disorders with concurrent cognitive features, which are discussed elsewhere, include mitochondrial disorders (Section 5.5.1), acid maltase deficiency (Section 5.5.3.1), Fabry's disease (Section 5.5.3.2), neurofibromatosis (Section 5.6.1), adult polyglucosan body disease (Section 5.5.6), and chronic inflammatory demyelinating polyneuropathy (Section 6.17).

10.1 Myotonic dystrophy

Myotonic dystrophies are classified on a genetic basis. Myotonic dystrophy type 1 (DM1) corresponds to classical dystrophia myotonica or Steinert's disease, and is associated with CTG trinucleotide repeat expansions in the 3′ untranslated region of the dystrophia myotonica protein kinase (DMPK) gene on chromosome 19q13 (OMIM#160900). Myotonic dystrophy type 2 (DM2), previously known as proximal myotonic myopathy (PROMM) or Ricker's syndrome, is associated with heterozygous expansion of a CCTG tetranucleotide repeat in intron 1 of the zinc finger protein-9 (ZNF9) gene on chromosome 3q (OMIM#602668) [2].

Despite the terminology, brain involvement is recognized in both DM1 and DM2, more so in the former [3,4]. A non-DM1 non-DM2 multisystem myotonic disorder with frontotemporal dementia has been described, for which the designation DM3 has been proposed [5].

10.1.1 Myotonic dystrophy type 1 (DM1; Steinert's disease)

Adult-onset DM1 is a pleiotropic disorder, one component of which may be cognitive impairment. Features such as cognitive dysfunction, visuospatial deficits, behavioral abnormalities, and hypersomnia are reported to be more prominent in DM1 than DM2 [6], concordant with the neuroimaging and neurophysiological findings of more severe brain involvement in DM1 [3].

The most commonly observed cognitive impairments in DM1 relate to executive dysfunction [7, 8], seen for example in performance of the Stroop color–word and phonemic verbal fluency tests [3], with lack of initiative and apathy despite preserved general intelligence. Features may be static or progressive, sometimes with temporal lobe (memory) impairments. Weber *et al.* [4] found pronounced impairments of nonverbal episodic memory in DM1. Decline in abilities over time, particularly linguistic and executive functions, was found in a follow-up study [9].

Atypical presentation of DM1 as apparent primary dementia may occur. There is noted to be a high risk of cognitive impairments in childhood-onset disease, particularly associated with maternal inheritance, whereas adult-onset disease is at lower risk. Wilson *et al.* [10] reported an adult patient with paternal inheritance and an 11-year decline in cognitive function, for which no cause other than DM1 was identified.

IQ has been reported to decline in DM1 as the size of the CTG expansion increases [11]. A correlation between cognitive deficits and CTG expansion size has also been reported [7,12,13]. However, other studies have found no correlation between cognitive impairment in DM1 and CTG repeat number or severity of muscle involvement [9,14,15], including progression of cognitive decline over time [9]. The explanation for these discrepant findings is currently unclear.

DM1 may be accompanied by white matter changes on magnetic resonance imaging (MRI) of the brain [16], which may [17] or may not [18] correlate with neuropsychological impairment. Weber *et al.* [4] found a correlation between the extent of white matter lesions and psychomotor speed. Sophisticated neuroimaging techniques indicate neocortical damage in DM1 brains even in the absence of white matter change [19], which might possibly be related to cognitive deficits. Voxel-based morphometry showed bilateral hippocampal volume reduction that correlated with episodic memory deficits [4].

Concurrent hypersomnia was excluded as a cause for impaired cognitive performance in DM1 in a study that examined both neuropsychological performance and polysomnography [8].

Neurofibrillary tangles (NFTs) comparable to those seen in Alzheimer's disease (AD) have been observed in DM1 brains [20], perhaps related to the altered splicing patterns of the tau gene in the DM1 brain [21]. One study found NFTs in the limbic system and brainstem of all cases examined, but no senile plaques [22]. Mutant DMPK transcripts were found to be widely expressed in discrete foci in the nuclei of cortical and subcortical neurons in DM1 [23].

10.1.2 Myotonic dystrophy type 2 (DM2; PROMM; Ricker's syndrome)

The cognitive phenotype of DM2 is less well characterized than DM1. Impaired visuospatial recall and construction has been noted, more prevalent than in DM1 [24]. Pronounced impairments of nonverbal episodic memory have also been reported in DM2, as in DM1, which correlate with hippocampal volume reduction [4]. NFTs were identified in a cognitively normal patient with DM2, suggesting that abnormal processing of tau isoforms may occur in DM2 as well as DM1 [25].

10.2 Limb-girdle muscular dystrophy (LGMD)

Limb-girdle muscular dystrophy (LGMD) is a heterogeneous group of muscular dystrophies characterized clinically by wasting and weakness of limb-girdle musculature with or without cardiac involvement. Over 20 genetic types have been defined to date. Of these, LGMD type 2I, due to mutations in the gene on chromosome 19q13.3 encoding fukutin-related protein (OMIM#607155), which is expressed in the brain and may be important in brain development, has been reported to be associated with deficits in executive function, visuospatial abilities, and visual memory [26].

10.3 Oculopharyngeal muscular dystrophy (OPMD)

Oculopharyngeal muscular dystrophy (OPMD) is an autosomal dominant muscle disorder characterized by late onset (fifth to sixth decade) of ptosis, dysphagia, and ophthalmoplegia, with characteristic muscle biopsy appearances of sarcoplasmic rimmed vacuoles with intranuclear filamentous/tubular inclusions. OPMD results from expansions of a trinucleotide repeat sequence (GCG) in the poly(A) binding protein II on chromosome 14q (OMIM#164300).

Cognitive decline has been recorded in some OPMD homozygotes, with the features of a subcortical dementia [27]. More recently, a study of heterozygotes has shown impaired executive function (reduced working memory, cognitive flexibility, and selective attention), with a negative correlation between cognitive function and trinucleotide expansion size, suggesting that this could be linked to the genetic defect possibly through a toxic gain-of-function mechanism, perhaps related to the intranuclear inclusions [28].

10.4 Spinal and bulbar muscular atrophy (Kennedy's syndrome)

Spinal and bulbar muscular atrophy (SBMA), also known as Kennedy's syndrome or bulbospinal neuronopathy, is an X-linked recessive syndrome of motor neuron dysfunction resulting from CAG trinucleotide repeat expansion in exon 1 of the gene encoding the androgen receptor on chromosome Xq12 (OMIM#313200). Unlike motor neuron disease (Section 2.3.1), with which it is sometimes confused clinically, SBMA is only slowly progressive with a generally good prognosis.

Neuropsychological deficits have been documented in SBMA, in both symptomatic patients and some female mutation carriers [29]. Subclinical deficits in verbal and nonverbal fluency, concept formation, working memory, and attentional mechanisms, suggesting impairment of frontotemporal cognitive functions, have been documented, indicating that extramotor as well as motor networks may be affected in this disorder [30].

10.5 McArdle's disease

McArdle's disease is due to myophosphorylase deficiency, an inborn error of metabolism, resulting from homozygous or compound heterozygous mutations in the gene encoding muscle glycogen phosphorylase (PYGM) on chromosome 11q13.1 (OMIM#232600). It is classified as glycogen storage disease type V (cf. acid maltase deficiency, glycogenosis type IIb; Section 5.5.3.1). Typical clinical features are exercise-induced muscle cramps and sometimes rhabdomyolysis in young adults, with almost invariably elevated blood creatine kinase levels [31].

The muscle isoform of glycogen phosphorylase is also expressed in astrocytes and may play a role in neuronal energy metabolism. A case of cognitive impairment in McArdle's disease has been reported, in which there was neuropsychological and functional neuroimaging evidence of frontal and prefrontal cortex dysfunction [32].

10.6 Myasthenia gravis

Myasthenia gravis (MG) is an antibody-mediated disorder of neuromuscular transmission causing painless fluctuating fatigable skeletal muscle weakness that worsens with exercise and improves with rest, affecting particularly extraocular, bulbar, and proximal limb muscles. Autoantibodies directed to the postsynaptic muscle nicotinic acetylcholine receptor (AChR) are the most commonly detected autoantibodies; antibodies directed against muscle-specific tyrosine kinase (MuSK) are found in some AChR seronegative MG patients. Cholinesterase inhibitors are effective symptomatic agents in MG patients, although treatment with immunomodulatory and disease-modifying agents may also be required [33].

A central cholinergic deficit, mirroring the peripheral (neuromuscular junction) cholinergic transmission deficit, has been suggested in myasthenia gravis, which might result in impaired memory [34,35]. Central cholinergic dysfunction is thought to be of central importance to the pathophysiology of cognitive deficits in AD and, possibly, dementia with Lewy bodies (Sections 2.1 and 2.4.2). Tucker *et al.* [34] found MG subjects to be impaired relative to both healthy controls and subjects with chronic nonneurological disease on the Boston Naming Test, WMS Logical Memory, and WMS Design Reproduction. Moreover, one patient with MG showed improvement in memory after treatment with plasmapheresis. A case control study found MG patients performed worse than controls on measures of response fluency, information processing, verbal and visual learning, but not on attention span or information retention [36]. A subsequent study by the same group found that increased subjective mental (but not physical) fatigue correlated with patient cognitive measures [37].

However, other researchers have found no evidence for memory impairments in MG patients in comparison with normal controls, and hence no support for the idea of impaired central cholinergic mechanisms [38–40]. Sleep abnormalities were suggested to be the cause of memory impairments noted in some studies of MG patients [39]. Impairments of attention, praxis, and frontal control observed in severe MG were found to be related to "general visual motor slowness" and other diseases, specifically diabetes mellitus and thyroid dysfunction [40].

A patient with anti-MuSK-positive MG and parkinsonism with cognitive impairment has been reported with the suggestion of a shared pathogenesis related to impaired cholinergic neurotransmission [41].

REFERENCES

[1] D'Angelo MG, Bresolin N. Cognitive impairment in neuromuscular disorders. *Muscle Nerve* 2006; 34: 16–33.

[2] Day J, Thornton C. Myotonic dystrophy. In: Karpati G, Hilton-Jones D, Bushby K, Griggs RC (eds.). *Disorders of Voluntary Muscle* (8th edn.). Cambridge: Cambridge University Press, 2010; 347–62.

[3] Romeo V, Pegoraro E, Ferrati C, *et al.* Brain involvement in myotonic dystrophies: neuroimaging and neurophysiological comparative study in DM1 and DM2. *J Neurol* 2010; 257: 1246–55.

[4] Weber YG, Roebling R, Kassubek J, *et al.* Comparative analysis of brain structure, metabolism, and cognition in myotonic dystrophy 1 and 2. *Neurology* 2010; 74: 1108–17.

[5] Le Ber I, Martinez M, Campion D, *et al.* A non-DM1, non-DM2 multisystem myotonic disorder with frontotemporal dementia: phenotype and suggestive mapping of the DM3 locus to chromosome 15q21–24. *Brain* 2004; 127: 1979–92.

[6] Harper PS, van Engelen B, Eymard B, Wilcox DE (eds.). *Myotonic Dystrophy: Present Management, Future Therapy.* Oxford: Oxford University Press, 2004.

[7] Sistiaga A, Urreta I, Jodar M, *et al.* Cognitive/personality pattern and triplet expansion size in adult myotonic dystrophy type 1 (DM1): CTG repeats, cognition and personality in DM1. *Psychol Med* 2010; 40: 487–95.

[8] Zalonis I, Bonakis A, Christidi F, *et al.* Toward understanding cognitive impairment in patients with myotonic dystrophy type 1. *Arch Clin Neuropsychol* 2010; 25: 303–13.

[9] Modoni A, Silvestri G, Vita MG, *et al.* Cognitive impairment in myotonic dystrophy type 1 (DM1): a longitudinal follow-up study. *J Neurol* 2008; 255: 1737–42.

[10] Wilson BA, Balleny H, Patterson K, Hodges JR. Myotonic dystrophy and progressive cognitive decline: a common condition or two separate problems? *Cortex* 1999; 35: 113–21.

[11] Turnpenny P, Clark C, Kelly K. Intelligence quotient profile in myotonic dystrophy, intergenerational

deficit, and correlation with CTG amplification. *J Med Genet* 1994; 31: 300–5.

[12] Perini GI, Menegazzo E, Ermani M, *et al.* Cognitive impairment and (CTG)n expansion in myotonic dystrophy patients. *Biol Psychiatry* 1999; 46: 425–31.

[13] Winblad S, Lindberg C, Hansen S. Cognitive deficits and CTG repeat expansion in classical myotonic dystrophy type 1 (DM1). *Behav Brain Funct* 2006; 2: 16.

[14] Rubinsztein JS, Rubinsztein DC, McKenna PJ, Goodburn S, Holland AJ. Mild myotonic dystrophy is associated with memory impairment in the context of normal general intelligence. *J Med Genet* 1997; 34: 229–33.

[15] Modoni A, Silvestri G, Pomponi MG, *et al.* Characterization of the pattern of cognitive impairment in myotonic dystrophy type 1. *Arch Neurol* 2004; 61: 1943–7.

[16] Di Costanzo A, Di Salle F, Santoro L, *et al.* Pattern and significance of white matter abnormalities in myotonic dystrophy type 1: an MRI study. *J Neurol* 2002; 249: 1175–82.

[17] Censori B, Provinciali L, Danni M, *et al.* Brain involvement in myotonic dystrophy: MRI features and their relationship to clinical and cognitive conditions. *Acta Neurol Scand* 1994; 90: 211–17.

[18] Sinforiani E, Sandrini G, Martelli A, *et al.* Cognitive and neuroradiological findings in myotonic dystrophy. *Funct Neurol* 1991; 6: 377–84.

[19] Giorgio A, Dotti MT, Battaglini M, *et al.* Cortical damage in brains of patients with adult-form of myotonic dystrophy type 1 and no or minimal MRI abnormalities. *J Neurol* 2006; 253: 1471–7.

[20] Kiuchi A, Otsuka N, Namba Y, Nakano I, Tomonaga M. Presenile appearance of abundant Alzheimer's neurofibrillary tangles without senile plaques in the brain in myotonic dystrophy. *Acta Neuropathol* 1991; 82: 1–5.

[21] Sergeant N, Sablonniere B, Schraen-Maschke S, *et al.* Dysregulation of human brain microtubule-associated tau mRNA maturation in myotonic dystrophy type 1. *Hum Mol Genet* 2001; 10: 2143–55.

[22] Oyamada R, Hayashi M, Katoh Y, *et al.* Neurofibrillary tangles and deposition of oxidative products in the brain in cases of myotonic dystrophy. *Neuropathology* 2006; 26: 107–14.

[23] Jiang H, Mankodi A, Swanson MS, Moxley RT, Thornton CA. Myotonic dystrophy type 1 is associated with nuclear foci of mutant RNA, sequestration of muscleblind proteins and deregulated alternative splicing in neurons. *Hum Mol Genet* 2004; 13: 3079–88.

[24] Meola G, Sansone V, Perani D, *et al.* Reduced cerebral blood flow and impaired visual-spatial function in proximal myotonic myopathy. *Neurology* 1999; 53: 1042–50.

[25] Maurage CA, Udd B, Ruchoux MM, *et al.* Similar brain tau pathology in DM2/PROMM and DM1/Steinert disease. *Neurology* 2005; 65: 1636–8.

[26] Palmieri A, Manara R, Bello L, *et al.* Cognitive profile and MRI findings in limb-girdle muscular dystrophy 2I. *J Neurol* 2011; 258: 1312–20.

[27] Blumen SC, Bouchard JP, Brais B, *et al.* Cognitive impairment and reduced life span of oculopharyngeal muscular dystrophy homozygotes. *Neurology* 2009; 73: 596–601.

[28] Dubbioso R, Moretta P, Manganelli F, *et al.* Executive functions are impaired in heterozygote patients with oculopharyngeal muscular dystrophy. *J Neurol* 2012; 259: 833–7.

[29] Guidetti D, Vescovini E, Motti L, *et al.* X-linked bulbar and spinal muscular atrophy, or Kennedy disease: clinical, neurophysiological, neuropathological, neuropsychological and molecular study of a large family. *J Neurol Sci* 1996; 135: 140–8.

[30] Soukup GR, Sperfeld AD, Uttner I, *et al.* Frontotemporal cognitive function in X-linked spinal and bulbar muscular atrophy (SBMA): a controlled neuropsychological study of 20 patients. *J Neurol* 2009; 256: 1869–75.

[31] Quinlivan R, Buckley J, James M, *et al.* McArdle disease: a clinical review. *J Neurol Neurosurg Psychiatry* 2010; 81: 1182–8.

[32] Mancuso M, Orsucci D, Volterrani D, Siciliano G. Cognitive impairment and McArdle disease: is there a link? *Neuromusc Disord* 2011; 21: 356–8.

[33] Sathasivam S, Larner AJ. Disorders of the neuromuscular junction. In: Sinclair A, Morley JE, Vellas B (eds.). *Pathy's Principles and Practice of Geriatric Medicine* (5th edn.). Chichester: Wiley, 2012; 769–78.

[34] Tucker DM, Roeltgen DP, Wann PD, Wertheimer RI. Memory dysfunction in myasthenia gravis: evidence for central cholinergic effects. *Neurology* 1988; 38: 1173–7.

[35] Davidov-Lusting M, Klinghoffer V, Kaplan DA, Steiner I. Memory abnormalities in myasthenia gravis: possible fatigue of central nervous system cholinergic circuits. *Autoimmunity* 1992; 14: 85–6.

[36] Paul RH, Cohen RA, Gilchrist JM, Aloia MS, Goldstein JM. Cognitive dysfunction in individuals with myasthenia gravis. *J Neurol Sci* 2000; 179: 59–64.

[37] Paul RH, Cohen RA, Gilchrist JM. Ratings of subjective mental fatigue relate to cognitive performance in patients with myasthenia gravis. *J Clin Neurosci* 2002; 9: 243–6.

[38] Glennerster A, Palace J, Warburton D, Oxbury S, Newsom-Davis J. Memory in myasthenia gravis: neuropsychological tests of cerebral cholinergic function before and after effective immunologic treatment. *Neurology* 1996; 46: 1138–42.

[39] Feldmann R, Kiefer R, Wiegard U, Evers S, Weglage J. Intelligence, attention, and memory in patients with myasthenia gravis [in German]. *Nervenarzt* 2005; 76: 960, 962–6.

[40] Marra C, Marsili F, Quaranta D, Evoli A. Determinants of cognitive impairment in elderly myasthenia gravis patients. *Muscle Nerve* 2009; 40: 952–9.

[41] Lanfranconi S, Corti S, Baron P, *et al.* Anti-MuSK-positive myasthenia gravis in a patient with parkinsonism and cognitive impairment. *Neurol Res Int* 2011; 2011: 859802.

Sleep-related disorders

The study and understanding of sleep-related disorders has been an area of major clinical advance over the last 20 to 30 years. Sleep disorders have been classified in the *International Classification of Sleep Disorders* (ICSD-2) into eight broad categories (with several subcategories) [1]:

- Insomnias;
- Sleep-related breathing disorders, such as sleep apnea syndromes;
- Hypersomnias of central origin, such as narcolepsy;
- Circadian rhythm sleep disorders;
- Parasomnias;
- Sleep-related movement disorders, such as restless legs syndrome;
- Isolated symptoms, apparently normal variants, and unresolved issues;
- Other sleep disorders.

There are also two appendices in ICSD-2, which list:

- Sleep disorders associated with conditions classifiable elsewhere, such as fatal familial insomnia (Section 2.5.3);

- Other psychiatric and behavioral disorders frequently encountered in the differential diagnosis of sleep disorders, such as somatoform disorders.

Sleep deprivation is recognized to have adverse consequences on cognitive function [2]. Poor sleep quality correlates with subjective memory complaint [3], and objectively measured sleep disturbance but not total sleep time is related to poorer cognition, suggesting that quality rather than quantity of sleep is the important factor affecting cognition [4].

Study of the cognitive impairments associated with sleep-related disorders is a developing area of clinical inquiry.

11.1 Sleep-related breathing disorders

Sleep-related breathing disorders include the sleep apnea syndromes. Sleep apnea refers to a temporary cessation or absence of breathing during sleep. Sleep apnea syndromes may be broadly divided into three categories: obstructive, central, and mixed [5,6].

11.1.1 Obstructive sleep apnea–hypopnea syndrome (OSAHS)

Obstructive sleep apnea-hypopnea syndrome (OSAHS) is caused by critical narrowing of the upper airway during sleep when reduced muscle tone leads to increased resistance to the flow of air, and partial obstruction often results in loud snoring. Sleep is restless due to successive episodes of apnea, often witnessed by the bed partner, which are relieved by brief arousal from sleep. A narrow pharyngeal anteroposterior diameter, obesity, high alcohol intake, and the male gender seem to be risk factors for the development of OSAHS. As a consequence of sleep fragmentation, the most common daytime symptom is excessive somnolence, manifest as a tendency to fall asleep in monotonous or inappropriate situations, a symptom which may be assessed with scales such as the Epworth Sleepiness Scale (ESS) [7]. OSAHS may be diagnosed using nocturnal polysomnography or, more practically in routine clinical work, pulse oximetry. The severity of OSAHS may be measured using the apnea/hypopnea index (AHI), or respiratory disturbance index (RDI), which is calculated from polysomnographic recordings as the number of apneas/hypopneas per hour of sleep: AHI or RDI of 10–20/hr indicates mild, 20–50/hr moderate, and >50/hr severe disease. With pulse oximetry, a desaturation index (DI) may be calculated as the number of desaturations (decrease in oxygen saturation by ≥4%) per hour of sleep or, if the recording is unattended, per time of recording. DI ≥5/hr may be used to define sleep-disordered breathing [8]. Treatment of OSAHS includes nocturnal continuous positive airway pressure (CPAP) via a mask. Surgery to palatal structures, such as uvulopalatopharyngoplasty, may sometimes have a place.

OSAHS may present with various neurological symptoms besides excessive daytime sleepiness, including blackouts and headache, sometimes with features suggestive of raised intracranial pressure, and may be mistaken for narcolepsy, epilepsy, and idiopathic intracranial hypertension, respectively. Apparent intellectual decline, which may be mistaken for dementia, is also reported as a recognized feature of OSAHS, which may improve after appropriate treatment of the underlying condition [6,9,10].

Findley et al. [11] found impairments in measures of attention, concentration, complex problem solving, and short-term recall of verbal and spatial information in OSAHS patients with hypoxemia as compared with OSAHS patients without hypoxemia; cognitive impairment did not correlate with measures of sleep fragmentation, suggesting that it was hypoxia rather than sleep disturbance that accounted for the cognitive deficits. A patient reported by Scheltens et al. [12], in whom cognitive impairment was the presenting feature of a sleep apnea syndrome, had impaired learning and retention, impaired sustained attention, impaired visuospatial reasoning, vulnerability to interference, impaired verbal fluency, but no aphasia, apraxia, or agnosia. Polysomnography showed mixed, central, and obstructive apneas in this patient. The authors suggested that both cerebral hypoxia and sleep fragmentation contributed to cognitive impairment, which reversed with nocturnal CPAP. Impairments in selective and continuous attention correlating with the degree of hypoxemia were documented in untreated OSAHS patients by Kotterba et al. [13]. A study in older persons (>65 years of age) at high risk for sleep-disordered breathing found that cognitive decline was associated with increased daytime sleepiness [14].

In a typical OSAHS patient (weight 140 kg; Body Mass Index (BMI) 40 kg/m^2; ESS 18/24; DI >60/hr; see reference [10], case 2 for further details), neuropsychological assessment showed mild impairment of cognitive function, with slight reductions in verbal reasoning and verbal comprehension performance, poor performance on tests of short-term memory and learning, reduced verbal fluency, and mild attentional problems, while nonverbal reasoning, language, and visuospatial and constructional functions were intact [15]. These impairments were more typical of those ascribed to subcortical rather than cortical pathology, and might reflect white matter change, as seen in "white matter dementias" such as multiple sclerosis (Section 6.1). Cerebral metabolic impairments have been identified in OSAHS using magnetic resonance spectroscopy, in association with white matter change [16]. Carrying the apolipoprotein E epsilon-4 allele, a risk factor for Alzheimer's disease (AD), may increase risk of memory impairment in OSAHS patients [17].

An overview of case-control studies of neuropsychological function in patients with sleep-disordered breathing found that impairment was generally greater with increasing severity of disease [9], recognizing that some tasks are more sensitive to hypoxemia, and others more sensitive to sleepiness. Comparing groups of patients with OSAHS and chronic obstructive pulmonary disease (COPD), Roehrs *et al.* [18] found that deficits in complex reasoning and memory were not specific to diagnosis, whereas sustained attention was worse in the OSAHS group, reflecting its sensitivity to sleepiness, while motor skills were worse in the COPD group, reflecting its sensitivity to hypoxemia. A study comparing OSAHS patients with AD, multi-infarct dementia, and COPD patients found a distinctive cognitive profile in OSAHS that was suggestive of subcortical damage [19].

Recently, Yaffe and colleagues reported that sleep-disordered breathing, defined as AHI ≥15/hr, was associated with an increased likelihood of developing mild cognitive impairment or dementia over a follow-up period ranging from two to six years. Measures of disordered breathing (elevated oxygen desaturation index, percentage of sleep time in apnea or hypopnea) were associated with increased risk, whereas measures of sleep fragmentation or sleep duration were not, suggesting that hypoxemia was the key factor predisposing to cognitive decline [20]. If confirmed, these data may have important implications for assessment and treatment of patients developing cognitive complaints. A large cross-sectional study found no association between OSAHS severity and cognitive function, although subjects in this study did not have significant daytime sleepiness [21]. It is possible that only subsets of individuals with OSAHS may have cognitive changes.

The current consensus is that sleep fragmentation and nocturnal hypoxemia and not apnea recurrence are the key determinants of cognitive dysfunction in OSAHS, with hypoxemia contributing to the executive impairment and sleep fragmentation influencing attention. It is suggested that OSAHS accelerates the process of brain ageing, hence mandating early treatment.

CPAP has frequently been reported to improve cognitive deficits in OSAHS [12,13,22,23], but not all patients benefit and complete reversal of attention and executive dysfunction may not occur. Identifying whether there are subgroups of OSAHS patients who are more likely to benefit from CPAP is required. Another approach has been to examine the utility of cholinesterase inhibitors. A trial of donepezil in AD patients with concurrent OSAHS showed an improvement in AHI and oxygen saturation as well as in ADAS-Cog scores at three months in the treatment group (n = 11) [24]. A more recent study of donepezil in non-AD OSAHS reported improved AHI, oxygen saturation and sleepiness measured by ESS after one month in the treatment group (n = 11). A possible role for cholinergic neurotransmission in the regulation of breathing in OSAHS patients was suggested [25].

11.1.2 Central sleep apnea

Central sleep apnea (CSA) is characterized by periodic apnea owing to loss of ventilatory motor output, because of an unstable ventilatory control system, resulting in lack of inspiratory muscle effort [5,6,26]. There are diverse causes of CSA, including congestive cardiac failure and neurological diseases such as stroke and multiple system atrophy, but some cases remain idiopathic.

A patient with CSA who presented with cognitive complaints had a neuropsychological profile that showed marked impairments in nonverbal reasoning and processing speed, indicative of a subcortical type of dementia, but the interpretation was confounded by prior radiotherapy for a malignant brain tumor [15].

11.2 Central hypersomnias

The central hypersomnias include narcolepsy with or without cataplexy, idiopathic hypersomnias, and hypersomnia due to a medical condition, drug, or substance [1].

11.2.1 Narcolepsy

Narcolepsy, or the narcoleptic syndrome, is characterized by excessive daytime sleepiness with brief "sleep attacks" lasting 10–20 minutes, often occurring in inappropriate circumstances such as when driving, eating, or talking. Additional features sometimes seen include cataplexy, sleep paralysis, hypnagogic (and/or hypnapompic) hallucinations, and insomnia. The pathogenesis relates to loss of hypothalamic hypocretin neurons in genetically predisposed individuals who carry the HLA DQB1*0602 allele [27].

Cognitive complaints are not uncommon in narcoleptics but detailed studies of cognitive function with correction for sleepiness/arousal are few. Naumann *et al.* [28] found impairments in continuously maintained selective attention, slowed information processing but with intact quality of performance, mild verbal memory deficits but with preserved visuospatial memory, and deficits in executive functions (verbal fluency, deficient inhibition, and high susceptibility to interference on the Hayling Sentence Completion Task). The overall pattern of cognitive performance was judged to be consistent with a limitation of cognitive processing resources [28].

Modafinil has proved efficacious for the sleep disorder in narcolepsy and has been reported to improve executive function [29]. There are anecdotal reports of the use of cholinesterase inhibitors in narcolepsy, predicated upon changes in the cholinergic system in this disorder [30]. For example, in two nondemented patients with narcolepsy treated with rivastigmine, improvements were noted in excessive daytime somnolence and in the ESS [31].

11.2.2 Kleine–Levin syndrome

Kleine–Levin syndrome is characterized by recurrent episodes of hypersomnia, typically occurring in adolescent males, in which episodes of hypersomnolence and bulimia last days to weeks. The etiology remains unknown and there is no effective treatment, although modafinil may reduce the duration of a symptomatic episode [32].

Cases of Kleine–Levin syndrome have been reported with short-term memory deficits during periods of remission, associated in some cases with frontotemporal hypoperfusion on single-photon emission computed tomography (SPECT) imaging [33]. Another patient with deficits of visual and verbal recall after remission of an episode was also found to have selective deficits of visual recall six months later [34].

11.3 Circadian rhythm sleep disorders

Circadian rhythm sleep disorders are characterized by desynchronization between internal circadian rhythms and external time, jet lag being an example [1]. Shift-workers are also at risk of circadian rhythm sleep disorder.

11.3.1 Shift-work sleep disorder (SWSD)

Shift-work sleep disorder (SWSD) is classified as a secondary circadian rhythm disorder resulting from exogenous factors. Poor sleep quality is commonplace in shift-workers [35], thus the observation of patients with SWSD presenting to cognitive clinics with subjective memory complaints but with no source amnesia [36] is perhaps not surprising, as poor sleep quality is recognized to be associated with subjective memory impairment [3].

11.4 Parasomnias

The parasomnias include sleep walking (somnambulism), night terrors (pavor nocturnus), sleep groaning (catathrenia), exploding head syndrome, and sleep-related eating disorders [1,37,38]. However, from the cognitive perspective, rapid eye movement (REM) sleep behavior disorder (REMBD) is the parasomnia that has attracted most attention, as this may be an early symptom of neurodegenerative disorders, in particular synucleinopathies such as dementia with Lewy bodies and multiple system atrophy (Sections 2.4.2 and 2.4.5), sometimes predating by decades the emergence of motor and cognitive symptoms [39].

11.4.1 REM sleep behavior disorder (REMBD)

REM sleep behavior disorder (REMBD) occurs when the physiological muscular atonia of sleep is lost, resulting in motor behaviors during sleep that are sometimes characterized as "dream enactment." Symptoms are often improved with clonazepam.

A distinction is drawn between idiopathic REMBD and REMBD associated with neurodegenerative diseases such as Parkinson's disease, dementia with Lewy bodies, and multiple system atrophy (Sections 2.4.1, 2.4.2, and 2.4.5).

Neuropsychological assessment of idiopathic REMBD cases has produced somewhat variable results in the cognitive profile, with the most affected domains typically being attention, executive functions, episodic verbal memory, and non-verbal learning [40–42], deficits that may persist at longitudinal follow-up [43]. Language and praxis appear to be well preserved. As far as visuospatial functions are concerned, matters are less certain, although deficits have been noted in some reports. For example, one study of 17 cases of idiopathic REMBD found impaired visuospatial constructional function (Rey-Osterrieth Figure copying) and visuospatial learning (Corsi Supraspan) compared to normal controls [40].

Whether these "idiopathic" cases in fact represent synucleinopathies with currently isolated REMBD remains to be determined [44]. Screening for mild cognitive impairment in REMBD may be possible using the Montreal Cognitive Assessment [45].

11.5 Sleep-related movement disorders

11.5.1 Restless legs syndrome (RLS)

Restless legs syndrome (RLS), or Ekbom's syndrome, is characterized clinically by an intense discomfort within the legs associated with a desire to move them, the discomfort being temporarily relieved by movement. Symptoms are often worse at rest or during the evening or night. RLS is a recognized cause of secondary insomnia and excessive daytime somnolence. RLS is frequently associated with periodic limb movement disorder (PLMD, also known as periodic limb movements of sleep, PLMS). RLS pathogenesis may be related to a central imbalance of serotoninergic and dopaminergic pathways, possibly at the level of the basal ganglia, linked in some way with disordered brain iron metabolism. A number of linked genetic loci have been defined in familial RLS [46].

The impact of RLS on sleep may also affect cognitive functions, particularly those thought to be mediated by the prefrontal cortex [47], producing deficits similar to those seen with sleep deprivation [2]. Presentation of RLS de novo to a cognitive clinic has been reported [48]. Possible associations of RLS with Parkinson's disease, essential tremor [49], and migraine [50] (Sections 2.4.1, 5.4.11, and 3.6.1, respectively) might also contribute to observed cognitive complaints.

REFERENCES

[1] American Academy of Sleep Medicine. *The International Classification of Sleep Disorders* (2nd edn.). Rochester: AASM, 2005.

[2] Durmer JS, Dinges DF. Neurocognitive consequences of sleep deprivation. *Semin Neurol* 2005; 25: 117–29.

[3] Hancock P, Larner AJ. Diagnostic utility of the Pittsburgh Sleep Quality Index in memory clinics. *Int J Geriatr Psychiatry* 2009; 24: 1237–41.

[4] Blackwell T, Yaffe K, Ancoli-Israel S, *et al*. Poor sleep is associated with impaired cognitive function in older women: the study of osteoporotic fractures. *J Gerontol A Biol Sci Med Sci* 2006; 61: 405–10.

[5] Abad VC, Guilleminault C. Neurological perspective on obstructive and nonobstructive sleep apnea. *Semin Neurol* 2004; 24: 261–9.

[6] Stradling JR, Craig SE. Sleep-related disorders of breathing. In: Warrell DA, Cox TM, Firth JD (eds.). *Oxford Textbook of Medicine* (5th edn.). Oxford: Oxford University Press, 2010; 3261–76.

[7] Johns MW. A new method for measuring daytime sleepiness: the Epworth Sleepiness Scale. *Sleep* 1991; 14: 540–5.

[8] Redline S, Kapur VK, Sanders MH, *et al*. Effects of varying approaches for identifying respiratory disturbances on sleep apnea assessment. *Am J Respir Crit Care Med* 2000; 161: 369–74.

[9] Engelman HM, Kingshott RN, Martin SE, Douglas NJ. Cognitive function in the sleep apnea/hypopnea syndrome (SAHS). *Sleep* 2000; 23: S102–8.

[10] Larner AJ. Obstructive sleep apnoea syndrome presenting in a neurology outpatient clinic. *Int J Clin Pract* 2003; 57: 150–2.

[11] Findley LJ, Barth JT, Powers DC, *et al*. Cognitive impairment in patients with obstructive sleep apnea and associated hypoxemia. *Chest* 1986; 90: 686–90.

[12] Scheltens P, Visscher F, Van Keimpema ARJ, *et al*. Sleep apnea syndrome presenting with cognitive impairment. *Neurology* 1991; 41: 155–6.

[13] Kotterba S, Rasche K, Widdig W, *et al*. Neuropsychological investigations and event-related potentials in obstructive sleep apnea syndrome before and during CPAP-therapy. *J Neurol Sci* 1998; 159: 45–50.

[14] Cohen-Zion M, Stepnowsky C, Marler M, *et al*. Changes in cognitive function associated with sleep disordered breathing in older people. *J Am Geriatr Soc* 2001; 49: 1622–7.

[15] Larner AJ, Ghadiali EJ. Cognitive findings in central sleep apnoea syndrome. www.acnr.co.uk/SO08/ACNRSO08CaseReport.pdf, 2008.

[16] Kamba M, Inoue Y, Higami S, *et al*. Cerebral metabolic impairments in patients with obstructive sleep apnoea: an independent association of obstructive sleep apnoea with white matter change. *J Neurol Neurosurg Psychiatry* 2001; 71: 334–9.

[17] O'Hara R, Schroder CM, Kraemer HC, *et al*. Nocturnal sleep apnea/hypopnea is associated with lower memory performance in APOE epsilon-4 carriers. *Neurology* 2005; 65: 642–4.

[18] Roehrs T, Merrion M, Pedrosi B, *et al*. Neuropsychological function in obstructive sleep apnea syndrome (OSAS) compared to chronic obstructive pulmonary disease (COPD). *Sleep* 1995; 18: 382–8.

[19] Antonelli Incalzi R, Marra C, Salvigni BL, *et al*. Does cognitive dysfunction conform to a distinctive pattern in obstructive sleep apnea syndrome? *J Sleep Res* 2004; 13: 79–86.

[20] Yaffe K, Laffan AM, Harrison SL, *et al*. Sleep-disordered breathing, hypoxia, and risk of mild cognitive impairment and dementia in older women. *JAMA* 2011; 306: 613–19.

[21] Quan SF, Chan CS, Dement WC, *et al*. The association between obstructive sleep apnea and neurocognitive performance – the Apnea Positive Pressure Long-term Efficacy Study (APPLES). *Sleep* 2011; 34: 303B–14B.

[22] Valencia-Flores M, Bliwise DL, Guilleminault C, Cilveti R, Clerk A. Cognitive function in patients with sleep apnea after acute nocturnal nasal continuous positive airway pressure (CPAP) treatment: sleepiness and hypoxaemia effects. *J Clin Exp Neuropsychol* 1996; 18: 197–210.

[23] Aloia MS, Ilniczky N, Di Pio P, *et al*. Neuropsychological changes and treatment compliance in older adults with sleep apnea. *J Psychosom Res* 2003; 54: 71–6.

[24] Moraes W, Poyares D, Sukys-Claudino L, Guilleminault C, Tufik S. Donepezil improves obstructive sleep apnea in Alzheimer disease: a double-blind, placebo-controlled study. *Chest* 2008; 133: 677–83.

[25] Sukys-Claudino L, Moraes W, Guilleminault C, Tufik S, Poyares D. Beneficial effect of donepezil on obstructive sleep apnea: a double-blind, placebo-controlled clinical trial. *Sleep Med* 2012; 13: 290–6.

[26] Badr MS. Central sleep apnea. *Prim Care* 2005; 32: 361–74.

[27] Akintomide GS, Rickards H. Narcolepsy: a review. *Neuropsychiatr Dis Treat* 2011; 7: 507–18.

[28] Naumann A, Bellebaum C, Daum I. Cognitive deficits in narcolepsy. *J Sleep Res* 2006; 15: 329–38.

[29] Becker PM, Schwartz JR, Feldman NT, Hughes RJ. Effect of modafinil on fatigue, mood and health-related quality of life in patients with narcolepsy. *Psychopharmacology (Berl)* 2004; 171: 133–9.

[30] Niederhofer H. Donepezil in the treatment of narcolepsy. *J Clin Sleep Med* 2006; 15: 71–2.

[31] Staszewski J, Stepien A. Efficacy of rivastigmine treatment in narcolepsy: report of 2 cases. *Eur J Neurol* 2009; 16(Suppl 3): 624 (abstract p. 2841).

[32] Huang YS, Lakkis C, Guilleminault C. Kleine-Levin syndrome: current status. *Med Clin N Am* 2010; 94: 557–62.

[33] Landtblom AM, Dige N, Schwerdt K, Safstrom P, Granerus G. Short-term memory dysfunction in Kleine-Levin syndrome. *Acta Neurol Scand* 2003; 108: 363–7.

[34] Körtner K, Hansen ML, Danker-Hopfe H, Neuhaus AH, Jockers-Scherübl MC. Persistent deficits of visual recall in Kleine-Levin syndrome. *J Clin Neurosci* 2011; 18: 439–40.

[35] Akerstedt T. Shift work and disturbed sleep/wakefulness. *Occup Med (Lond)* 2003; 53: 89–94.

[36] Larner AJ. Shift-work sleep disorder presenting in the cognitive disorders clinic. *Eur J Neurol* 2010; 17(Suppl 3): 213 (abstract P1359).

[37] Reading P. Parasomnias: the spectrum of things that go bump in the night. *Pract Neurol* 2007; 7: 6–15.

[38] Thorpy MJ, Plazzi G (eds.). *The Parasomnias and Other Sleep-Related Movement Disorders*. Cambridge: Cambridge University Press, 2010.

[39] Boeve BF, Silber MH, Saper CB, *et al.* Pathophysiology of REM sleep behaviour disorder and relevance to neurodegenerative disease. *Brain* 2007; 130: 2770–88.

[40] Ferini-Strambi L, Di Gioia MR, Castronovo V, *et al.* Neuropsychological assessment in idiopathic REM sleep behaviour disorders (RBD): does the idiopathic form of RBD really exist? *Neurology* 2004; 62: 41–5.

[41] Terzaghi M, Sinforiani E, Zucchella C, *et al.* Cognitive performance in REM sleep behaviour disorder: a possible early marker of neurodegenerative disease? *Sleep Med* 2008; 9: 343–51.

[42] Massicotte-Marquez J, Decary A, Gagnon J, *et al.* Executive dysfunction and memory impairment in idiopathic REM sleep behavior disorder. *Neurology* 2008; 70: 1250–7.

[43] Fantini M, Faini E, Ortelli P, *et al.* Longitudinal study of cognitive function in idiopathic REM sleep behaviour disorder. *Sleep* 2011; 34: 619–25.

[44] Boeve BF, Ferman TJ. Neuropsychological characterization of evolving cognitive decline in idiopathic REM sleep behaviour disorder is important, but not easy. *Sleep* 2011; 34: 561–2.

[45] Gagnon J-F, Postuma RB, Joncas S, Desjardins C, Latreille V. The Montreal Cognitive Assessment: a screening tool for mild cognitive impairment in REM sleep behavior disorder. *Mov Disord* 2010; 25: 936–40.

[46] Hening WA, Allen RP, Chokroverty S, Earley CJ (eds.). *Restless Legs Syndrome*. Philadelphia, PA: Saunders Elsevier, 2009.

[47] Pearson VE, Allen RP, Dean T, *et al.* Cognitive deficits associated with restless legs syndrome (RLS). *Sleep Med* 2006; 7: 25–30.

[48] Davies M, Larner AJ. Sleep-related disorders presenting in the Cognitive Function Clinic. www.acnr.co.uk/JA09/ACNRJA09_case%20report.pdf, 2009.

[49] Larner AJ, Allen CMC. Hereditary essential tremor and restless legs syndrome. *Postgrad Med J* 1997; 73: 254.

[50] Cannon PR, Larner AJ. Migraine and restless legs syndrome: Is there an association? *J Headache Pain* 2011; 12: 405–9.

Psychiatric disorders in the cognitive function clinic

Disorders with impaired cognitive function transcend the classical professional boundaries of neurology and psychiatry, all being brain disorders, so it is not surprising that patients with what may be labeled as "psychiatric disorders" [1] present to cognitive clinics. While the psychiatric symptoms that may be encountered in neurological diseases are well described [2–4], the neuropsychological deficits in psychiatric disorders that may result in their presentation to cognitive clinics are perhaps less well authenticated [5]. This scenario may present a very significant challenge to cognitive neurologists who may have received little if any training in the art of psychiatric assessment and diagnosis. While some clinics enjoy the presence of both psychiatrists and neurologists jointly undertaking patient assessment, this is by no means universal.

The observations in this chapter are necessarily those of a neurologist, and may lack the knowledge and subtlety of those familiar with the art of psychiatry. The classification used here follows that outlined in the *Diagnostic and Statistical Manual of Mental Disorders*, 4th edition, text revision (DSM-IV-TR) [1]. Disorders that are classified in DSM-IV but considered elsewhere in this volume include dementia syndromes of neurodegenerative or vascular etiology (see Chapters 2 and 3, respectively), substance-related disorders including alcohol (Section 8.3.1), and sleep disorders including narcolepsy (Section 11.2.1).

12.1 Delirium

Delirium, or acute confusional state, enters the differential diagnosis of cognitive disorders because, by definition, one of the phenotypic features of delirium is change in cognition (e.g., disorientation, language impairment, memory deficit, perceptual disturbance) not better accounted for by dementia [1]. Impairments of consciousness, a *sine qua non* for the diagnosis of delirium, may be subtle.

Delirium and dementia may overlap, neuro-degenerative brain disease being a recognized pre-disposing factor for the development of delirium [6]. Indeed, delirium may be the presenting feature of an underlying dementia syndrome [7,8], presumably because cerebral reserve is reduced, and hence the brain is less able to cope with additional precipitating factors, of which infection or metabolic derangement are the most common ("toxic-metabolic encephalopathy") [6]. Furthermore, one study found that around one-quarter of Alzheimer's disease (AD) patients had an episode of delirium during the course of their illness [9]. Guidelines for the prevention, diagnosis, and treatment of delirium have been published [10–13].

12.2 Schizophrenia

Kraepelin originally designated the disorder now known as schizophrenia as "dementia praecox," implying an early onset of cognitive decline. Subsequently, the psychiatric features of schizophrenia became the focus of clinical definition and management [1], especially Schneider's first-rank symptoms [14], but interest in cognitive features has been rekindled in recent years [15–21].

It is evident that schizophrenia is associated with cognitive impairments affecting attention, memory (both verbal and nonverbal), language ("schizopha-sia"), and executive function. Reviews and meta-analyses of large numbers of studies have confirmed pervasive memory impairment in schizophrenics (sometimes said to resemble an amnesic syndrome [22]) independent of disease duration (i.e., present in the first episode of psychotic illness as well as in chronic disease), medication use, and premorbid intelligence. These deficits may precede the onset of symptoms, as noted by examination of high-risk groups (especially executive function and working memory), but become more apparent once the diagnosis is established.

What currently remains less clear is whether these deficits change over time. Although some studies report progressive cognitive decline in later life [23],

there is also a view that following a drop in cognitive function early in the illness, there is little substantial change thereafter [24]. Certainly, the cognitive profile in schizophrenia differs from that in AD.

A schizophrenia-like psychosis has been reported in some patients with very early onset frontotemporal dementia (Section 2.2), and has been interpreted as the presenting feature of neurodegenerative disease [25]. An interictal schizophrenia-like psychosis may also occur in the context of epilepsy, most commonly left-sided temporal lobe epilepsy (Section 4.2.2.1) [26].

12.3 Mood disorders

12.3.1 Depression

Depression may be characterized as a disorder of mood, behavior, sleep, and cognition. It is associated with both subjective complaints and objective measures of cognitive dysfunction, which at their extreme resemble a dementia syndrome, hence use of the term pseudodementia [27–29], or the "dementia syndrome of depression," or "depression-related cognitive dysfunction."

The pattern of cognitive deficits in individuals with depression is typified by bradyphrenia (sometimes labeled psychomotor retardation), with impairments in attention, memory (episodic and recognition), visuospatial skills, and executive function including phonemic verbal fluency (possibly as a result of overall global cognitive slowing) [30–33]. The profile often most closely resembles that seen in so-called subcortical dementias. A meta-analytic study found depression had the largest effect on measures of encoding and retrieval from episodic memory, with intermediate effect sizes on tests of psychomotor speed and sustained attention, with relative sparing of semantic and working memory [34]. In addition, there may be an apparent lack of effort and application when performing cognitive screening tests with frequent "No" or "Don't know" answers, approximate answers (Ganser phenomenon or *vorbereiden*), as well as evidence of mood disturbance (tearfulness). Memory loss for recent and distant events may be equally severe (cf. the temporal gradient of memory loss in dementia; e.g., due to AD). On recognition memory testing, depressed patients are said to produce more false negatives than AD patients who produce more false positives or intrusions.

To ascertain with certainty whether manifest cognitive decline, particularly in elderly patients, results from depression or from an underlying neurodegenerative disorder, or both, is one of the greatest challenges facing the clinician in the memory clinic [35], a task further complicated by the frequency of depression in mild cognitive impairment and dementia [36], one review suggesting that depressive symptoms may occur in up to 40% of AD patients [37]. Depression and impaired cognition may reflect a shared pathogenesis, or may coexist independently. Elderly depressed patients may risk being incorrectly labeled with dementia, or the latter diagnosis may be overlooked if symptoms are ascribed entirely to depression. Searching for symptoms and signs of affective disorder, therefore, is critical in assessing cognitive complaints [27–29]. Provisional criteria for the identification of depression in AD have been published [38].

Neuropsychological assessment may not discriminate dementia and depression reliably, as both conditions may be associated with poor performance with overlapping profiles. Some cognitive screening instruments have been claimed to facilitate differential diagnosis, such as the CANTAB-PAL computerized battery [39] and the Addenbrooke's Cognitive Examination [40] (although other studies have not confirmed the latter finding [41]). A 22-item checklist to help differentiate pseudodementia from AD has been described, based on clinical history, behavior, and mental status [28]. Use of brief depression rating scales, such as the Patient Health Questionnaire-9 (PHQ-9), may help to identify patients attending cognitive clinics who might benefit from a trial of antidepressant medication [42].

An empirical trial of antidepressant medication may be given to patients with suspected depression-related cognitive dysfunction, but response is variable. Even clinical improvement may not absolutely establish the diagnosis of depression, and prolonged follow-up may be required. Depression with executive dysfunction has been reported to have a poor response to antidepressants [43]. Some patients may progress to an irreversible dementia, suggesting that depression may be the prodrome of dementia in some cases [30].

12.3.2 Bipolar disorder

Bipolar disorder is a severe and common mental disorder causing mood shifts (mania, depression), various subtypes of which are recognized [1]. Cognitive disturbances have increasingly been noted as phenotypic features of bipolar disorder, even during remission [44,45]. Deficits in attention, learning and memory, and executive function have been documented, particularly in the bipolar I subtype, but no unique profile of neuropsychological function has emerged. A meta-analysis found that cognitive function was consistently better in patients with bipolar disorder compared to patients with schizophrenia [46]. Bipolar disorder enters the differential diagnosis of pseudodementia. Whether bipolar disorder represents a risk factor for development of dementia is even less clear than is the case with depression.

12.4 Anxiety disorders

12.4.1 Obsessive-compulsive disorder (OCD); Tourette syndrome

Obsessive-compulsive disorder (OCD) is characterized by recurrent obsessions or compulsions that are severe enough to be time consuming or cause marked distress or impairment [1]. There is a high concordance of OCD with Tourette syndrome (TS) of multiple vocal and motor tics [47,48].

Neuropsychological function is impaired in OCD [49]. One review found evidence for memory dysfunction and executive deficits [50]. Other studies have reported visual-constructive and verbal fluency deficits that are apparently specific to OCD, whereas spatial learning deficits are also seen in panic disorder [51]. Although findings are variable across studies, the memory deficit appears to be principally nonverbal and related to encoding and/or retrieval difficulties, with recall worse than recognition. There may be poor organization of information at the encoding stage, perhaps related to difficulties in inhibitory functions [52] or in sustaining attention and forming internal representations of stimuli. Impairments in initiating encoding strategies, but not in implementing them once initiated, have been suggested [49]. Dysfunction in orbitofrontolimbic networks (orbitofrontal cortex, anterior cingulate cortex, striatum) is postulated to underlie these cognitive impairments, consistent with a disease model of corticostriatal dysfunction [49,53].

Tourette syndrome is thought to result from dysfunction in frontostriatal networks [47,48], and the documented neuropsychological features of the condition correspond with this, specifically visuomotor integration problems, impaired fine motor skill, and executive dysfunction [54,55]. A correlation between OCD symptoms and performance on the Wisconsin Card Sorting Test has been noted in children with TS [56]. A Tourette-like syndrome of vocal motor tics has also been reported in frontotemporal dementia (Section 2.2), responding to clonidine [57].

12.5 Dissociative disorders

Dissociative disorders are characterized by disruption in the usually integrated functions of consciousness, memory, identity, and perception [1]. Of the various conditions falling within this rubric, psychogenic or dissociative amnesia is perhaps the most likely to be encountered in cognitive disorders clinics.

12.5.1 Psychogenic amnesia

Psychogenic amnesia is one of a number of terms used to describe medically unexplained amnesia, other labels including dissociative amnesia (as in DSM-IV [1]) and functional amnesia. Psychogenic amnesia enters the differential diagnosis of transient global amnesia (Section 3.6.2) and transient epileptic amnesia (Section 4.3.1). The term encompasses transient or discrete episodes of anterograde and/or retrograde memory loss, which may be global, as in psychogenic fugue or psychogenic retrograde focal amnesia, or situation-specific as in amnesia for offences or arising in posttraumatic stress disorder. Predisposing factors for psychogenic amnesia include emotional stress (e.g., relationship, financial), depressed mood, and a history of transient organic amnesia [58].

In psychogenic retrograde focal amnesia (cf. Section 1.1.3), all retrograde memories are lost (e.g., identity) whereas anterograde memory is entirely or largely spared, such that patients can relearn personal semantic knowledge. The repetitive questioning typical of organic amnesias is replaced by a *belle indifference* to the predicament. Interview under sedation (amytal interview, abreaction) may help to recover memories in psychogenic amnesia, according to some authorities [58].

12.6 Disorders of uncertain etiology

For want of a better place, disorders of uncertain etiology are included here. Whatever its ultimate pathogenesis, fibromyalgia is a pain disorder, which is a category in DSM-IV even though fibromyalgia per se is not mentioned.

12.6.1 Fibromyalgia

Patients with a diagnostic label of fibromyalgia, a syndrome of widespread musculoskeletal or soft tissue pain with multiple tender points, may be encountered in cognitive clinics with complaints of poor memory. Studies suggest poor performance on memory tests (immediate and delayed recall) and sustained concentration compared to controls, with correlations between performance and measures of pain and anxiety [59]. While some authors have found that a history of major depressive disorder is associated with poor memory [60], others maintain that cognitive impairments cannot be attributed solely to concomitant psychiatric conditions such as depression and poor sleep, although they do seem to be related to the level of pain [61]. Pain is recognized as a potential confounder of neuropsychological testing, as in mild traumatic brain injury or headache [62], perhaps impacting on attentional control [61]. Certainly, the apparent perception of memory problems is often greater than objective deficits [61].

REFERENCES

[1] American Psychiatric Association. *Diagnostic and Statistical Manual of Mental Disorders, Fourth Edition, Text Revision (DSM-IV-TR)*. Washington, DC: American Psychiatric Association, 2000.

[2] Cummings JL, Mega MS. *Neuropsychiatry and Behavioral Neuroscience*. Oxford: Oxford University Press, 2003.

[3] Lyketsos CG, Rabins PV, Lipsey JR, Slavney PR (eds.). *Psychiatric Aspects of Neurologic Diseases. Practical Approaches to Patient Care*. New York, NY: Oxford University Press, 2008.

[4] Moore DP. *Textbook of Clinical Neuropsychiatry* (2nd edn.). London: Hodder Arnold, 2008.

[5] Wood SJ, Allen NB, Pantelis C (eds.). *The Neuropsychology of Mental Illness*. Cambridge: Cambridge University Press, 2009.

[6] Lindesay J, Rockwood K, Macdonald A (eds.). *Delirium in Old Age*. Oxford: Oxford University Press, 2002.

[7] Robertsson B, Blennow K, Gottfries CG, Wallin A. Delirium in dementia. *Int J Geriatr Psychiatry* 1998; 13: 49–56.

[8] Rockwood K, Cosway S, Carver D, *et al.* The risk of dementia and death following delirium. *Age Ageing* 1999; 28: 551–6.

[9] Baker FM, Wiley C, Kokmen E, Chandra V, Schoenberg BS. Delirium episodes during the course of clinically

diagnosed Alzheimer's disease. *J Natl Med Assoc* 1999; 91: 625–30.

[10] American Psychiatric Association. *Practice Guidelines for the Treatment of Patients with Delirium*. Washington, DC: American Psychiatric Association, 1999.

[11] Royal College of Psychiatrists. *Who Cares Wins: Improving the Outcome for Older People Admitted to the General Hospital. Report of a Working Group for the Faculty of Old Age Psychiatry*. London: Royal College of Psychiatrists, 2005.

[12] Royal College of Physicians. *The Prevention, Diagnosis and Management of Delirium in Older People*. London: Royal College of Physicians, 2006.

[13] National Institute for Health and Clinical Excellence. *Delirium: Diagnosis, Prevention and Management*. London: NICE, 2010.

[14] Mellors CS. First-rank symptoms of schizophrenia. *Br J Psychiatry* 1970; 117: 15–23.

[15] Aleman A, Hijman R, de Haan EHF, Kahn RS. Memory impairment in schizophrenia. A meta-analysis. *Am J Psychiatry* 1999; 156: 1358–66.

[16] Cirillo MA, Seidman LJ. Verbal declarative memory dysfunction in schizophrenia: from clinical assessment to genetics and brain mechanisms. *Neuropsychol Rev* 2003; 13: 43–77.

[17] Fioravanti M, Carlone O, Vitale B, *et al.* A meta-analysis of cognitive deficits in adults with a diagnosis of schizophrenia. *Neuropsychol Rev* 2005; 15: 73–95.

[18] Rajji TK, Mulsant BH. Nature and course of cognitive function in late-life schizophrenia: a systematic review. *Schizophr Res* 2008; 102: 122–40

[19] Barnett JH, Fletcher PC. Cognition in schizophrenia. In: Cappa SF, Abutalebi J, Démonet JF, Fletcher PC, Garrard P (eds.). *Cognitive Neurology: A Clinical Textbook*. Oxford: Oxford University Press, 2008: 419–46.

[20] Testa R, Wood SJ, Pantelis C. Schizophrenia. In: Wood SJ, Allen NB, Pantelis C (eds.). *The Neuropsychology of Mental Illness*. Cambridge: Cambridge University Press, 2009; 378–88.

[21] Waters F, Almeida OP. Schizophrenia, cognitive impairment and dementia. In: Ames D, Burns A, O'Brien J (eds.). *Dementia* (4th edn.). London: Hodder Arnold, 2010; 713–17.

[22] McKenna PJ, Tamlyn D, Lund CE, *et al.* Amnesic syndrome in schizophrenia. *Psychol Med* 1990; 20: 967–72.

[23] Morrison G, O'Carroll R, McCreadie R. Long-term course of cognitive impairment in schizophrenia. *Br J Psychiatry* 2006; 189: 556–7.

[24] Szoke A, Trandafir A, Dupont ME, *et al.* Longitudinal studies of cognition in schizophrenia: meta-analysis. *Br J Psychiatry* 2008; 192: 248–57.

[25] Velakoulis D, Waltefang M, Mocellin R, Pantelis C, McLean C. Frontotemporal dementia presenting as schizophrenia-like psychosis in young people: clinico-pathological series and review of cases. *Br J Psychiatry* 2009; 194: 298–305.

[26] Nathaniel-James DA, Brown RG, Maier M, *et al.* Cognitive abnormalities in schizophrenia and schizophrenia-like psychosis of epilepsy. *J Neuropsychiatry Clin Neurosci* 2004; 16: 472–9.

[27] Kiloh L. Pseudodementia. *Acta Psychiatr Scand* 1961; 37: 336–51.

[28] Wells CE. Pseudodementia. *Am J Psychiatry* 1979; 136: 895–900.

[29] Fischer P. The spectrum of depressive pseudo-dementia. *J Neural Transm Suppl* 1996; 47: 193–203.

[30] Shizuko Morimoto S, Shanmugham B, Kelly RE Jr, Alexopoulos G. Depression with cognitive impairment. In: Ames D, Burns A, O'Brien J (eds.). *Dementia* (4th edn.). London: Hodder Arnold, 2010; 703–12.

[31] Fossati P, Deweer B, Raoux N, Allilaire JF. Deficits in memory retrieval: an argument in favor of frontal subcortical dysfunction in depression [in French]. *Encéphale* 1995; 21: 295–305.

[32] Henry J, Crawford JR. A meta-analytic review of verbal fluency deficits in depression. *J Clin Exp Neuropsychol* 2005; 27: 78–101.

[33] Mesholam-Gately RI, Giuliano AJ, Zillmer EA, *et al.* Verbal learning and memory in older adults with minor and major depression. *Arch Clin Neuropsychol* 2012; 27: 196–207.

[34] Zakzanis KK, Leach L, Kaplan E. On the nature and pattern of neurocognitive function in major depressive disorder. *Neuropsychiatry Neuropsychol Behav Neurol* 1998; 11: 111–19.

[35] Christensen H, Griffiths K, MacKinnon A. A quantitative review of cognitive deficits in depression and Alzheimer-type dementia. *J Int Neuropsychol Soc* 1997; 3: 631–51.

[36] Potter GG, Steffens DC. Contribution of depression to cognitive impairment and dementia in older adults. *Neurologist* 2007; 13: 105–17.

[37] Wragg RE, Jeste DV. Overview of depression and psychosis in Alzheimer's disease. *Am J Psychiatry* 1989; 146: 577–87.

[38] Olin JT, Schneider LS, Katz IR, *et al.* Provisional diagnostic criteria for depression of Alzheimer disease. *Am J Geriatr Psychiatry* 2002; 10: 125–8.

[39] Swainson R, Hodges JR, Galton CJ, *et al.* Early detection and differential diagnosis of Alzheimer's disease and depression with neuropsychological tests. *Dement Geriatr Cogn Disord* 2001; 12: 265–80.

[40] Dudas RB, Berrios GE, Hodges JR. The Addenbrooke's Cognitive Examination (ACE) in the differential diagnosis of early dementias versus affective disorder. *Am J Geriatr Psychiatry* 2005; 13: 218–26.

[41] Stokholm J, Vogel A, Johannsen P, Waldemar G. Validation of the Danish Addenbrooke's Cognitive Examination as a screening test in a memory clinic. *Dement Geriatr Cogn Disord* 2009; 27: 361–5.

[42] Hancock P, Larner AJ. Clinical utility of Patient Health Questionnaire-9 (PHQ-9) in memory clinics. *Int J Psychiatry Clin Pract* 2009; 13: 188–91.

[43] Alexopoulos GS, Kiosses DN, Heo M, *et al.* Executive dysfunction and the course of geriatric depression. *Biol Psychiatry* 2005; 58: 204–10.

[44] Savitz J, Solms M, Ramesar R. Neuropsychological dysfunction in bipolar affective disorder: a critical opinion. *Bipolar Disord* 2005; 7: 216–35.

[45] Sole B, Bonnin CM, Torrent C, *et al.* Neurocognitive impairment across the bipolar spectrum. *CNS Neurosci Ther* 2012; 18: 194–200.

[46] Krabbendam L, Arts B, van Os J, Aleman A. Cognitive functioning in patients with schizophrenia and bipolar disorder: a quantitative review. *Schizophr Res* 2005; 80: 137–49.

[47] Robertson MM. Gilles de la Tourette syndrome: the complexities of phenotype and treatment. *Br J Hosp Med* 2011; 72: 100–7.

[48] Jankovic J, Kurlan R. Tourette syndrome: evolving concepts. *Mov Disord* 2011; 26: 1149–56.

[49] Deckersbach T, Savage CR, Rauch SL. Neuropsychology of obsessive compulsive disorder. In: Wood SJ, Allen NB, Pantelis C (eds.). *The Neuropsychology of Mental Illness.* Cambridge: Cambridge University Press, 2009; 342–52.

[50] Kuelz AK, Hohagen F, Voderholzer U. Neuropsychological performance in obsessive-compulsive disorder: a critical review. *Biol Psychol* 2004; 65: 185–236.

[51] Boldrini M, Del Pace L, Placidi GP, *et al.* Selective cognitive deficits in obsessive-compulsive disorder compared to panic disorder with agoraphobia. *Acta Psychiatr Scand* 2005; 111: 150–8.

[52] Chamberlain SR, Blackwell AD, Fineberg NA, Robbins TW, Sahakian BJ. The neuropsychology of obsessive compulsive disorder: the importance of failures in cognitive and behavioural inhibition as candidate endophenotypic markers. *Neurosci Biobehav Rev* 2005; 29: 399–419.

[53] Aycicegi A, Dinn WM, Harris CL, Erkmen H. Neuropsychological function in obsessive-compulsive disorder: effects of comorbid conditions on task performance. *Eur Psychiatry* 2003; 18: 241–8.

[54] Como PG. Neuropsychological function in Tourette syndrome. *Adv Neurol* 2001; 85: 103–11.

[55] Eddy CM, Rizzo R, Cavanna AE. Neuropsychological aspects of Tourette syndrome: a review. *J Psychosom Res* 2009; 67: 503–13.

[56] Bornstein RA. Neuropsychological correlates of obsessive characteristics in Tourette syndrome. *J Neuropsychiatry Clin Neurosci* 1991; 3: 157–62.

[57] Stewart JT, Williams LS. Tourette's-like syndrome and dementia. *Am J Psychiatry* 2003; 160: 1356–7.

[58] McKay GCM, Kopelman MD. Psychogenic amnesia: when memory complaints are medically unexplained. *Adv Psychiatr Treat* 2009; 15: 152–8.

[59] Landro NI, Stiles TC, Sletvold H. Memory functioning in patients with primary fibromyalgia and major depression and healthy controls. *J Psychosom Res* 1997; 42: 297–306.

[60] Grace GM, Nielson WR, Hopkins M, Berg MA. Concentration and memory deficits in patients with fibromyalgia syndrome. *J Clin Exp Neuropsychol* 1999; 21: 477–87.

[61] Glass JM. Review of cognitive dysfunction in fibromyalgia: a convergence on working memory and attentional control impairments. *Rheum Dis Clin North Am* 2009; 35: 299–311.

[62] Nicholson K, Martelli MF, Zasler ND. Does pain confound interpretation of neuropsychological test results? *NeuroRehabilitation* 2001; 16: 225–30.

Index

Printed in the United States
By Bookmasters